PREHOSPITAL PROVIDERS' GUIDE TO MEDICATION

PREHOSPITAL PROVIDERS' GUIDE TO MEDICATION

ALAN J. AZZARA, JD, EMT-P

QUALITY ASSURANCE COORDINATOR
NORTH EAST MOBILE HEALTH SERVICES
TOPSHAM, MAINE

MEDICAL CONSULTANT:
Matthew Sleeth, MD
Director of Emergency Services
St. Andrew's Hospital
Boothbay Harbor, Maine

WITH CONTRIBUTIONS BY:
Sarah Mosher Skolfield, BA, EMT-1
Freeport, Maine

W.B. SAUNDERS COMPANY
A Division of Harcourt Brace & Company
Philadelphia   London   Toronto   Sydney

W.B. SAUNDERS COMPANY
A Division of Harcourt Brace & Company

The Curtis Center
Independence Square West
Philadelphia, Pennsylvania 19106

Library of Congress Cataloging-in-Publication Data

Azzara, Alan J.
Prehospital providers' guide to medication / Alan J.
Azzara. — 1st ed.

p.   cm.

ISBN 0–7216–1136–2

1. Drugs.   2. Emergency medical technicians.
I. Title.   [DNLM: 1. Drug Therapy.   2. Emergency
Medical Technicians.   3. Pharmaceutical Preparations.
4. Pharmacology.   QV 55 A999p 1999]

RM300.A99 1999   615'.1—dc21

DNLM/DLC   99–21429

PREHOSPITAL PROVIDERS' GUIDE TO MEDICATION
ISBN 0–7216–1136–2

Printed in the United States of America.

Last digit is the print number: 9 8 7 6 5 4 3 2 1

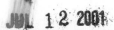

DEDICATION

To family and friends

To health care providers everywhere, particularly those who understand that much of what we do goes well beyond the bounds of science and who know that sometimes we can best assess the status of our patients' hearts, not by listening with our stethoscopes but by listening with our own hearts

In memory of the late Charles Ernest Baker, MD, physician and friend, who first made me appreciate the distinction between curing and healing

ABOUT THE AUTHOR

Alan Azzara has been involved in emergency medical services since 1977 when he first became a basic emergency medical technician with the Locust Valley Fire Department on Long Island, New York. Since that time he has been associated with six services in three states at every level, from basic EMT to paramedic. In addition to providing patient care, Alan has been active in EMS administration and has served as chief, director of operations, director of administration, and training coordinator. He was an EMS instructor/coordinator for many years in New York and is now active instructing EMS programs in Maine. He has also been both a BLS and ACLS instructor for the American Heart Association for the past fifteen years.

Alan is also well known as an author and lecturer. His articles have appeared in *Emergency, Family Practice, Physicians Practice Digest,* and the *Maine EMS Journal,* and he was a member of the editorial advisory board of *Emergency Magazine* for two years. He is the coauthor, with Bruce Cohn, of *Legal Aspects of Emergency Medical Services,* published by the W.B. Saunders Company in 1998. He regularly lectures on a variety of EMS topics and has presented programs at EMS conferences throughout the Northeast.

He currently resides on Westport Island off the coast of Maine.

FOREWORD

As an emergency department physician, I am privileged to interact on a regular basis with prehospital emergency personnel from both paid and volunteer services. Over the years I have developed enormous respect for these individuals, who daily, for little or no compensation, perform acts requiring skill, compassion, and courage. Those of us who work in the hospital under controlled conditions and with many available resources sometimes forget how different circumstances are in the field. We never have to treat our patients in rainstorms or in below freezing temperatures; we don't have to struggle to gain access to seriously injured accident victims or start IVs in overturned cars; and we don't carry patients down narrow flights of stairs while trying to maintain effective CPR.

Clearly, prehospital care is not for everyone. In addition to the physical ability obviously needed to perform the job effectively, prehospital personnel must have a solid understanding of emergency medical concepts and be able to make rapid and effective decisions, often with limited or incomplete data on hand. The old axiom "first do no harm" must be balanced with the knowledge that to "do nothing" will often result in the worsening of the patient's condition and sometimes death.

An area of knowledge that is most important in the assessment and treatment of the patient and which can be particularly challenging is pharmacology. EMS personnel must have a good understanding and knowledge of both the medications that are administered in the field as well as those taken by the patient at home. Such information is invaluable to the provider and emergency department personnel. Knowing what medications the patient takes often provides an important diagnostic clue. It also helps prevent the administration, both in the field and in the hospital, of medications that might result in dangerous interactions or that cause severe adverse reactions. Knowledge of the drugs carried on board the ambulance is essential if prompt and safe treatment is to be administered to the patient.

Alan Azzara is an outstanding paramedic with many years of field experience in New York and Maine. He has put together a book that I believe will serve as an invaluable aide for emergency personnel. It will provide them with a useful tool that can be easily referenced in the field when medication information must be readily accessible. A number of medication books have been written for EMS personnel but they essentially deal with the medications that are administered in the field. While such information is thoroughly covered in the *Prehospital Providers' Guide to Medication,* what I find particularly impressive about the book is its comprehensive and easily understood coverage of the medications that patients take at home.

The essence of emergency medicine, in order to be most effective, must be a team effort. When done with care, knowledge, and diligence, it represents the best aspects of society working together for the benefit of the individual in need. I believe that the *Prehospital Providers' Guide to Medication* can help make the EMS provider a more effective member of the team.

MATTHEW SLEETH, MD
Director of Emergency Services
St. Andrews Hospital
Boothbay Harbor, Maine

PREFACE

Years ago, as a paramedic student, I recall being over-whelmed by the quantity of material that I was expected to learn to pass the course and then apply in the field. Particularly intimidating was the seemingly endless amount of medication data that I would have to absorb if I ever hoped to become a competent paramedic. There was the long list of medications that I would carry on the ambulance, with their various indications, con-traindications, precautions, and dosages. And then there was the staggering number of medications that I would find my patients were already taking at home, which I would have to understand in order to do my job safely and effectively. Two facts became apparent: (1) it was go-ing to be impossible to memorize all of this infor-mation so that I would always have it available to me in the field; and (2) new medications were continually being developed that would be prescribed to patients I would see in the field, and additions and deletions to my paramedic drug box would be a never-ending process.

Once I started to practice, I searched for a book that might be a good resource for medication information that I would need in the field. There were a number of books on the market that were useful but not really comprehensive. Most dealt only with the medications that we administered in the field but ignored those that our patients took at home. The more time I spent in the field, the more I realized how important these medi-cations were to my assessment and treatment. Of course, I could have carried around the *Physicians' Desk Reference,* but anyone who has ever seen this book knows that its mere size makes it impractical to do so. And so, after due consideration, I decided to write my own book and to put into it exactly what I thought would be useful to me in the field.

With so many things that we do, the final product is a far cry from what was originally intended and the book that has emerged after two years is certainly different and, I hope, better than what I thought it would be. Everywhere I went I asked providers at every level what information they thought might be useful to include in the book. I consulted with emergency department physicians, pharmacists, and nurses, and I benefited from their many useful suggestions. I solicited comments over the Internet and received valuable ideas from all over the United States, as well as from Canada, Germany, Australia, and Saudi Arabia.

Prehospital Providers' Guide to Medication is essentially designed to be used as a reference in the field, although some may find that it serves other purposes as well. It should not be considered a text on pharmacology, and where more detailed information is needed the reader should consult one of the many available texts on that subject.

Chapter 1 is a brief overview of pharmacokinetics and pharmacodynamics that refreshes some of the basic concepts of drug administration, absorption, and elimination that were originally learned in our EMS courses.

Chapter 2 is a guide to patient medication. It includes suggestions on obtaining information from patients about the medications they take, discusses some of the medication-related problems that may be encountered in the field, and outlines treatment interventions where appropriate.

Chapter 3 is a guide to the medications that providers administer in the field and includes actions, indications, contraindications, precautions, dosage information, and signs and symptoms of toxicity or overdose, along with appropriate treatment interventions. The reader will undoubtedly find many more drugs in this chapter than are included in the average drug box. The drugs included reflect a compilation of drug lists obtained from services around the country.

Chapter 4 presents a discussion of the administration of drugs in the prehospital setting and focuses on a review of the various routes of administration and a step-by-step guide to the actual processes associated with the administration of medication.

Chapter 5 reviews the various intravenous fluids used in the field, including indications for each fluid, contraindications, precautions, and dosage. Also included is a review of the formula used to calculate drip rates.

Chapter 6 is a discussion of the major classifications of drugs of abuse, including narcotics, stimulants, barbiturates, hallucinogens, and alcohol. The chapter focuses on the assessment and treatment of the patient suffering from an overdose or other abuse of these drugs.

Chapter 7 presents some of the more common emergencies encountered in the field, such as difficulty breathing, chest pain, and seizures. It reviews the signs and symptoms commonly associated with each emergency, basic treatment objectives, and emergency interventions, with a focus on possible medications that can be used to treat the emergency.

Also included at the end of the book are a number of appendices that will be useful to providers in the field, including a list of most of the available prescription and over-the-counter medications presented alphabetically by both generic and trade names.

The preparation of this book has been a long and arduous process. It is hard to imagine, unless you have actually gone through the process, the amount of time and effort that is necessary to bring a project such as this from the initial idea to completion. But if the reader finds that this book has given him or her a better understanding of medication and greater confidence in being able to deal with medication-related issues in the field, all my efforts will have been worthwhile.

ALAN J. AZZARA, JD, EMT-P

ACKNOWLEDGMENTS

Though I am credited as the author of this book, it would be naïve and unrealistic of me to claim full credit for the final product. Anyone who has ever written a book knows that the author is but one of many individuals who contribute their time, their creativity, their talent, and their support all on behalf of a common goal.

Accordingly, I wish to acknowledge and extend my sincerest thanks to the following individuals at the W.B. Saunders Company: Selma Kasczuk, my original editor, for her encouragement and support; Rachel Kelly, editorial assistant, for her ideas, her kindness, and her wonderful accent; Shirley Kuhn, my current editor, for her creative input and friendship; Kathy Maccioca, for her kindness and patience; the many people in the editorial and production departments, whose names I don't know, for their creative input and assistance; and the anonymous peer reviewers who made many valuable suggestions that have been incorporated into the book.

Special thanks to Matthew Sleeth, MD, my medical editor and consultant, for his many thoughtful suggestions and his photography, but mostly for his friendship; Sarah Skolfield, my contributing writer, for her remarkable research and writing assistance; and Kathy Miller, pharmacist at Midcoast Hospital, for her assistance with research and photography.

I thank you all for making this a much better book than it would have been without your contributions.

ALAN J. AZZARA, JD, EMT-P

CONTENTS

CHAPTER*ONE*
PHARMACOKINETICS AND
PHARMACODYNAMICS   1

CHAPTER*TWO*
UNDERSTANDING PATIENT
MEDICATIONS   9

CHAPTER*THREE*
GUIDE TO PREHOSPITAL
MEDICATION   45

CHAPTER*FOUR*
ADMINISTRATION OF PREHOSPITAL
MEDICATIONS   227

CHAPTER*FIVE*
INTRAVENOUS FLUID
ADMINISTRATION   249

CHAPTER*SIX*
DRUGS OF ABUSE   265

CHAPTER*SEVEN*
PREHOSPITAL TREATMENT OF
COMMON EMERGENCIES   277

APPENDIX*A*
PRESCRIPTION AND OVER-THE-
COUNTER MEDICATIONS—
GENERIC NAMES   301

APPENDIX *B*
PRESCRIPTION AND OVER-THE-
COUNTER DRUGS—TRADE NAMES   337

APPENDIX *C*
COMMON HERBAL PREPARATIONS   425

APPENDIX *D*
EARLY MANAGEMENT OF PATIENTS
WITH CHEST PAIN AND POSSIBLE
ACUTE MI   431

APPENDIX *E*
WEIGHT CONVERSION TABLE   435

APPENDIX *F*
TEMPERATURE CONVERSION TABLE   437

APPENDIX *G*
ALGORITHM: ASYSTOLE TREATMENT   439

APPENDIX *H*
APGAR SCORING SYSTEM   443

APPENDIX *I*
GLASGOW COMA SCALE   445

APPENDIX *J*
REVISED TRAUMA SCALE   447

APPENDIX *K*
COMMON CAUSES OF COMA   449

APPENDIX *L*
GUIDE TO DIAGNOSTIC SIGNS   451

APPENDIX _M_
CONSENSUS FORMULA FOR
FLUID REPLACEMENT IN
BURN MANAGEMENT   453

APPENDIX _N_
COMMONLY USED MEDICAL AND
PHARMACOLOGICAL ABBREVIATIONS   455

APPENDIX _O_
ALGORITHM: VENTRICULAR
FIBRILLATION/PULSELESS
VENTRICULAR TACHYCARDIA   463

APPENDIX _P_
ALGORITHM: TACHYCARDIA   467

GLOSSARY OF
PHARMACOLOGICAL TERMS   471

INDEX   475

NOTICE

Emergency Medical Services is an ever-changing field. Standard safety precautions must be followed, but as new research and clinical experience broaden our knowledge, changes in treatment and drug therapy become necessary or appropriate. Readers are advised to check the product information currently provided by the manufacturer of each drug to be administered to verify the recommended dose, the method and duration of administration, and the contraindications. It is the responsibility of the treating physician, relying on experience and knowledge of the patient, to determine dosages and the best treatment for the patient. Neither the publisher nor the editor assumes any responsibility for any injury and/or damage to persons or property.

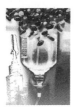

CHAPTER *ONE*

PHARMACOKINETICS AND PHARMACODYNAMICS

Although the prehospital provider does not need to have the same level of knowledge of medication as does a physician or pharmacist, it is important to have at least a basic understanding of how drugs work in the body and how they achieve their desired effects. This knowledge affords the provider with a greater level of confidence in the performance of his or her job.

The two basic concepts that the provider should understand are pharmacokinetics and pharmacodynamics. Though closely related, these concepts are very different from one another. *Pharmacokinetics* is the study of how drugs are absorbed, how they reach their site of action, the means of their distribution in the body, and the manner in which they are excreted. *Pharmacodynamics* is the study of the action or influence that drugs have on living organisms.

PHARMACOKINETICS

Pharmacokinetics involves four basic processes: absorption, distribution, biotransformation, and excretion or elimination.

Absorption. Absorption is the movement of a drug from its point of entry into the body to the systemic circulation. Rate of absorption is a particularly important aspect and is a function of several factors, including solubility, concentration, site of absorption, pH of the drug, circulation to the site of absorption, and the nature of the absorbing surface area.

Solubility is one of the more important factors in absorption. The greater the solubility, the faster the rate of absorption. Drugs dissolved in water or isotonic solutions tend to be absorbed more quickly than do drugs dissolved in oil-based solutions.

The concentration of the drug is also important in determining the rate of absorption. As a general rule, the higher the concentration, the more rapid the rate of absorption.

The pH of a drug refers to its relative acidic or alkaline qualities. Drugs can vary significantly in pH. A drug that is acidic will generally be absorbed rapidly when it is introduced into an acidic environment such as the stomach, whereas an alkaline drug will absorb rapidly in an alkaline environment such as the kidneys. Both the pH of the drug and the pH of the absorbing environment affect absorption.

To reach the systemic circulation, a drug must pass through various anatomical components at the site of absorption. The rate of absorption will obviously be quite rapid if the drug is passing through a single layer of cells such as the intestinal epithelium. As the thickness of the cell layers increases, the rate of absorption decreases. Absorption through structures such as the skin is very slow. In some cases, a slower absorption rate is desirable (see Chapter 4, Administration of Prehospital Medications).

The surface area of the site of absorption also affects the absorption rate. The larger the surface area, the faster the rate of absorption. Absorption of inhaled medications such as albuterol is typically very rapid due to the extensive surface area of the pulmonary epithelium.

Circulation or blood supply to the site of absorption

also helps determine the rate of absorption. A drug administered at a site with a rich blood supply is generally absorbed quickly. Such sites include the sublingual area and the vasculature. Where blood supply is poor, the absorption rate is diminished.

Distribution. Distribution refers to the manner by which a drug is transported from the site of absorption to the site of action. The main factors that influence distribution include cardiovascular function, drug reservoirs, and physiological distribution barriers.

Cardiovascular function is particularly important in the distribution process, since drugs ultimately make their way to the site of action through the bloodstream. If circulation is impaired for any reason, such as shock, myocardial infarction, or congestive heart failure, the resulting decrease in cardiac output will interfere with drug distribution.

Drug reservoirs are locations within the body at which drugs can accumulate by binding to certain types of tissue. The two storage reservoirs that influence the distribution process are tissue reservoirs and plasma reservoirs. Once a drug enters the bloodstream, it frequently attaches or binds itself to plasma proteins. The result is a drug-protein complex. The degree to which this binding takes place significantly influences the distribution of the drug. The portion of drug bound to plasma becomes pharmacologically inactive and is considered a drug reservoir. The unbound portion is considered the active portion. As the free drug is eliminated from the body, additional supplies of the drug can be released from the reservoir and become active. Different drugs have different potentials for binding. This potential is referred to as the binding capacity. Additional reservoirs also exist in bone and fat tissue. Drugs stored in such tissues are distributed very slowly.

3

Distribution is also influenced by certain physiological barriers. The two primary barriers are the blood-brain barrier and the placenta barrier. The blood-brain barrier is composed of specialized cells that line the walls of the vessels that enter the central nervous system. These cells severely restrict the types of drugs that can enter the brain and central nervous system. Drugs that are fat-soluble can generally be distributed to the brain. Similarly, the placenta barrier prevents many drugs from passing from the maternal into the fetal circulation.

Biotransformation. Biotransformation, also known as metabolism, is the process by which drugs are inactivated or detoxified and converted into a form that can be eliminated from the body. This inactive form is known as a metabolite. With some drugs, biotransformation takes place very rapidly, while with others, the process can be quite slow. When biotransformation takes place rapidly, it may be necessary to administer the drug at frequent intervals. Epinephrine, for example, metabolizes very quickly and must be readministered every 3 to 5 minutes in cases of cardiac arrest. The liver plays the most significant role in metabolism. Accordingly, a patient with liver disease may have very delayed metabolism. In such cases, drugs may accumulate in the liver, causing untoward cumulative effects. The health provider with knowledge of poor liver function sometimes must consider reducing a drug's usual dosage to avoid such complications.

Excretion. Drugs or their inactive metabolites are excreted or eliminated from the body primarily through the kidneys, but other structures such as the lungs, liver, intestines, and sweat, salivary, and mammary glands also play a role. When drugs are eliminated through the kidneys, they are excreted as urine, whereas intestinal elimination takes place through fecal material. The liver eliminates drugs through bile and the lungs through expired air. The sweat, salivary, and mammary glands excrete drug metabolites through sweat, saliva, and breast milk, respectively.

PHARMACODYNAMICS

A fundamental knowledge of pharmacodynamics is useful to the prehospital provider because it explains the effect that a drug has on living tissue. Simply stated, pharmacodynamics tells us how a drug works and how we can expect the body to respond to administration of the drug.

Although there are several different ways by which drugs can exercise an influence or effect on body tissue, the most common and most important is through interaction with drug receptors. In most cases, drug receptors are protein coatings found on the outer surface of the cell membrane. The relationship between a drug and a receptor is often referred to as a "lock and key" relationship. The receptor is the lock, and the drug is the key. A drug can interact with a particular receptor, or open the lock, only if it has the appropriate chemical structure. Generally, when a drug binds or attaches to a receptor site, a chemical reaction occurs that initiates the desired response. Drugs that attach to and cause a receptor site to produce a desired response are known as *agonists*. Certain drugs produce their desired effect in a completely different manner. These drugs, known as *antagonists,* compete with and oppose other drugs or chemicals in attempting to bind with and activate receptor sites. An example of drug *antagonism* can be seen in the relationship between morphine and naloxone (Narcan). Morphine or other narcotic drugs ordinarily occupy and activate specific receptor sites. But naloxone, because it has a greater affinity or attraction to those same receptor sites

5

than does morphine, effectively blocks or interferes with morphine's ability to cause the normal narcotic-like response. In the field, we see the principle of antagonism demonstrated by a reversal of the typical signs and symptoms of narcotic overdose, particularly respiratory depression and diminished level of consciousness.

DRUG ACTIONS AND INTERACTIONS

The principle of antagonism demonstrates one manner in which drugs can act or interact and have an effect on the body and on each other. The prehospital provider should also be aware of and understand several other concepts regarding the ways that drugs act when administered into the body.

Synergism. Synergism is the joint action of two drugs that produces an effect neither drug could produce alone.

Potentiation. Potentiation is an increased or enhanced action of two drugs in which the total effect is greater than the sum of the independent effects of the two drugs. This is demonstrated in the field when promethazine (Phenergan) is administered with morphine. The effect of the morphine is enhanced, or potentiated, by the promethazine.

Cumulative action. Cumulative action refers to the toxic effects that result from repeated doses of the same drug that accumulate in the body. This occurs when repeated doses are administered before the prior doses are eliminated from the body.

Drug tolerance. Drug tolerance is the progressive decrease in the effectiveness of a drug on the body. In the field, we might see this principle demonstrated when we administer morphine for pain to a patient who has been using morphine for some time. Where we might have expected a dose of 5 mg of morphine to have a significant analgesic effect, we find that the patient receives little or no relief because he or she has become tolerant to morphine as a result of frequent use. This patient will require a larger dose than normal to achieve the desired result or, in many cases, administration of a different drug.

Habituation. Habituation is the act or process of becoming accustomed to a drug as a result of frequent use. Physical tolerance and dependence develop. The drug is no longer taken for its therapeutic effect but rather to avoid the unpleasant effects that can occur when the patient is denied the drug.

Idiosyncrasy. Idiosyncrasy is an unusual and unanticipated response to a drug that typically manifests itself as an accelerated, toxic, or inappropriate response to the usual therapeutic dose.

A basic understanding of the foregoing concepts will make the provider feel more confident and more comfortable in administering medication in the field.

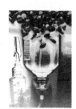

CHAPTER*TWO*

UNDERSTANDING PATIENT MEDICATIONS

Anyone who has ever taken an EMS training course has been told that it is important to inquire about the medications being taken by patients. This information is useful to both prehospital and hospital personnel in the following ways:

1. Such information can provide an important key to assessment both in the field and in the hospital.
2. Medication information can be useful in formulating a plan of treatment. Knowledge of what the patient is taking helps prevent drug interactions or overdoses, which might result from the administration of medication in the field or in the hospital.
3. Medication information allows for the continuity of care by ensuring that the patient continues to receive all necessary and appropriate medications while confined to the hospital. If the hospital is unaware that the patient is taking certain medications, the treatment of conditions unrelated to the present emergency may be interrupted or delayed, possibly with serious consequences.

If EMS personnel do not obtain medication information at the scene, such information may not otherwise be available to emergency department personnel.

This chapter will first discuss the various ways patient medication information can be obtained and then explain how medication information may be used to assist with patient assessment. The chapter will conclude with a description of some of the more common classes of medications that EMS providers are likely to encounter in the field. For each class, the indications, common side effects, signs and symptoms of overdose, and field treatment for overdose are presented, followed by a list of the generic and trade names for the more commonly prescribed medications in each class.

OBTAINING MEDICATION INFORMATION

Information about patient medication may be obtained in several ways. If the patient is conscious and alert, he or she will probably be the best source of such information, but this is not always the case. Some patients, even though fully competent, honestly do not know what they are taking. Such patients may be aware that they are taking a pill for high blood pressure but will not know the name of the medication or the dose. The way to begin is by carefully questioning the patient. If the patient is unable to communicate or is unreliable, information can often be obtained from a family member, a friend, or a home health aide. Appropriate questions might include the following:

1. *Are you currently taking any medication that has been prescribed for you by a physician? Ask about inhalers, medication patches, birth control pills, eye drops, and topical preparations such as creams or ointments. Some patients will overlook certain medications unless you ask about them specifically.*
2. *What are the names of these medications?*
3. *Why are you taking them? How often do you take them?*
4. *Have you recently completed taking any medication? What are the names of these medications? Why were you taking them?*

5. Are you taking any over-the-counter medications or any medication that was not prescribed for you by a doctor? (Sometimes a patient may be taking a medication prescribed for a friend or family member.)
6. When did you last take your medications? Did you take them today?
7. Have you been taking your medications according to the directions stated on the container? If not, how have you been taking them?
8. Are any of your medications new? Is this the first time that you have taken any of them?
9. Have you experienced any side effects, discomfort, or illness that you believe may have been caused by any of your medications? Have you reported any such problems to your doctor?
10. Are you taking any herbal, natural, or homeopathic preparations?

Depending on the answers that you receive to these questions, other questions will undoubtedly come to mind. Ask to see the medication containers, since the label can provide a great deal of useful information that the patient may not know. Often patients store their medication in a plastic container that has a compartment for each day of the week. If this is the case, try to obtain the original medication containers. If the patient or a family member is unable to help you locate medications, check the medicine chest, the bedroom, and the kitchen, since these are the places where medications are most likely to be kept. When you do locate a medication container, check the name on the container to ensure that it belongs to the patient and not another family member. Keep in mind that more than one person in the family may have the same name (father and son, for example).

At times it may be useful to bring all of the medication to the hospital. If you do so, try to ensure that it is left with a responsible person because medication can easily be lost in a busy emergency department and replacement can be very costly.

1. **Patient's Name.** As noted above, it is important to make sure that the container belongs to the patient and not to someone else. Where the identification of the patient is uncertain, the medication container may sometimes assist in establishing identity, particularly if found on or in the immediate vicinity of the patient.

2. **Name of the Medication.** The name may appear as either a trade or a generic name. If you are unfamiliar with the drug, look it up in the appendix, the *PDR* (*Physicians' Desk Reference*), or other medication reference book so that you will be familiar with the drug the next time you encounter it on an ambulance call.

3. **Purpose of the Medication.** The label often states the purpose of the drug such as "for pain."

4. **The Date the Prescription was Filled.** The date can sometimes be important in determining the number of pills that the patient has taken and whether or not the medication has expired or is still effective.

5. **Number of Pills.** How many pills came in the container? This is also important in determining possible overdose or general noncompliance.

6. **Strength or Dose.** This is particularly useful to hospital personnel to ensure that the patient continues to receive his or her normal medications in the proper doses.

7. **Name of the Prescribing Physician.** Knowing the name of the physician will provide the emergency

department staff with someone who can provide a medical history and other important patient information.

8. **Name of the Pharmacy.** This can also be a resource for the emergency department staff to obtain additional information about the patient.

9. **Directions for Use.** The label will provide directions for patient use such as "twice daily," "every 4 hours," or "as needed for pain." This information will help determine patient compliance.

10. **Expiration Date.** This date will help determine the efficacy of the medication.

Also remember to check the secondary labels that often appear on prescription bottles. These labels can provide information such as "to be taken with food," "take on an empty stomach," or "may cause drowsiness." A patient complaining of abdominal distress may simply have failed to follow these directions and taken his or her pills on an empty stomach when the secondary label indicated that they should be taken with food.

Patient Medication As An Assessment Tool

Knowing what medications have been prescribed for or are being used by a patient will provide a basis for determining a number of different assessment possibilities.

Condition for Which the Medication Is Being Taken. Identifying the reason why the patient is using a particular medication can sometimes be the most useful assessment key that you will have, particularly if the patient is unresponsive or incompetent. Many medications are so specific in their indications that they will immediately point to the fact that the patient has a certain condition such as diabetes, heart disease, or asthma. If, for example, you observe a bottle of insulin

13

at the home of a patient, you can quickly assume that the patient has diabetes. Similarly, a patient taking gabapentin (Neurontin) is probably suffering from a seizure disorder. But keep in mind that many medications have a variety of uses and it will be more difficult to reach any conclusions without further inquiry. The beta blocker propranolol (Inderal), for example, while commonly used to treat hypertension or irregular heart rhythms, is sometimes used for patients suffering from migraine headaches. It is also important to understand that while medication is often a clue to assessment, it is also possible that the patient's present emergency may be completely unrelated to the medication he or she is taking; it is still necessary to conduct a full assessment.

CASE SCENARIO

You arrive at the home of a 78-year-old woman who has been complaining of weakness and nausea for several hours. While your partner takes a set of vitals, you observe several medication bottles on the table near the patient's bed. These medications are glyburide, Lanoxin, and Cardizem.

What can you conclude from these medications? Glyburide is an oral diabetic agent, Lanoxin (digoxin) is generally used to help regulate an irregular heartbeat, and Cardizem (diltiazem) is most commonly used to treat hypertension or angina. So, without even seeing the patient you know that she is a diabetic and that she probably has a history of hypertension and an underlying cardiac condition. This information, combined with the results of your assessment and patient history, will prove most useful in determining the true nature of the patient's current problem and will assist you and the hospital in formulating a plan of treatment.

Medication Overdose. Patients commonly overdose on medication for various reasons, including simple absentmindedness, misunderstanding of instructions, the desire to enhance or increase the action of the drug, or to commit suicide. In some cases, a patient may be taking the same medication in both generic form and as a trade preparation without realizing it. It is always wise to ask the patient if more than one physician is treating the same condition.

CASE SCENARIO

You respond to the home of a 64-year-old woman who has experienced a syncopal episode and now feels weak and dizzy. She has a pulse rate of 46. In questioning this patient you discover that she regularly takes atenolol, a beta blocker, for hypertension. She had forgotten to take her pills for 3 days, and this morning she took 3 at one time to try to "catch up." Shortly thereafter she began to feel weak and lightheaded. It is very probable that this patient is experiencing the effect of a beta blocker overdose.

A medication overdose may present with a wide variety of signs and symptoms. Assessment can be as simple as asking the patient how many pills she took. If the overdose was accidental, the patient may be truthful, but responses from a suicidal patient may be unreliable. If the medication container is available, it will be useful in determining the amount of medication taken. The label will generally state the number of pills that were originally contained in the bottle, the date the prescription was filled, and the directions for use. Suppose we find that there were 60 pills in the original prescription when filled 2 days ago and that the patient was directed to take 1 pill every 6 hours for pain. If the bottle now contains only 8 pills, we should consider the possibility of an overdose.

Medication Underdose. In some cases a patient will experience a problem caused by a medication underdose.

This typically occurs when the patient fails to take his or her medication or takes an amount inadequate to achieve the desired therapeutic result. Sometimes this is simply an oversight, whereas at other times the patient may have discontinued the medication or reduced the amount of the dose because he or she either felt good and believed it was not

needed or perhaps to minimize side effects. As in the case of a possible overdose, careful questioning of the patient and family members and examining medication containers are useful in assessing a problem of this nature.

A common example of underdosing seen by EMS personnel is when diabetics fail to take insulin according to schedule.

Side Effects/Adverse Effects. Side effects or adverse effects are undesired consequences that can sometimes occur as a result of using a medication. Such effects are generally known to the manufacturer and are listed in the product literature and in references such as the *PDR*. In some cases, these effects will occur rarely, whereas at other times they may be quite common. Some of the more commonly seen side effects include nausea, vomiting, drowsiness, headache, and lightheadedness. The headache associated with the use of sublingual nitroglycerin is a common example of a medication adverse effect. Patients who experience an adverse or side effect will sometimes erroneously claim that they are allergic to the medication.

Some effects manifest themselves almost immediately, whereas others may not occur for hours or days. In assessing the patient, ascertain if any medications are new. Quite often, a troubling adverse effect that has prompted a request for an ambulance will be caused by a new medication. Ask if the patient has ever felt this way before when he or she took any of these medications and whether or not any such effect was reported to the physician.

CASE SCENARIO

A 59-year-old man has called for the ambulance and is complaining of heart palpitations and a "racing heart." His pulse is 122. In questioning the patient, you discover that only 2 days ago the patient received a prescription for albuterol to assist him with his emphysema. He used this medication for the first time about 20 minutes before he started feeling the palpitations. Both palpitations and tachycardia are known adverse effects of albuterol, and this patient's problem is most likely the direct result of his use of the medication.

Allergic Reactions. Allergic reactions are hypersensitive reactions that may be characterized by hives, itching, watery eyes, tachycardia, nausea, wheezing, laryngeal edema, and bronchospasm. Such reactions generally occur within a short time after the medication has been used, although some reactions can be delayed for much longer. Patients commonly confuse allergic reactions with adverse effects, but a true allergic reaction is far more serious and may quickly lead to death if not treated promptly. An allergy to almost any medication is possible, but those more commonly implicated are antibiotics, opiates, muscle relaxers, and vaccines. An assessment finding of allergic reaction is usually reached by evaluating the patient's signs and symptoms and obtaining a good history.

Medication Interactions. Interactions occur when a patient takes two or more medications or takes a medication with another substance such as food or alcohol. Such reactions will manifest themselves in a variety of ways. In some cases, the end result is greatly reduced effi-

cacy of one or both of the medications, but such reactions rarely generate a request for an ambulance. On the other hand, some medications can interact in very dangerous ways, causing severe effects or toxicity. Pharmacists are generally good at identifying possible interactions between the patient's various medications, but in many cases a patient will fill prescriptions at more than one pharmacy.

Interactions are not easily assessed in the field, making it all the more important to provide the hospital with as much detailed medication information as possible and to bring along any available medication bottles. Do not overlook the possibility of an interaction with an over-the-counter medication, food product, alcohol, or herbal preparation.

As an EMS provider, when dealing with any possible

medication-related problem, the best source of assistance is often your local poison control center.

COMMON MEDICATION CLASSIFICATIONS

In this section, some of the more commonly encountered classes of medications are listed, along with a brief explanation of how they work, their indications, common side effects, signs and symptoms of overdose or toxicity, and treatment for overdose. A basic knowledge of these common medications helps in effective assessment and treatment and will make the reader feel more comfortable in handling medication problems that arise in the field. Also included is a list of the more common drugs in each class that EMS providers will frequently find among their patients' prescription and over-the-counter medications. These lists are by no means exhaustive, and, in some cases, many more medications exist than have been listed. Only the more commonly used medications have been included. For a more complete list of any class of medication, the reader is referred to the PDR.

ACE INHIBITORS

ACE is an abbreviation for angiotensin converting enzyme. ACE inhibitors act by preventing the hormone angiotensin I from converting into angiotensin II, a potent vasoconstrictor. In preventing this conversion, ACE inhibitors relax blood vessels and help reduce blood pressure. They also make it easier for the heart to pump, thereby assisting in the relief of congestive heart failure.

| INDICATIONS | Hypertension and as an adjunctive treatment for congestive heart failure |

SIDE EFFECTS	Dizziness, fatigue, headache, nausea, persistent cough, tachycardia
SIGNS AND SYMPTOMS OF OVERDOSE/ TOXICITY	Most significant manifestation is severe hypotension with dizziness and syncope
TREATMENT OF OVERDOSE	Induce vomiting if the patient is fully alert and follow with activated charcoal once vomiting has stopped; consider intravenous (IV) fluid challenge; administer oxygen and provide general supportive measures; contact poison center for additional options

Commonly Prescribed ACE Inhibitors
benazepril (Lotensin)
captopril (Capoten)
enalapril (Vasotec)
fosinopril (Monopril)
lisinopril (Prinivil, Zestril)
quinapril (Accupril)
ramipril (Altace)
spirapril (Renormax)

ANTIDEPRESSANTS (SEROTONIN RE-UPTAKE INHIBITORS)

While there are a number of different classes of antidepressants, serotonin re-uptake inhibitors are among the more commonly prescribed preparations in recent years. As their name suggests, these medications work by blocking the uptake of serotonin, a substance naturally present in certain neurons in the brain that are believed to play a role in depression, into human platelets. Tricyclic antidepressants, another popular class of antidepressants, are discussed later in this chapter.

INDICATIONS	Treatment of depression and a variety of obsessive-compulsive disorders
SIDE EFFECTS	Headache, hot flashes, insomnia, dizziness, anxiety, palpitations, rash, sweating, nausea, chills, chest pain, loss of appetite
SIGNS AND SYMPTOMS OF OVERDOSE/ TOXICITY	Nausea and vomiting, tachycardia, severe agitation, hypotension
TREATMENT OF OVERDOSE	General supportive measures; administer oxygen; contact poison control or medical control for option of emesis and/or activated charcoal; establish IV access and consider fluid challenge for hypotension

Commonly Prescribed Serotonin Re-Uptake Inhibitors
fluoxetine (Prozac)
nefazodone (Serzone)
paroxetine (Paxil)
sertraline (Zoloft)
venlafaxine (Effexor)

ANTIDIABETIC AGENTS (ORAL)

Oral antidiabetic agents work by stimulating the release of insulin from functioning beta cells in the pancreas. This process results in a lowering of blood glucose levels.

21

One oral agent, metformin, works by lowering sugar production and improving the body's response to existing insulin.

INDICATIONS	To reduce and maintain blood glucose levels in patients with Type II diabetes; sometimes used as an adjunct in insulin-dependent diabetes
SIDE EFFECTS	Anorexia, nausea, diarrhea, dizziness, hypoglycemia
SIGNS AND SYMPTOMS OF OVERDOSE/ TOXICITY	Symptomatic hypoglycemia, tingling of the lips and tongue, nausea, lethargy, confusion, sweating, tremors, tachycardia, convulsions, coma
TREATMENT OF OVERDOSE	General supportive measures; oxygen; IV fluids; administer oral glucose if the patient is conscious and alert; otherwise consider 50% dextrose (D50) by IV route

Commonly Prescribed Antidiabetic Agents
acarbose (Precose)
acetohexamide (Dymelor)
chlorpropamide (Diabinese)
glipizide (Glucotrol)
glyburide (DiaBeta, Micronase)
metformin (Glucophage)
tolazamide (Tolinase)
tolbutamide (Orinase)
troglitazone (Rezulin)

Antihistamines are taken by everyone at one time or another and are commonly available as both prescription and over-the-counter preparations. These medications work by competing with histamines for H_1 receptor sites on the smooth muscle of the bronchi, the gastrointestinal (GI) tract, the uterus, and large blood vessels. They suppress histamine-induced allergic symptoms.

INDICATIONS	Management of seasonal and perennial allergies; adjunctive therapy in anaphylaxis; prevention and treatment of motion sickness; insomnia
SIDE EFFECTS	Drowsiness, sedation, dizziness, dry mouth, headache, hypotension, nausea, vomiting, cough
SIGNS AND SYMPTOMS OF OVERDOSE/ TOXICITY	Drowsiness, dilated pupils, GI symptoms, seizures, respiratory depression, hypotension, coma
TREATMENT OF OVERDOSE	General supportive measures; administer oxygen and be prepared to support ventilations; establish IV access and consider fluid challenge for hypotension; if patient is conscious and alert, contact medical control for options of syrup of ipecac and/or activated charcoal; treat seizures with diazepam (Valium)

Commonly Prescribed Antihistamines

astemizole (Hismanal)
azatadine (Optimine)
brompheniramine (Bromfed, Diamine)
chlorpheniramine (Atrohist Pediatric, Chlorspan, Chlor-Trimeton)
clemastine (Tavist)
cyproheptadine (Periactin)
diphenhydramine (Benadryl)
loratadine (Claritin)
methdilazine (Tacaryl)
promethazine (Phenergan)
terfenadine (Seldane)
trimeprazine (Temaril)
tripolidine (Myidyl)

NOTE: Antihistamines are also available as over-the-counter preparations such as Benadryl and can be found in a number of cold, cough, and allergy preparations such as Actifed, Comtrex, and Sinutab.

BENZODIAZEPINES

Benzodiazepines are a large class of medications made up of antianxiety agents, muscle relaxants, anticonvulsants, and sedatives. They act by depressing the central nervous system.

INDICATIONS	Management of anxiety disorders; reduction of skeletal muscle spasm; management of convulsive disorders; insomnia
SIDE EFFECTS	Confusion, depression, drowsiness, hypotension,

	bradycardia, respiratory depression
SIGNS AND SYMPTOMS OF OVERDOSE/ TOXICITY	Severe hypotension, bradycardia, slurred speech, confusion, impaired coordination, coma
TREATMENT OF OVERDOSE	General supportive measures; administer oxygen and be prepared to support ventilations and intubate, if necessary; consider IV fluid challenge for hypotension; contact medical control for option of flumazenil to reverse effects of benzodiazepines; contact medical control for further options such as atropine for symptomatic bradycardia

Commonly Prescribed Benzodiazepines
alprazolam (Xanax)
clonazepam (Klonopin)
clorazepate (Tranxene)
diazepam (Valium)
estazolam (ProSom)
flurazepam (Dalmane)
halazepam (Paxipam)
lorazepam (Ativan)
midazolam (Versed)
oxazepam (Serax)
prazepam (Centrax)
quazepam (Doral)
temazepam (Restoril)
triazolam (Halcion)

Beta blockers are a particularly useful class of drugs with a number of diverse indications. They are used to treat hypertension, angina, and various tachyarrhythmias, particularly supraventricular tachycardia. EMS personnel frequently encounter patients who are taking beta blockers for various reasons. These medications block the beta adrenergic receptors in the heart, thereby decreasing significantly the influence of the sympathetic nervous system. The overall effect is to decrease myocardial excitability, cardiac workload, and oxygen consumption. Beta blockers also have what is referred to as a membrane-stabilizing effect that, in part, is responsible for their antiarrhythmic capabilities.

In the field it is important to be aware of the fact that patient use of beta blockers can sometimes alter the body's normal response to certain medical conditions. For example, patients in the early stage of shock, hypovolemia, or hypoglycemia would normally be expected to have a rapid heart rate. Beta blocker use may modify this anticipated response by maintaining the heart rate in the normal range.

INDICATIONS	Hypertension; management of angina and certain cardiac arrhythmias, including supraventricular tachycardia, atrial fibrillation, and atrial flutter; management of migraine headaches
SIDE EFFECTS	Lethargy, fatigue, dizziness, hypotension, bradycardia, nausea, vomiting, diarrhea,

	hypoglycemia, pulmonary edema
SIGNS AND SYMPTOMS OF OVERDOSE/ TOXICITY	Severe hypotension, congestive heart failure, symptomatic bradycardia, bronchospasm
TREATMENT OF OVERDOSE	General supportive measures; administer oxygen and be prepared to support ventilations; establish IV access and consider fluid challenge for severe hypotension; contact medical control for the option of emesis and/or activated charcoal if the patient is conscious and alert; consider atropine for bradycardia and furosemide or other diuretic for congestive heart failure

Commonly Prescribed Beta Blockers

acebutolol (Sectral)
atenolol (Tenormin)
betaxolol (Kerlone)
bisoprolol (Zebeta)
carteolol (Cartrol)
labetalol (Normodyne)
metoprolol (Lopressor)
nadolol (Corgard)
penbutolol (Levatol)
propranolol (Inderal)
sotalol (Betapace)
timolol (Blocadren)

NOTE: The generic names of all beta blockers end in -lol.

Most bronchodilators achieve their desired effect by selectively stimulating beta 2 adrenergic receptors in the lungs and vascular smooth muscle. This stimulation results in relaxation of bronchial smooth muscle, reduction in airway resistance, and bronchodilation. These medications are generally available as tablets or inhalers. A number of bronchodilators are available as over-the-counter medications.

INDICATIONS	Prevention and relief of reversible bronchospasm associated with asthma, emphysema, or other obstructive airway disease; prevention of exercise-induced bronchospasm
SIDE EFFECTS	Anxiety, restlessness, nausea, arrhythmias (particularly tachyarrhythmias), palpitations, sweating, paradoxical bronchospasm
SIGNS AND SYMPTOMS OF OVERDOSE/ TOXICITY	Arrhythmias, angina, diaphoresis, hypertension, seizures
TREATMENT OF OVERDOSE	General supportive measures; administer oxygen and establish IV access; treat arrhythmias as per current advanced cardiac life support (ACLS) guidelines or as directed by medical control; consider diazepam for seizures

Commonly Prescribed Bronchodilators

albuterol (Proventil, Ventolin) (salbutamol, Volmax in Canada)
aminophylline (Amoline, Somophylline)
bitolterol (Tornalate)
ephedrine (Vicks Vatronol)
epinephrine (Bronkaid Mist, Primatene)
ipratropium (Atrovent)
ipratropium and albuterol (Combivent)
isoetharine (Bronkosol)
metaproterenol (Alupent, Metaprel)
oxtriphylline (Choledyl)
pirbuterol (Maxair)
salmeterol (Serevent)
terbutaline (Brethine)
theophylline (Theobid, Theo-Dur, Uniphyl)

CALCIUM CHANNEL BLOCKERS

Calcium channel blockers inhibit the transport of calcium ions across the membranes of cardiac and vascular smooth muscle cells; the result is dilation and relaxation of cardiac and systemic arteries; decreased peripheral vascular resistance, afterload, and systemic blood pressure; and inhibited coronary artery spasms.

INDICATIONS	Treatment of hypertension, angina, tachyarrhythmias
SIDE EFFECTS	Dizziness, lightheadedness, headache, nausea, diarrhea, constipation, peripheral edema, bradycardia, nasal congestion
SIGNS AND SYMPTOMS OF OVERDOSE/ TOXICITY	Overdose usually consists of an exaggeration of side effects; more serious cases involve

	heart blocks, symptomatic bradycardia, and profound hypotension
TREATMENT OF OVERDOSE	General supportive measures; administer oxygen and be prepared to support ventilations; establish IV access; treat arrhythmias as per current ACLS guidelines or as directed by medical control; consider atropine for bradycardia and fluid challenge and/or vasopressors for hypotension; contact medical control for option of calcium preparations

Commonly Prescribed Calcium Channel Blockers

amlodipine (Norvasc)
bepridil (Vascor)
diltiazem (Cardizem, Cardizem CD, Dilacor)
felodipine (Plendil)
isradipine (DynaCirc)
nicardipine (Cardene)
nifedipine (Adalat, Procardia)
verapamil (Calan, Isoptin)

CHOLESTEROL-LOWERING AGENTS

Cholesterol-lowering agents, also known as antilipid agents, are now very commonly prescribed for patients with elevated cholesterol levels. They are particularly common in patients who have already been diagnosed with cardiovascular disease, have had a myocardial infarction, or have other significant cardiac risk factors.

Most drugs in this class work by inhibiting the hepatic enzyme that is essential to cholesterol synthesis.

INDICATIONS	Reduction of total cholesterol and low-density lipids (LDL) in patients with levels that present a risk for cardiovascular disease
SIDE EFFECTS	Abdominal pain or cramping, constipation, headache, dizziness, rash, flushing
SIGNS AND SYMPTOMS OF OVERDOSE/ TOXICITY	Overdoses of cholesterol-lowering medications are uncommon; intestinal obstruction has occurred in rare cases
TREATMENT OF OVERDOSE	General supportive measures; monitor airway, breathing, and circulation (ABCs); contact medical control or poison control for further advice

Commonly Prescribed Cholesterol-Lowering Agents
cerivastatin (Baycol)
cholestyramine (Questran)
colestipol (Colestid)
fluvastatin (Lescol)
gemfibrozil (Lopid)
lovastatin (Mevacor)
niacin
pravastatin (Pravachol)
simvastatin (Zocor)

Diuretics make up a very large classification of drugs that may be divided into several sub-classifications. Thiazide diuretics inhibit the reabsorption of sodium and chloride in the distal renal tubules, resulting in the increased excretion of sodium, chloride, and water. Loop diuretics inhibit sodium and chloride reabsorption both in the renal tubules and in the loop of Henle; for this reason they are considered more potent than thiazide diuretics. Potassium-sparing diuretics promote the excretion of sodium and water but retain potassium. Osmotic diuretics actually draw fluid directly out of the tissues; they are generally used in the hospital and are only rarely prescribed for patient use at home.

INDICATIONS	Prevention and management of edema associated with congestive heart failure; liver or renal disease, or steroid therapy; management of hypertension (often used in conjunction with other anti-hypertensive agents)
SIDE EFFECTS	Dizziness, headache, nausea and vomiting, constipation, dry mouth, hypotension, irregular heartbeat, muscle weakness, blurred vision
SIGNS AND SYMPTOMS OF OVERDOSE/ TOXICITY	Severe dehydration, nausea and vomiting, electrolyte imbalance, arrhythmias, severe hypotension

TREATMENT OF OVERDOSE	General supportive measures; administer oxygen and establish IV access; monitor vitals frequently; consider fluid challenge and/or vasopressors for hypotension; treat arrhythmias as per current ACLS guidelines or as directed by medical control

Commonly Prescribed Diuretics

Thiazide Diuretics

bendroflumethiazide (Naturetin)

benzthiazide (Exna)

chlorothiazide (Diuril)

chlorthalidone (Hygroton)

hydrochlorothiazide (HydroDIURIL)

hydroflumethiazide (Diucardin)

indapamide (Lozol)

methyclothiazide (Enduron)

metolazone (Zaroxolyn)

polythiazide (Renese)

quinethazone (Hydromox)

trichlormethiazide (Diurese)

Loop Diuretics

bumetanide (Bumex)

ethacrynic acid (Edecrin)

furosemide (Lasix)

torsemide (Demadex)

Potassium-Sparing Diuretics

amiloride (Midamor)

spironolactone (Aldactone)

triamterene (Dyrenium)

This class includes narcotic preparations that are derived from opium, as well as synthetic drugs, known as opioids, whose actions mimic those of opium-derived drugs such as morphine. Narcotics are most commonly used for the relief of pain but also have antidiarrheal, antitussive, and sedative effects. They achieve their desired effect by acting as agonists at opioid receptor sites in the central nervous system. Because of the high potential for abuse and addiction, narcotic drugs are classified as Schedule II and may only be administered pursuant to a physician's order.

INDICATIONS	Relief of moderate to severe pain; relief of diarrhea and cough
SIDE EFFECTS	Lightheadedness, dizziness, sedation, nausea, vomiting, dry mouth, hypotension, bradycardia, respiratory depression, urinary retention
SIGNS AND SYMPTOMS OF OVERDOSE/ TOXICITY	Exaggeration of side effects; respiratory depression, miosis (pinpoint pupils), severe hypotension, bradycardia, convulsions
TREATMENT OF OVERDOSE	General supportive measures; administer oxygen and be prepared to assist ventilations and/or intubate; establish IV access and consider IV fluid challenge for hypotension; for ingested narcotics, consider ipecac and/or activated

charcoal; administer naloxone (Narcan) to reverse respiratory depression; contact medical control for further options

Commonly Prescribed Narcotics
codeine (Empirin with Codeine, Tylenol with Codeine)
difenoxine (Motofen)
diphenoxylate (Lomotil)
fentanyl (Duragesic transdermal patch)
hydrocodone (Lortab, Vicodin)
hydromorphone (Dilaudid)
levorphanol (Levo-Dromoran)
meperidine (Demerol)
methadone (Dolophine)
morphine (Duramorph, Roxanol)
oxycodone (Roxicodone, Tylox)
oxycodone with acetaminophen (Percocet)
oxycodone with aspirin (Percodan)
oxymorphone (Numorphan)
pentazocine (Talwin)
propoxyphene (Darvon, Darvocet-N)

Cough Medications with Narcotics
Dimetane-DC
Phenergan with Codeine
Tussionex Pennkinetic
Tussi-Organidin
Tylenol with Codeine

NONSTEROIDAL ANTI-INFLAMMATORY DRUGS (NSAIDs)

NSAIDs are a rapidly growing class of drugs primarily used for their analgesic, anti-inflammatory, and antipyretic effects. They are believed to work, at least in part, by inhibiting the synthesis of prostaglandin.

NSAIDs are commonly available in both prescription and over-the-counter preparations.

INDICATIONS	Relief of moderate to severe pain; relief of discomfort associated with inflammation; reduction of fever
SIDE EFFECTS	Headache, dizziness, constipation, diarrhea, nausea, vomiting, edema
SIGNS AND SYMPTOMS OF OVERDOSE/ TOXICITY	Drowsiness, stupor, paresthesia, vomiting, abdominal pain, sweating, dyspnea, cyanosis, nystagmus (constant involuntary movement of the eyeball)
TREATMENT OF OVERDOSE	General supportive measures; administer oxygen and be prepared to assist ventilations; establish IV access; consider emesis with syrup of ipecac followed by activated charcoal; contact medical control or poison control for further options

Commonly Prescribed/Used NSAIDs
diclofenac (Voltaren)
etodolac (Lodine)
fenoprofen (Nalfon)
flurbiprofen (Ansaid)
ibuprofen (Advil, Motrin, Nuprin)
indomethacin (Indocin)
ketoprofen (Orudis)
ketorolac (Toradol)

meclofenamate (Meclomen)
mefenamic acid (Ponstel)
nabumetone (Relafen)
naproxen (Naprosyn)
oxaprozin (Daypro)
piroxicam (Feldene)
sulindac (Clinoril)
tolmetin (Tolectin)

TRICYCLIC ANTIDEPRESSANTS

Although the exact mechanism of action is unknown, tricyclic antidepressants are often effective in relieving depression when other classes of antidepressants have been unsuccessful. Some of these drugs are also used in the treatment of certain obsessive-compulsive disorders and chronic pain. Side effects are numerous, and patients must be carefully monitored.

INDICATIONS	Treatment of depression, obsessive-compulsive disorders, and chronic pain
SIDE EFFECTS	Dizziness, sedation, blurred vision, dry mouth, constipation, nausea, sweating, hypotension, abdominal cramping
SIGNS AND SYMPTOMS OF OVERDOSE/ TOXICITY	Agitation, confusion, seizures, dilated pupils, hypothermia, arrhythmias, cyanosis, severe hypotension; severity of toxicity is sometimes indicated by a widening of the QRS complex

TREATMENT OF OVERDOSE	General supportive measures; monitor ABCs and administer oxygen; establish IV access and consider fluid challenge for hypotension; consider emesis and activated charcoal if patient is conscious and alert; consider diazepam for seizures and physostigmine, if available, to reverse the effects of tricyclics; treat arrhythmias as per current ACLS guidelines or as directed by medical control

Commonly Prescribed Tricyclics

amitriptyline (Elavil)
amoxapine (Asendin)
clomipramine (Anafranil)
desipramine (Norpramin)
doxepin (Sinequan)
imipramine (Tofranil)
maprotiline (Ludiomil)
nortriptyline (Pamelor)
protriptyline (Triptil, Vicatil)
trimipramine (Surmontil)

QUICK ASSESSMENT GUIDE

EMS providers obtain medication information from patients, family members, and friends of the patient, as well as finding medication containers at the scene. As noted earlier, these medications can often provide the key that will lead to an accurate assessment of the patient's current problem. In this Quick Assessment Guide, the reader will find lists of some of the more common medications used by patients suffering from medical conditions that frequently require EMS treatment and transportation. If the provider locates one or more of the patient's medications on any of these lists, it will strongly suggest that the patient is suffering from the subject condition. The generic form of each drug is listed on the left, in lowercase letters, and the trade name is on the right, in parentheses.

SEIZURE DISORDERS

A person found to be taking any of the following may be suffering from epilepsy or some other seizure disorder.

carbamazepine (Tegretol)
clonazepam (Klonopin)
diazepam (Valium)
divalproex sodium (Depakote)
felbamate (Felbatol)
gabapentin (Neurontin)
lamotrigine (Lamictal)
phenobarbital (Solfoton)
phenytoin (Dilantin)
primidone (Mysoline)
valproic acid (Depakene)

DIABETES

A patient taking any of the following medications may generally be presumed to be a diabetic.

acarbose (Precose)
acetohexamide (Dymelor)
chlorpropamide (Diabinese)
glimepiride (Amaryl)
glipizide (Glucotrol)

glucagon
glyburide (DiaBeta, Micronase)
insulin (Humulin, Lente, Novolin, NPH)
metformin (Glucophage)
tolazamide (Tolinase)
tolbutamide (Orinase)
troglitazone (Rezulin)

RESPIRATORY DISEASE

A patient taking any of the following medications can generally be presumed to be suffering from a respiratory condition such as asthma, emphysema, or chronic bronchitis.

albuterol (Proventil, Ventolin)
aminophylline (Amoline)
bitolterol (Tornalate)
ephedrine (Vicks Vatronol)
epinephrine (Bronkaid Mist)
ipratropium (Atrovent)
ipratropium and albuterol (Combivent)
isoetharine (Bronkosol)
metaproterenol (Alupent, Metaprel)
oxtriphylline (Choledyl)
pirbuterol (Maxair)
salmeterol (Serevent)
terbutaline (Brethine)
theophylline (Theobid, Theo-Dur)

CARDIOVASCULAR DISEASE

A patient taking any of the following medications may be suffering from a cardiac condition such as angina, arrhythmia, recent myocardial infarction, or a cardiac-related condition such as hypertension or congestive heart failure.

ACE Inhibitors—used to treat hypertension and congestive heart failure

benazepril (Lotensin)	lisinopril (Prinivil, Zestril)
captopril (Capoten)	quinapril (Accupril)
enalapril (Vasotec)	ramipril (Altace)
fosinopril (Monopril)	spirapril (Renormax)

Beta Blockers—used to treat hypertension, angina, and cardiac arrhythmias such as atrial fibrillation, atrial flutter, and supraventricular tachycardia

acebutolol (Sectral)	metoprolol (Lopressor)
atenolol (Tenormin)	nadolol (Corgard)
betaxolol (Kerlone)	penbutolol (Levatol)
bisoprolol (Zebeta)	propranolol (Inderal)
carteolol (Cartrol)	timolol (Blocadren)

Calcium Channel Blockers—used to treat hypertension, angina, and tachyarrhythmias

amlodipine (Norvasc)	isradipine (DynaCirc)
bepridil (Vascor)	nicardipine (Cardene)
diltiazem (Cardizem)	nifedipine (Adalat, Procardia)
felodipine (Plendil)	verapamil (Calan, Isoptin)

Cholesterol-Lowering Agents—used to reduce cholesterol levels that present a risk of heart disease

cholestyramine (Questran)	lovastatin (Mevacor)
colestipol (Colestid)	niacin
fluvastatin (Lescol)	pravastatin (Pravachol)
gemfibrozil (Lopid)	simvastatin (Zocor)

Diuretics—used to treat congestive heart failure and hypertension

amiloride (Midamor)

bendroflumethiazide (Naturetin)

benzthiazide (Exna)
bumetanide (Bumex)

chlorothiazide (Diuril)

chlorthalidone (Hygroton)

ethacrynic acid (Edecrin)

furosemide (Lasix)

hydrochlorothiazide (HydroDIURIL)

hydroflumethiazide (Diucardin)

indapamide (Lozol)

methyclothiazide (Enduron)

metolazone (Zaroxolyn)

polythiazide (Renese)

quinethazone (Hydromox)

spironolactone (Aldactone)

torsemide (Demadex)

triamterene (Dyrenium)

trichlormethiazide (Diurese)

Antiarrhythmics—used to treat arrhythmias, including atrial fibrillation, atrial flutter, and supraventricular tachycardia

amiodarone (Cordarone)

digoxin (Lanoxin)

disopyramide (Norpace)

flecainide (Tambocor)

mexiletine (Mexitil)

moricizine (Ethmozine)

phenytoin (Dilantin)

propafenone (Rythmol)

quinidine (Quinidex)

sotalol (Betapace)

tocainide (Tonocard)

NOTE: Beta blockers and calcium channel blockers are also used to treat arrhythmias.

In using this guide, it is always important to remember that many medications have more than one use. Always look past the obvious and avoid forming any conclusions until you have completed your assessment and taken a detailed patient history.

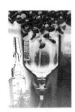

CHAPTER *THREE*

GUIDE TO PREHOSPITAL MEDICATION

There is little doubt that the administration of medication in the field by paramedics and other advanced life support providers has been among the most significant developments in prehospital emergency care and has had a remarkable, positive impact on patient outcome. Thousands of times each day, symptoms are improved, pain is relieved, and lives are saved by the use of medication. Much of the promise of the future of medicine and prehospital care will be the product of new medications. Newly discovered drugs are constantly being added to the prehospital arsenal and old ones removed to reflect current trends in medical research and treatment. A thorough working knowledge of medication is therefore essential for any prehospital provider who hopes to maintain his or her status as a competent and respected health care professional who is fully capable of delivering the highest standard of patient care.

This chapter provides the reader with a quick reference to the medications most commonly used in the prehospital environment. Many of these medications, such as epinephrine or nitroglycerin, are routinely carried in most paramedic drug boxes, while others are carried in services with specialized needs or with an active interfacility transfer component.

Every effort has been made to present medication information in a manner that reflects national standards such as the American Heart Association's Advanced Cardiac Life

Support (ACLS) guidelines and data obtained from texts and references that are generally accepted as standards within the prehospital community. Notwithstanding the foregoing, the reader will find that the information presented may occasionally vary from that contained in local protocols. Because medicine is not an exact science but one that is subject to varying opinions among experts, indications, dosages, precautions, routes of administration, and other considerations will not always be the same in every jurisdiction. It is the reader's responsibility to be fully familiar with the medication standards in his or her own system. Obviously, where differences occur, the provider is obliged to follow the local standards established by written protocol, standing orders, or the direction of the on-line medical control physician.

HOW TO USE THIS CHAPTER

The medications discussed in this chapter appear alphabetically according to generic name. The information for each drug is presented in a way that will hopefully reduce the confusion and frustration often encountered in studying medications.

The information for each drug is presented in the following manner:

Drug Name. The name appearing in bold, capital letters is the generic name. It is followed, parenthetically, by the most popular trade name or names.

EXAMPLE   FUROSEMIDE (Lasix)

If the medication is known by another name in Canada, that name appears on the next line, followed by the abbreviation *Can* in parentheses.

Class. In this section, the medication is categorized by its pharmacological classification, its therapeutic classification, or both. Where a particular medication has several therapeutic classifications, the one with the most relevant prehospital applications is indicated.

> **EXAMPLE** **Epinephrine:** Pharmacologically classified as a sympathomimetic and therapeutically classified as a bronchodilator, a vasopressor, or a cardiac stimulant.

Actions. The actions of the medication refer to the chemical and/or physiological mechanisms by which the medication's desired therapeutic effects are produced.

> **EXAMPLE** **Nitroglycerin:** relaxes vascular smooth muscle, which results in vasodilation. This has the effect of reducing preload, increasing coronary blood flow, and decreasing myocardial oxygen demand.

Indications. Indications are the medical conditions for which the subject medication is usually administered.

> **EXAMPLE** **Morphine:** Relief of moderate to severe pain
> **Naloxone:** Used to reverse adverse symptoms of narcotic overdose

In certain cases, indications for a particular medication may differ based on local protocol.

Contraindications. This section sets forth the conditions under which the subject drug should not be administered based on a determination that use of the medication would be unsafe.

EXAMPLE **Morphine:** Contraindicated in patients with undiagnosed abdominal pain.

Precautions. This section alerts the provider to circumstances under which the use of a medication may possibly be dangerous to the patient.

EXAMPLE **Adenosine:** May cause cardiac arrhythmias. Be prepared to treat.

Side Effects. Almost all medications have the potential to produce undesired or adverse effects. This section presents some of the more common undesired effects associated with the use of each drug under emergency, prehospital conditions. Side effects that are more commonly associated with long-term use of a particular medication are not included.

EXAMPLE **Nitroglycerin:** Headache, hypotension

Significant Interactions. Listed here are those medications which may produce undesirable effects when used concomitantly or concurrently with the subject medication.

EXAMPLE **Morphine:** Concomitant use with other narcotics, sedatives, barbiturates, tranquilizers, or alcohol may result in increased central nervous system (CNS) depression.

Dosage. Presented in this section are the standard dosages for each medication. These dosages have been compiled from nationally recognized texts, manuals, and other sources and reflect dosages generally used in the prehospital setting. Of course, local protocols may differ from these dosages in certain cases, and where differences do occur, local protocols should be followed.

Pediatric Dosage. This presents the standard pediatric dosages of each drug. It is important to check local protocols regarding pediatric dosages.

Route. This section describes the manner in which the medication is generally introduced into the body. In many cases, there will be more than one route of administration.

EXAMPLE IV, IM

Overdose or Toxicity Presentation. Contained in this section are the signs and symptoms typically associated with an overdose or toxic level of the drug. This refers to toxicity that might arise as a result of administration of the drug in the field or, in certain cases, personal use by the patient.

Treatment of Overdose or Other Adverse Reactions. This section contains treatment considerations for patients experiencing overdose, adverse reactions, or toxic reactions to the subject medication. In the case of any such reactions, providers are encouraged to contact online medical control.

Special Considerations. Any considerations deserving special attention by the provider are contained in this section. These include unusual side effects, special administration information, or a reminder to have certain drugs or equipment available before use of the drug.

> **EXAMPLE** **Dextrose 50%:** Obtain a blood glucose level before administration and obtain a pre-dextrose blood sample for hospital use.

At the conclusion of this section are three pages where the reader can place information concerning additional medications that may be currently used in his or her service or that may be added at a later date.

MEDICATIONS INCLUDED IN THIS SECTION

Medication	Page
Activated charcoal	53
Adenosine	55
Albuterol	58
Alteplase tPA	60
Aminophylline	63
Amrinone	65
Amyl nitrite	67
Aspirin	69
Atropine	71
Bretylium	75
Bumetanide	77
Butorphanol	79
Calcium chloride/gluconate	81

Medication	Page
Chlorpromazine	84
Dexamethasone	86
Dextrose 50%	87
Diazepam	89
Diazoxide	92
Digoxin	94
Diltiazem	96
Dimenhydrinate	98
Diphenhydramine	100
Dobutamine	101
Dopamine	106
Droperidol	109
Epinephrine 1:10,000	111
Epinephrine 1:1000	113
Epinephrine, racemic	116
Flumazenil	118
Fosphenytoin	120
Furosemide	122
Glucagon	125
Haloperidol	126
Hydralazine	128
Hydrocortisone	130
Hydromorphone	132
Insulin	134

Medication	Page
Ipecac	136
Isoetharine	139
Isoproterenol	141
Labetalol	143
Lidocaine	145
Lorazepam	149
Magnesium sulfate	150
Mannitol	153
Meperidine	155
Methylprednisolone	157
Metoprolol	159
Midazolam	161
Morphine sulfate	163
Nalbuphine	166
Naloxone	168
Nifedipine	171
Nitroglycerin	173
Nitroprusside	176
Nitrous oxide	178
Norepinephrine	180
Oxygen	183
Oxytocin	185
Pancuronium	188

Medication	Page
Pentazocine	190
Phenobarbital	191
Phenytoin	193
Physostigmine	196
Pralidoxime	198
Procainamide	200
Promethazine	203
Proparacaine	205
Propranolol	206
Sodium bicarbonate	208
Streptokinase	210
Succinylcholine	212
Terbutaline	215
Thiamine	217
Vecuronium	219
Verapamil	220

ACTIVATED CHARCOAL (Actidose-Aqua, Insta-Char)

CLASS	Adsorbent; antidote
ACTIONS	Binds to and adsorbs many ingested poisons and inhibits absorption into the gastrointestinal tract

INDICATIONS	Ingested poisoning, drug overdose
CONTRAINDICATIONS	Generally contraindicated in patients who have ingested cyanide, mineral acids, methanol, or caustic acids and bases; contact medical control for advice
PRECAUTIONS	Can sometimes induce vomiting; be prepared to protect the patient's airway
SIDE EFFECTS	Vomiting, diarrhea, constipation
SIGNIFICANT INTERACTIONS	Milk products decrease the effectiveness of activated charcoal.
DOSAGE	Usual dose is 1 g/kg. Powder is mixed in water to make a slurry.
PEDIATRIC DOSAGE	Same as for adults
ROUTE	Orally or through a nasogastric tube
OVERDOSE OR TOXICITY PRESENTATION	Overdose and toxicity are rare; if present, may consist of nausea and repeated vomiting
TREATMENT OF OVERDOSE OR OTHER ADVERSE REACTIONS	Generally only supportive measures are necessary.

| SPECIAL CONSIDERATIONS | Most effective if administered within 30 minutes after ingestion of toxin |

ADENOSINE (Adenocard)

| CLASS | Antiarrhythmic; a nucleoside |

| ACTIONS | Slows conduction through the atrioventricular (AV) node; inhibits re-entry through the AV node |

| INDICATIONS | Conversion of paroxysmal supraventricular tachycardia (PSVT) to regular sinus rhythm |

| CONTRAINDICATIONS | Second- or third-degree heart block, sick sinus syndrome |

| PRECAUTIONS | May produce new arrhythmias such as bradycardia, tachycardia, heart blocks, premature ventricular contractions (PVCs), or asystole; usually transient but be prepared to treat |

| SIDE EFFECTS | In addition to arrhythmias, may produce dyspnea, flushing, chest pain or |

pressure, dizziness, headache, palpitations, and feelings of impending doom

SIGNIFICANT INTERACTIONS

- Should not be used for patients taking carbamazepine (Tegretol) or dipyridamole (Persantine) because these drugs may potentiate and prolong adenosine's effect. If used in the presence of these two drugs, the dose of adenosine may have to be reduced. Contact medical control for options.
- Theophylline and related drugs can reduce the effectiveness of adenosine, and larger doses may be necessary. Contact medical control for options.

DOSAGE

6 mg IV push administered over 1 to 3 seconds. Use most proximal medication port in the IV line and flush immediately with 10 to

20 mL of saline. Elevate the arm to promote rapid introduction of the drug into the systemic circulation. If PSVT is not converted in 1 to 2 minutes, consider a second dose of 12 mg. If still unsuccessful, contact medical control for option of additional 12 mg dose.

PEDIATRIC DOSAGE

Generally not indicated for pediatric use

ROUTE

IV only

OVERDOSE OR TOXICITY PRESENTATION

Since the half life of adenosine is less than 10 seconds, any toxic or adverse effects usually resolve almost immediately. Occasionally, heart blocks, bradycardia, or PVCs may persist for a brief period.

TREATMENT OF OVERDOSE OR OTHER ADVERSE REACTIONS

Administer oxygen and treat any remaining effects symptomatically. Consider atropine for symptomatic bradycardia and lidocaine for PVCs per current ACLS guidelines.

- Monitor patient in the record mode during the administration of adenosine to capture any change in rhythm that results from the drug.
- Advise patient before administration of drug that resulting chest pain, flushing, or feelings of impending doom are normal and usually transitory.

ALBUTEROL SULFATE (Proventil, Ventolin)
Salbutamol (Can)

CLASS	Sympathomimetic
ACTIONS	Dilates bronchial smooth muscle, selectively stimulates beta 2 adrenergic receptors of bronchial smooth muscle and lungs
INDICATIONS	Asthma, bronchospasm associated with chronic obstructive pulmonary disease (COPD)
CONTRAINDICATIONS	Hypersensitivity to the drug, symptomatic tachyarrhythmias
PRECAUTIONS	Use with caution in patients with

tachyarrhythmias, cardiac disease, or severe hypertension.

SIDE EFFECTS

Dizziness, headache, arrhythmias, palpitations, diaphoresis, chest pain, or anxiety

SIGNIFICANT INTERACTIONS

Use with epinephrine or other sympathomimetics may increase risk of toxicity; beta blockers may inhibit bronchodilation effects of albuterol.

DOSAGE

Nebulizer with oxygen aerosolization: 0.5 mL (2.5 mg) in 2 to 3 mL of sodium chloride given over 5 to 10 minutes; may be repeated in cases of severe bronchospasm as per medical control or local protocol
Metered dose inhaler: 1 to 2 inhalations; may be repeated in 15 minutes

PEDIATRIC DOSAGE

Same as for adult unless otherwise directed by medical control

ROUTE

Inhalation

OVERDOSE OR TOXICITY PRESENTATION

Exaggeration of common side effects; angina, hypertension, seizures, and arrhythmias

TREATMENT OF OVERDOSE OR OTHER ADVERSE REACTIONS	Discontinue use of drug; focus on immediate life threats; administer oxygen, establish IV access if not yet available; treat arrhythmias per current ACLS guidelines or as directed by medical control.
SPECIAL CONSIDERATIONS	Monitor heart rate closely during albuterol administration because tachyarrhythmias frequently develop.

ALTEPLASE tPA (Tissue Plasminogen Activator)

CLASS	Thrombolytic; enzyme
ACTIONS	Catalyzes the conversion of plasminogen to plasmin, which dissolves thrombi (clots) associated with acute myocardial infarction (MI)
INDICATIONS	Treatment of acute MI also used in the treatment of cerebrovascular accident (CVA) but not in the prehospital setting
	Inclusion Criteria for Alteplase • Chest pain lasting between 20 minutes and 6 hours

- Pain unrelieved by nitroglycerin
- S-T elevation of 1 mm or more in two adjacent leads
- Systolic blood pressure greater than 80 mm Hg

Exclusion Criteria for Alteplase
- Surgery within the past 2 months
- History of CVA within the past 6 months
- History of bleeding disorder
- Severe hypertension
- Prolonged cardiopulmonary resuscitation (CPR) chest compressions

Check local protocols for additional or different inclusion or exclusion criteria.

CONTRAINDICATIONS	See exclusion criteria.
PRECAUTIONS	Use cautiously in patients over the age of 75.
SIDE EFFECTS	Intracranial and gastrointestinal (GI) bleeding, headache, arrhythmias, nausea, vomiting

SIGNIFICANT INTERACTIONS	Use with anticoagulants such as warfarin (Coumadin).
DOSAGE	Usual dose is a total of 100 mg administered as follows:

- 10 mg by IV bolus over 1 to 2 minutes
- 50 mg over the first hour
- 20 mg over the second hour
- 20 mg over the third hour

	Check local protocols for possible alternate dosing.
PEDIATRIC DOSAGE	Not used for pediatric patients in the field
ROUTE	IV only
OVERDOSE OR TOXICITY PRESENTATION	Intracranial, GI, or other bleeding problems; arrhythmias; severe nausea and vomiting
TREATMENT OF OVERDOSE OR OTHER ADVERSE REACTIONS	Discontinue drug immediately at first signs of bleeding; provide general supportive measures; administer oxygen; give IV fluids. Treat arrhythmias per current ACLS guidelines. Contact medical control for further options.

SPECIAL CONSIDERATIONS	• Monitor vitals continuously during administration.
	• Watch carefully for signs of bleeding.
	• Be prepared to treat arrhythmias.
	• Check patency of IV lines before administration of the drug.
	• If possible, start a second IV line.
	• Do not administer any IM injections before or during alteplase administration.

AMINOPHYLLINE

CLASS	Bronchodilator; smooth muscle relaxant
ACTIONS	Relaxes and dilates bronchial smooth muscle, mild diuretic
INDICATIONS	Bronchial asthma and COPD refractory to front-line medications, used in rare instances to treat congestive heart failure (CHF)
CONTRAINDICATIONS	Hypersensitivity to aminophylline, cardiac arrhythmias

PRECAUTIONS	Use cautiously in patients with history of cardiac disease, hypertension, or seizures; rapid administration may cause hypotension.
SIDE EFFECTS	Arrhythmias, seizures, nausea, vomiting, dizziness
SIGNIFICANT INTERACTIONS	Use with beta blockers or erythromycin may result in toxic effects. Use with sympathomimetic drugs increases the likelihood of CNS and cardiovascular side effects.
DOSAGE	250 to 500 mg of aminophylline diluted in 50 to 100 mL of 5% dextrose in water (D_5W); standard dose is 5 to 6 mg/kg infused over 30 minutes.
PEDIATRIC DOSAGE	Contact medical control for concentration and rate of infusion.
ROUTE	IV infusion
OVERDOSE OR TOXICITY PRESENTATION	Serious manifestations include arrhythmias (particularly ventricular fibrillation), seizures, and vomiting.

TREATMENT OF OVERDOSE OR OTHER ADVERSE REACTIONS

Monitor airway, breathing, and circulation (ABCs); give supportive care and administer oxygen; treat arrhythmias per current ACLS guidelines or as directed by medical control; seizures may be treated with benzodiazepine; if vomiting does not quickly subside, contact medical control for option of promethazine or other antiemetic drug.

SPECIAL CONSIDERATIONS

If patient has used theophylline preparation within the last 24 hours, aminophylline dose may need to be reduced.

AMRINONE (Inocor)

CLASS

Inotropic agent; vasodilator

ACTIONS

Increases the force of contraction and cardiac output, relaxes vascular smooth muscle

INDICATIONS

Treatment of severe CHF that has not responded to diuretics and vasodilators

65

CONTRAINDICATIONS	Hypersensitivity to amrinone or bisulfite drugs
PRECAUTIONS	Use very cautiously in presence of acute MI or ischemic disease.
SIDE EFFECTS	Arrhythmias, hypotension, nausea, vomiting
SIGNIFICANT INTERACTIONS	Amrinone and furosemide form a precipitate when mixed; do not inject furosemide into an IV line if amrinone is being infused.
DOSAGE	• 0.75 mg/kg administered over 2 to 3 minutes; may be followed by maintenance dose of 5 to 10 mg/kg/minute. • Prepare infusion by adding 100 mg of amrinone to 500 mL of normal saline.
PEDIATRIC DOSAGE	Not recommended in the field
ROUTE	IV only
OVERDOSE OR TOXICITY PRESENTATION	Severe hypotension, arrhythmias

TREATMENT OF OVERDOSE OR OTHER ADVERSE REACTIONS	Give general supportive measures; administer oxygen; administer IV fluids but do so carefully in the presence of CHF; consider vasopressors for hypotension.
SPECIAL CONSIDERATIONS	• Monitor vitals, particularly blood pressure, frequently. • Use smallest dose possible to achieve desired effect.

AMYL NITRITE (Vaporole)

CLASS	Nitrate; cyanide poisoning adjunct; vasodilator
ACTIONS	Converts hemoglobin to methemoglobin, which reacts with cyanide and decreases its toxicity
INDICATIONS	Treatment of cyanide poisoning in the field, also used for treatment of angina but rarely in the field
CONTRAINDICATIONS	None, in cases of cyanide poisoning
PRECAUTIONS	Use cautiously in pregnant women and in patients with

hypotension; place patient in recumbent or sitting position, since sudden hypotension may occur; amyl nitrite is highly flammable. **Do not administer amyl nitrite to patients who have recently taken the anti-impotence drug Viagra. Contact medical control for advice.**

SIDE EFFECTS

Hypotension, tachycardia, headache, palpitations, dizziness, nausea, vomiting

SIGNIFICANT INTERACTIONS

Severe hypotension may result if amyl nitrite is used concomitantly with beta blockers or other antihypertensives.

DOSAGE

1 or 2 ampules containing 0.3 mL of amyl nitrite. Ampules should be crushed and inhaled by the patient for 15 to 30 seconds. Repeat every 60 to 90 seconds until arrival at the emergency department. Administer oxygen between doses.

PEDIATRIC DOSAGE	1 ampule only; otherwise follow procedure for adults
ROUTE	Inhalation only
OVERDOSE OR TOXICITY PRESENTATION	Overdose or toxicity usually consists of an exaggeration of known side effects such as hypotension, tachycardia, syncope, vomiting, and coma.
TREATMENT OF OVERDOSE OR OTHER ADVERSE REACTIONS	Give general supportive measures; monitor vitals and cardiac rhythms; administer oxygen and start IV with normal saline or lactated Ringer's. Treat hypotension with fluid challenge; elevate legs. Contact medical control for further options.
SPECIAL CONSIDERATIONS	Amyl nitrite is often used illegally to enhance sexual pleasure.

ASPIRIN (ASA)

CLASS	Platelet inhibitor; anti-inflammatory; analgesic
ACTIONS	Impedes clotting action and platelet aggregation

by blocking prostaglandin synthetase action

INDICATIONS

Onset of recent chest pain suggestive of MI, signs and symptoms of recent CVA

CONTRAINDICATIONS

Recent history of GI bleeding or ulcers, patients with known bleeding disorders, known sensitivity to aspirin

PRECAUTIONS

Use cautiously in patients with history of asthma, pregnancy, or recent surgery. Contact medical control before use in patients taking warfarin (Coumadin) or other anticoagulants.

SIDE EFFECTS

Nausea, vomiting, heartburn, bronchospasm, dizziness, occult bleeding

SIGNIFICANT INTERACTIONS

Use with anticoagulants such as warfarin may potentiate the platelet-inhibiting effects of aspirin and increase the risk of occult bleeding.

DOSAGE

160 to 325 mg (Use of chewable children's

aspirin is frequently
recommended.)

PEDIATRIC DOSAGE

Generally not used in the
field for children

ROUTE

PO

**OVERDOSE OR
TOXICITY
PRESENTATION**

Overdose or toxicity is
very rare with the
recommended therapeutic
dose; if toxicity occurs, it
will usually consist of an
exaggeration of side
effects such as nausea,
vomiting, heartburn, or
bronchospasm.

**TREATMENT OF
OVERDOSE OR OTHER
ADVERSE REACTIONS**

Give general supportive
measures; monitor vitals;
administer oxygen; if
bronchospasm occurs,
consider use of albuterol;
contact medical control
for additional
considerations.

**SPECIAL
CONSIDERATIONS**

Inquire if patient has had
recent surgery, since
aspirin can promote
bleeding at the surgical
site.

ATROPINE SULFATE

CLASS

Parasympatholytic;
antiarrhythmic;
anticholinergic

ACTION	Decreases action of the parasympathetic nervous system, increases conduction velocity and heart rate, enhances conduction through the AV junction
INDICATIONS	Symptomatic bradycardia, bradyarrhythmias, asystole, organophosphate poisoning
CONTRAINDICATIONS	None when used for asystole, symptomatic bradycardia, or organophosphate poisoning
PRECAUTIONS	Use cautiously in patients with known or suspected MI because it may increase the size of the infarct or promote arrhythmias. Administer rapidly; if administered too slowly or in too small a dose, paradoxical profound bradycardia may result.
SIDE EFFECTS	Palpitations, headache, blurred vision, tachycardia, dry mouth, dilated pupils, drowsiness, anxiety

SIGNIFICANT INTERACTIONS

Use of atropine with other anticholinergics may result in additive effects.

DOSAGE

Bradycardia: 0.5 to 1.0 mg IV every 3 to 5 minutes until desired heart rate is achieved— total dose should not exceed 2 mg.
Asystole: 1.0 mg IV every 3 to 5 minutes to a maximum of 2 mg; 2.0 to 2.5 mg endotracheal tube (ET) every 3 to 5 minutes to a maximum of 5 mg. Dilute with 5 to 10 mg of normal saline or sterile water.
Organophosphate poisoning: 2.0 to 3.0 mg IV; may be repeated in 20 to 30 minutes
OR
2.0 mg IM and 1.0 mg IV.

PEDIATRIC DOSAGE

Bradycardia or asystole: 0.02 mg/kg IV, IM, or IO; minimum pediatric single dose is 0.1 mg; maximum pediatric single dose is 0.5 mg. Double dose when using ET route.
Organophosphate poisoning: 0.05 mg/kg

	IV, IM, IO; repeat until improvement is noted.
ROUTES	IV, IM, ET, or IO (children 6 and under). When using ET route, use 2 to 2 1/2 times the normal dose.
OVERDOSE OR TOXICITY PRESENTATION	Tachycardia, palpitations, angina, hallucinations, disorientation, agitation, coma, flushed skin, excessive dryness
TREATMENT OF OVERDOSE OR OTHER ADVERSE REACTIONS	Monitor ABCs; administer oxygen; give general supportive measures; treat arrhythmias per current ACLS guidelines or as directed by medical control; if available, consider physostigmine (Antilirium). **Adults:** 0.5 to 2.0 mg by slow IV bolus **Pediatric:** 0.02 mg/kg by slow IV bolus
SPECIAL CONSIDERATIONS	If paradoxical bradycardia develops, wait 2 to 3 minutes before initiating any corrective treatment, since bradycardia often resolves quickly.

BRETYLIUM TOSYLATE (Bretylol)
Bretylate (Can)

CLASS	Adrenergic blocking agent; antiarrhythmic
ACTIONS	Increases the ventricular fibrillation threshold, may occasionally successfully convert ventricular fibrillation or pulseless ventricular tachycardia without electric shock and for this reason has been called the "chemical defibrillator"
INDICATIONS	Ventricular fibrillation, pulseless ventricular tachycardia, less commonly used as a third-line drug for refractory ventricular tachycardia with a pulse
CONTRAINDICATIONS	None in the presence of life threatening arrhythmias
PRECAUTIONS	When administered in cases of non-cardiac arrest, infuse slowly because severe nausea, vomiting, or hypotension may occur.
SIDE EFFECTS	In conscious patients, nausea, vomiting,

dizziness, syncope, or
hypotension possible

**SIGNIFICANT
INTERACTIONS**

Interactions are of no
significance in the
presence of ventricular
fibrillation or pulseless
ventricular tachycardia;
in conscious patients,
severe hypotension may
occur when used with
procainamide or other
antiarrhythmics.

DOSAGE

**Ventricular fibrillation
or pulseless ventricular
tachycardia:** 5 mg/kg
IV bolus followed by 1
minute of CPR and
then electric shock;
if condition persists,
increase dose to
10 mg/kg after 5
minutes; maximum
dose should not exceed
30 mg/kg
OR
Follow current ACLS
guidelines
**Refractory ventricular
tachycardia with a
pulse:** 5 to 10 mg/kg IV
infusion administered
over a period of 8 to 10
minutes; may be
followed by a continuous

	infusion of 1 to 2 mg/minute
PEDIATRIC DOSAGE	Same as for adults
ROUTE	IV
OVERDOSE OR TOXICITY PRESENTATION	Severe hypotension
TREATMENT OF OVERDOSE OR OTHER ADVERSE REACTIONS	Give general supportive measures; monitor vitals; administer oxygen; consider IV fluid challenge and vasopressors such as dopamine; elevate the legs.
SPECIAL CONSIDERATIONS	In ventricular fibrillation, bretylium is second-line agent to lidocaine.

BUMETANIDE (Bumex)

CLASS	Potent loop diuretic; antihypertensive
ACTIONS	Inhibits the reabsorption of sodium and chloride in the kidney and promotes excretion of water, sodium, potassium, and chloride; decreases peripheral vascular resistance

INDICATIONS	Pulmonary edema and CHF; secondary medication for hypertension
CONTRAINDICATIONS	Hypersensitivity to the drug, severe dehydration, hypotension
PRECAUTIONS	Use cautiously in diabetic or pregnant patients.
SIDE EFFECTS	Dizziness, headache, vomiting, diarrhea, dehydration, hypotension, electrocardiographic (ECG) changes (arrhythmias)
SIGNIFICANT INTERACTIONS	Use with other diuretics may cause increased hypotension and fluid depletion; use with NSAIDs may inhibit diuretic effects.
DOSAGE	0.5 to 1.0 mg by IV bolus over 1 to 2 minutes or by IM injection; repeat dose rarely given in prehospital setting; daily dose should not exceed 10 mg.
PEDIATRIC DOSAGE	Pediatric use not recommended in the field

ROUTES	IV, IM
OVERDOSE OR TOXICITY PRESENTATION	Most common manifestation of toxicity or overdose is severe fluid depletion; severe hypotension, vomiting, and arrhythmias are also possible.
TREATMENT OF OVERDOSE OR OTHER ADVERSE REACTIONS	Give general supportive measures; monitor vitals and administer oxygen; replace fluids but use caution in the presence of pulmonary edema or CHF. Treat lingering arrhythmias per current ACLS guidelines or as directed by medical control. In cases of severe vomiting, consider use of promethazine (Phenergan) 12.5 to 25 mg IV or IM.
SPECIAL CONSIDERATIONS	Monitor blood pressure frequently because severe hypotension may develop.

BUTORPHANOL (Stadol)

CLASS	Synthetic analgesic
ACTIONS	Binds to opiate receptors in the CNS and reduces sensitivity to pain

INDICATIONS	Treatment of moderate to severe pain
CONTRAINDICATIONS	Hypersensitivity to the drug, head injury, narcotic addiction
PRECAUTIONS	Use with caution in patients with respiratory depression or history of seizure disorder. Elderly patients may be more sensitive to the drug and may require a smaller dose than usual. Naloxone (Narcan) should be available if respiratory depression or respiratory arrest occurs.
SIDE EFFECTS	Hypotension or hypertension, respiratory depression, headache, flushing, palpitations, nausea, vomiting
SIGNIFICANT INTERACTIONS	Narcotics, barbiturates, alcohol, tranquilizers, tricyclic antidepressants
DOSAGE	0.5 to 2.0 mg IV or 1 to 4 mg IM; may be repeated in 3 to 4 hours
PEDIATRIC DOSAGE	Not recommended for pediatric use
ROUTE	IV or IM

OVERDOSE OR TOXICITY PRESENTATION	Respiratory depression, severe hypotension, vomiting, palpitations
TREATMENT OF OVERDOSE OR OTHER ADVERSE REACTIONS	Give general supportive measures; monitor vitals; consider oxygen therapy and IV access. Consider naloxone to reverse effects of drug. Support ventilations; intubate, if necessary. Treat hypotension with fluid challenge; elevate legs. If necessary, consider vasopressors.
SPECIAL CONSIDERATIONS	Monitor vitals frequently when using butorphanol because hypotension and/or respiratory depression may occur.

CALCIUM CHLORIDE
CALCIUM GLUCONATE

CLASS	Electrolyte
ACTION	Calcium is an essential component for the proper functioning of the nervous, muscular, skeletal, and endocrine systems; it increases the strength of myocardial contractions.

INDICATIONS	Hypocalcemia; hyperkalemia; antidote for overdose of magnesium sulfate; treatment of certain insect bites and stings, particularly black widow spiders and scorpions; treatment of calcium channel blocker overdose; cardiac arrest when hyperkalemia is suspected
CONTRAINDICATONS	Hypercalcemia, digitalis toxicity, ventricular fibrillation
PRECAUTIONS	Use with caution in patients with renal insufficiency or history of cardiac disease.
SIDE EFFECTS	Cardiac arrhythmias, headache, dizziness, hypotension, nausea and vomiting
SIGNIFICANT INTERACTIONS	Avoid mixing with sodium bicarbonate because a precipitate may form; use of calcium with digoxin can cause increased cardiac irritability.
DOSAGE	**Calcium chloride:** 4 to 12 mg/kg by slow IV

82

bolus at a rate of 0.5 to 2.0 mL/minute; 1 mL of a 10% solution equals 100 mg of calcium chloride; repeat in 10 minutes if needed.
Calcium gluconate: 5 to 8 mL by slow IV bolus at a rate of 0.5 to 2.0 mL/minute; repeat in 10 minutes if needed.

PEDIATRIC DOSAGE

Calcium chloride: 5 to 7 mg/kg by slow IV bolus; repeat in 10 minutes if needed.
Calcium gluconate: not recommended in the field

ROUTE

IV only in the field

OVERDOSE OR TOXICITY PRESENTATION

Cardiac arrhythmias, vomiting, hypotension, and confusion

TREATMENT OF OVERDOSE OR OTHER ADVERSE REACTIONS

Give general supportive measures; administer oxygen; monitor vitals and cardiac rhythms.
Arrhythmias: Treat arrhythmias per current ACLS guidelines or as directed by medical control.
Hypotension: Consider fluid challenge; elevate legs.

SPECIAL CONSIDERATIONS

- Monitor vitals and cardiac rhythms closely during use.
- Slow injection will reduce the chances of adverse side effects.

CHLORPROMAZINE (Thorazine)
Chlor-Promanyl, Largactil (Can)

CLASS	Antipsychotic; tranquilizer
ACTIONS	Blocks postsynaptic dopamine receptors in the brain and CNS; results in antipsychotic effect
INDICATIONS	Acute psychotic episodes, mild alcohol withdrawal
CONTRAINDICATIONS	Hypersensitivity to the drug, coma, CNS depression, severe hypotension
PRECAUTIONS	Use cautiously in patients with history of cardiac arrhythmias, seizures, or respiratory disease.
SIDE EFFECTS	Headache, tachycardia, hypotension, nausea, vomiting
SIGNIFICANT INTERACTIONS	Additive CNS depression can occur if used with

other tranquilizers, sedatives, barbiturates, or alcohol; additive effect of both drugs when used with beta blockers; increased risk of symptomatic tachycardia if used with epinephrine

DOSAGE 25 mg; may be repeated in 1 hour

PEDIATRIC DOSAGE 0.5 mg/kg

ROUTE IM injection only

OVERDOSE OR TOXICITY PRESENTATION Coma, hypotension or hypertension, seizures, arrhythmias

TREATMENT OF OVERDOSE OR OTHER ADVERSE REACTIONS Give general supportive measures; obtain IV access if not yet available; administer oxygen, monitor vitals.
Coma: Maintain airway; support ventilations and be prepared to intubate; maintain body temperature; administer IV fluids.
Arrhythmias: treat per current ACLS guidelines or as directed by medical control.
Seizures: consider use of diazepam or barbiturates (phenobarbital).

| SPECIAL CONSIDERATIONS | • Assess vital signs every 5 minutes. |
| | • Administer by deep IM injection. |

DEXAMETHASONE (Decadron)
Dexasone (Can)

CLASS	Anti-inflammatory; steroid
ACTIONS	Suppresses inflammation, suppresses immune system
INDICATIONS	Cerebral edema associated with head injury, occasionally used as an adjunct in the treatment of shock
CONTRAINDICATIONS	Generally, no contraindications for single-dose use in the field
PRECAUTIONS	Use with caution in patients with seizures, hypertension, or CHF
SIDE EFFECTS	Hypertension, headache, edema, nausea, vomiting
SIGNIFICANT INTERACTIONS	Use with barbiturates or phenytoin may reduce the effectiveness of dexamethasone.
DOSAGE	10 mg by slow IV bolus

PEDIATRIC DOSAGE	0.25 to 0.50 mg/kg by slow IV bolus
ROUTE	IV
OVERDOSE OR TOXICITY PRESENTATION	Toxic effects of any significance are rare but when present usually consist of exaggeration of side effects such as hypertension, headache, edema, or nausea.
TREATMENT OF OVERDOSE OR OTHER ADVERSE REACTIONS	Give general supportive measures; monitor vitals.
SPECIAL CONSIDERATIONS	Protect from heat; dexamethasone is very sensitive to warm temperatures.

DEXTROSE 50%

CLASS	Carbohydrate; sugar
ACTIONS	Rapidly elevates blood glucose levels
INDICATIONS	Treatment of hypoglycemia, used to rule out hypoglycemia in coma of unknown origin, also used to treat seizures of unknown cause or where hypoglycemia is suspected as a cause of the seizure.

CONTRAINDICATIONS	No significant contraindications in the emergency setting
PRECAUTIONS	Check patency of IV line as D50 can cause local venous irritation and/or tissue necrosis; in cases of known or suspected CVA or intracranial hemorrhage, check with medical control before administration; consider administration of thiamine before D50, especially in known or suspected alcoholics, in order to avoid possible neurological consequences associated with Wernicke's encephalopathy.
SIDE EFFECTS	Venous irritation and CNS consequences as noted above
SIGNIFICANT INTERACTIONS	None in the field
DOSAGE	25 g administered slowly
PEDIATRIC DOSAGE	0.5 to 1 g/kg administered slowly
ROUTE	IV only
OVERDOSE OR TOXICITY PRESENTATION	Overdose is very rare and of little significance in the field.

TREATMENT OF OVERDOSE OR OTHER ADVERSE REACTIONS

Any adverse reactions usually require general supportive measures. If signs of fluid overload are present, slow or discontinue IV fluid administration. If infiltration occurs during administration of D50, discontinue administration immediately.

SPECIAL CONSIDERATIONS

- Obtain blood glucose level, when possible, before administration; obtain pre-D50 blood sample for hospital use.
- Never withhold D50 if severe hypoglycemia is suspected.

DIAZEPAM (Valium) Meval, Vivol (Can)

CLASS

Tranquilizer

ACTIONS

Reduces anxiety, suppresses seizure activity, induces amnesia, relaxes skeletal muscle

INDICATIONS

Generalized seizures and status epilepticus, acute anxiety, premedication

	before cardioversion, relax skeletal muscle
CONTRAINDICATIONS	Known sensitivity to the drug, respiratory depression from any source, patients who have taken sedatives or alcohol, severe hypotension
PRECAUTIONS	Short duration of effect, avoid mixing with other drugs because of potential to precipitate, possibility of local venous irritation
SIDE EFFECTS	Respiratory depression, drowsiness, hypotension, apnea
SIGNIFICANT INTERACTIONS	Narcotics, barbiturates, alcohol, antidepressants
DOSAGE	• **Status epilepticus:** 5 to 15 mg IV • **Acute anxiety:** 2 to 10 mg IV or IM • **Cardioversion:** 5 to 15 mg IV
PEDIATRIC DOSAGE	0.5 to 2.0 mg IV slowly as per medical control
ROUTES	• IV or IM; may also be administered rectally for pediatric patients with seizures

- ET is no longer considered an appropriate route for diazepam.

OVERDOSE OR TOXICITY PRESENTATION

Hypotension, respiratory depression, bradycardia, coma, confusion, slurred speech

TREATMENT OF OVERDOSE OR OTHER ADVERSE REACTIONS

Discontinue drug; monitor vital signs; monitor cardiac rhythm; administer oxygen and support ventilations as necessary. Be prepared to intubate.

Significant hypotension: Consider fluid challenge and/or dopamine (2 to 5 μg/kg/min).

Flumazenil: A diazepam antagonist, it may reverse adverse effects, but the drug is not generally available in the prehospital setting.

Apparent allergic reaction: Consider epinephrine 1:1000 (0.3 to 0.5 mg by subcutaneous injection) or diphenhydramine (Benadryl) (25 to 50 mg IV or IM).

| SPECIAL CONSIDERATIONS | Thoroughly flush the IV line before and after using diazepam because it frequently precipitates with other drugs. |

DIAZOXIDE (Hyperstat)

CLASS	Antihypertensive; peripheral vasodilator
ACTIONS	Relaxes arterial smooth muscle, resulting in vasodilation and a decrease in blood pressure
INDICATIONS	Malignant hypertension; hypertensive crisis
CONTRAINDICATIONS	Known sensitivity to the drug or to other thiazide medications
PRECAUTIONS	Use cautiously in patients with compromised cardiovascular function; monitor blood pressure every 5 minutes after administration; keep patient lying down until blood pressure is stable.
SIDE EFFECTS	Dizziness, headache, hypotension, arrhythmias, nausea, vomiting

SIGNIFICANT INTERACTIONS	Use with other antihypertensive agents may produce significant additive effects.
DOSAGE	1 to 3 mg/kg by rapid IV bolus with a maximum dose of 150 mg; may repeat in 5 to 15 minutes if necessary.
PEDIATRIC DOSAGE	Same as for adults
ROUTE	IV only in the field
OVERDOSE OR TOXICITY PRESENTATION	Severe hypotension, hyperglycemia, arrhythmias
TREATMENT OF OVERDOSE OR OTHER ADVERSE REACTIONS	Discontinue drug; monitor vitals and heart rhythm; administer oxygen. **Hypotension:** Consider IV fluid challenge and elevation of legs for hypotension; consider vasopressors if conservative treatment is unsuccessful. **Arrhythmias:** Treat arrhythmias per current ACLS guidelines, local protocols, or as directed by medical control. **Hyperglycemia:** Administer insulin, if available.

| SPECIAL CONSIDERATIONS | Diazoxide frequently causes pain and burning at the IV site; check IV site for infiltration. |

DIGOXIN (Lanoxin)

CLASS	Antiarrhythmic; inotropic agent; digitalis glycoside
ACTION	Increases the force and velocity of myocardial contractions, slows conduction through the AV node
INDICATIONS	Atrial fibrillation and flutter, supraventricular tachycardia, CHF (rarely used for this in the field)
CONTRAINDICATIONS	Hypersensitivity to the drug, ventricular fibrillation, digitalis toxicity, patients already on therapeutic dose
PRECAUTIONS	Use with caution in patients with MI, second- and third-degree heart blocks, and renal failure.
SIDE EFFECTS	Headache, confusion, bradycardia and other arrhythmias, nausea and vomiting, blurred vision
SIGNIFICANT INTERACTIONS	Use with loop diuretics such as furosemide or IV

	calcium preparations may cause increased incidence of arrhythmias. Use with beta blockers can cause symptomatic bradycardia.
DOSAGE	Initial dose: 0.25 to 0.50 mg by slow IV push (5 to 8 minutes)
PEDIATRIC DOSAGE	Not recommended for pediatric use in the field
ROUTE	IV only in the field
OVERDOSE OR TOXICITY PRESENTATION	Cardiac disturbances including lethal arrhythmias such as ventricular fibrillation, asystole, and heart blocks; vomiting; visual disturbances
TREATMENT OF OVERDOSE OR OTHER ADVERSE REACTIONS	Give general supportive measures; administer oxygen; maintain airway and support ventilations as necessary; discontinue drug. **Arrhythmias:** Treat arrhythmias per current ACLS guidelines or as directed by medical control; consider antiarrhythmic medications such as lidocaine, atropine, or procainamide.

SPECIAL CONSIDERATIONS	• Monitor vitals and heart rhythms continuously.
	• Obtain information from patient about any recent digoxin use.
	• Do not cardiovert a patient with possible digitalis toxicity (consult medical control for options).

DILTIAZEM (Cardizem)

CLASS	Calcium channel blocker
ACTIONS	Inhibits the movement of calcium ions across cardiac muscle cells, decreases conduction velocity and ventricular rate
INDICATIONS	Symptomatic atrial fibrillation and atrial flutter
CONTRAINDICATIONS	Hypotension below 90 mm Hg, second- or third-degree heart block, hypersensitivity to the drug
PRECAUTIONS	Use cautiously in patients with renal failure or CHF.
SIDE EFFECTS	Headache, nausea, vomiting, bradycardia, hypotension

SIGNIFICANT INTERACTIONS	CHF may result if used concomitantly with beta blockers.
DOSAGE	• 0.25 mg/kg by IV bolus administered over 2 minutes; if response is not adequate, repeat in 15 minutes with a dosage of 0.35 mg/kg over 2 minutes. • Bolus may be followed with infusion of 5 to 10 mg/hour.
PEDIATRIC DOSAGE	Not recommended
ROUTE	IV only in the field
OVERDOSE OR TOXICITY PRESENTATION	Generally consists of exaggeration of side effects, including severe hypotension and symptomatic bradycardia
TREATMENT OF OVERDOSE OR OTHER ADVERSE REACTIONS	Give general supportive measures; monitor vitals, administer oxygen. **Hypotension:** Consider IV fluid challenge with lactated Ringer's or normal saline; elevate legs; consider vasopressors. **Bradycardia:** Consider atropine (0.5 to 1.0 mg); if necessary, consider pacing.

Contact medical control
for option of calcium
preparations, if available.
Treat other arrhythmias
per current ACLS
guidelines or as directed
by medical control.

SPECIAL CONSIDERATIONS	Carefully monitor vitals before, during, and after administration.

DIMENHYDRINATE (Dramamine) Travamine (Can)

CLASS	Antihistamine; antiemetic; anti-vertigo agent
ACTIONS	Depresses sensitivity of the labyrinth apparatus, blocks synapses in the vomiting center
INDICATIONS	Treatment of nausea and vomiting, to potentiate the effects of narcotics, treatment of motion sickness
CONTRAINDICATIONS	Hypersensitivity to the drug or to other antiemetic antihistamines such as diphenhydramine
PRECAUTIONS	Use with caution in patients with asthma or seizure disorders.

SIDE EFFECTS	Drowsiness, headache, seizures, hypotension, blurred vision
SIGNIFICANT INTERACTIONS	Significant CNS depression may occur when used concomitantly with alcohol, barbiturates, tranquilizers, or narcotics.
DOSAGE	• 25 to 100 mg by slow IV bolus or IM. • For IV administration, dilute 50 mg of the drug in 10 mL of normal saline and inject over 2 to 3 minutes.
PEDIATRIC DOSAGE	12.5 to 50 mg by IV bolus or IM
ROUTES	IV or IM
OVERDOSE OR TOXICITY PRESENTATION	Severe CNS depression, seizures, dilated pupils
TREATMENT OF OVERDOSE OR OTHER ADVERSE REACTIONS	Give general supportive measures; monitor vitals and cardiac rhythms; administer oxygen. Consider diazepam (Valium) or phenytoin (Dilantin) for seizures.

| SPECIAL CONSIDERATIONS | • Monitor vitals during administration.
• Check patency of IV line because drug can cause local irritation. |

DIPHENHYDRAMINE (Benadryl)

CLASS	Antihistamine; sedative
ACTIONS	Blocks the effects of histamines
INDICATIONS	As an adjunct to epinephrine in treating severe allergic reactions, including anaphylactic shock; may be used independently in cases of mild to moderate allergic reactions
CONTRAINDICATIONS	Asthma or COPD attacks, late-stage pregnancy, lactation
PRECAUTIONS	Use cautiously in patients with narrow-angle glaucoma, heart disease, and hypertension.
SIDE EFFECTS	Drowsiness, headache, confusion, wheezing, palpitations, tachycardia, hypotension, nausea, vomiting
SIGNIFICANT INTERACTIONS	Additive CNS depression may occur when used

	together with alcohol, tranquilizers, or sedatives.
DOSAGE	10 to 50 mg
PEDIATRIC DOSAGE	2 to 5 mg/kg by IV bolus or deep IM injection
ROUTES	IV or deep IM
OVERDOSE OR TOXICITY PRESENTATION	Severe hypotension, seizures, or coma may infrequently occur.
TREATMENT OF OVERDOSE OR OTHER ADVERSE REACTIONS	Give general supportive measures; monitor vitals; administer oxygen; consider diazepam for seizures and vasopressors such as dopamine for hypotension.
SPECIAL CONSIDERATIONS	Elderly patients are particularly sensitive to diphenhydramine; monitor closely and observe for hypotension and seizure activity.

DOBUTAMINE (Dobutrex)

CLASS	Adrenergic; beta 1 agonist; inotropic agent
ACTIONS	Increases cardiac contractility and stroke volume but causes little, if any, increase in heart rate

INDICATIONS	Short-term management of CHF and cardiogenic shock
CONTRAINDICATIONS	Hypersensitivity to the drug, bradycardia, severe hypotension
PRECAUTIONS	Use cautiously in presence of myocardial infarction or tachyarrhythmias.
SIDE EFFECTS	Tachycardia, hypertension, chest pain, palpitations, nausea, vomiting, dyspnea
SIGNIFICANT INTERACTIONS	Concomitant use with beta blockers can result in ineffectiveness of dobutamine; use with nitroprusside may result in higher cardiac output.
DOSAGE	**Usual adult rate:** 2.5 to 10 μg/kg/minute by IV infusion; administration is titrated to patient's response; occasionally, larger dosages may be needed. **Infusion:** Prepare by adding 250 mg of dobutamine to 250 mL of D_5W or normal saline

OR

500 mg of dobutamine to 500 mL. Either will produce a concentration of 1000 μg/mL. Adding 250 mg of dobutamine to 500 mL of fluid will produce a concentration of 500 μg/mL. See following infusion chart.

PEDIATRIC DOSAGE

Rarely, if ever, used in the field for children

ROUTE

IV infusion only

OVERDOSE OR TOXICITY PRESENTATION

Stated side effects, nervousness, and fatigue

TREATMENT OF OVERDOSE OR OTHER ADVERSE REACTIONS

Give general supportive measures; administer oxygen. Most adverse reactions resolve fairly rapidly if dobutamine is discontinued. Treat any lingering effects symptomatically; treat cardiac manifestations per current ACLS guidelines or as directed by medical control.

SPECIAL CONSIDERATIONS

- Monitor vitals continuously.
- If hypovolemia is present, treat with volume expanders

DOBUTAMINE INFUSION CHART

Based on a concentration of 1000 μg/mL. This may be achieved by mixing 250 mg of dobutamine in 250 mL of normal saline or D$_5$W or 500 mg in 500 mL. Administration should be with a microdrip set. 60 gtt = 1 mL.

WEIGHT (kg)	40	45	50	55	60	65	70	75	80	85	90	95	100	105
DOSAGE (μg/kg/hr)					RATE IN mL/hr OR gtt/min (MICRODRIP)									
1.0	2	3	3	3	4	4	4	5	5	5	5	6	6	6
1.5	4	4	5	5	5	6	6	7	7	8	8	9	9	9
2.0	5	5	6	7	7	8	8	9	10	10	11	11	12	13
2.5	6	7	8	8	9	10	11	11	12	13	14	14	15	16
3.0	7	8	9	10	11	12	13	14	14	15	16	17	18	19

	8	9	11	12	13	14	15	16	17	18	19	20	21	22
3.5	8	9	11	12	13	14	15	16	17	18	19	20	21	22
4.0	10	11	12	13	14	16	17	18	19	20	22	23	24	25
4.5	11	12	14	15	16	18	19	20	22	23	24	26	27	28
5.0	12	14	15	17	18	20	21	23	24	26	27	29	30	32
5.5	13	15	17	18	20	21	23	25	26	28	30	31	33	35
6.0	14	16	18	20	22	23	25	27	29	31	32	34	36	38
7.0	17	19	21	23	25	27	29	32	34	36	38	40	42	44
8.0	19	22	24	26	29	31	34	36	38	41	43	46	48	50
9.0	22	24	27	30	32	35	38	41	43	46	49	51	54	57
10.0	24	27	30	33	36	39	42	45	48	51	54	57	60	63
12.0	29	32	36	40	43	47	50	54	58	61	65	68	72	76
15.0	36	41	45	50	54	55	63	69	72	77	81	86	90	95
16.0	38	43	48	53	58	52	67	72	77	82	86	91	96	101

before administration
of dobutamine.
- Administer with
infusion pump to
control rate.

DOPAMINE (Intropin)
Revimine (Can)

CLASS   Sympathomimetic agent

ACTIONS   Stimulates both alpha
                       and beta receptors in the
                       sympathetic nervous
                       system; effects are
                       dose dependent. Low
                       to moderate doses
                       of dopamine (1 to
                       10 μg/kg/minute)
                       produce cardiac
                       stimulation and renal
                       and mesenteric
                       vasodilation; higher
                       doses produce increased
                       peripheral vascular
                       resistance and renal
                       vasoconstriction.

INDICATIONS   Hypotension associated
                       with cardiogenic shock
                       or bradycardia, treatment
                       of hypovolemic shock
                       after fluid replacement

CONTRAINDICATIONS   Uncorrected
                       tachyarrhythmias,
                       pheochromocytoma (a
                       usually benign tumor

that produces
epinephrine and causes
hypertension),
hypovolemic shock,
unless substantial fluid
replacement has taken
place

PRECAUTIONS

Use with extreme caution
in patients with ischemic
cardiac disease or history
of occlusive vascular
disease.

SIDE EFFECTS

Ectopic heart beats,
tachyarrhythmias,
bradycardia, angina,
nausea and vomiting,
hypertension, headache

**SIGNIFICANT
INTERACTIONS**

Use with sodium
bicarbonate may
deactivate dopamine. Use
with phenytoin can result
in significant hypotension
and bradycardia. MAO
inhibitors may prolong
and intensify the effects
of dopamine (dosage may
need to be reduced).

DOSAGE

2 to 5 μg/kg/minute by
IV infusion; may be
increased gradually to
achieve therapeutic effect;
maximum dose is usually
20 μg/kg/minute. Consult

medical control for dosage instructions. **Infusion:** Dilute 200 mg of dopamine in 250 mL of D_5W for a concentration of 800 μg/mL or 400 mg in 250 mL for a concentration of 1600 μg/mL.

PEDIATRIC DOSAGE	1 to 20 μg/kg/minute; titrate to therapeutic effect.
ROUTE	IV infusion only
OVERDOSE OR TOXICITY PRESENTATION	Hypertension, arrhythmias, nausea, vomiting, severe headache
TREATMENT OF OVERDOSE OR OTHER ADVERSE REACTIONS	Give general supportive measures; monitor vitals and heart rhythm; administer oxygen; discontinue dopamine or reduce dose as directed by medical control. **Arrhythmias:** Treat per current ACLS guidelines or as directed by medical control.
SPECIAL CONSIDERATIONS	• Vitals and cardiac rhythm must be monitored continuously during

administration of
dopamine.
- Discontinue dopamine
  gradually to avoid
  severe hypotension.

Dosage-Related Responses to Dopamine

1 to 2 μg/kg/minute	Results in dilation of renal, mesenteric, and cerebral arteries; no effect on blood pressure
2 to 10 μg/kg/minute	Increase in cardiac output (beta 1)
10 to 20 μg/kg/minute	Renal, mesenteric, and peripheral vasoconstriction

DROPERIDOL (Inapsine)

CLASS	Antiemetic; tranquilizer
ACTIONS	Produces sedation by blocking subcortical receptors, antiemetic effect results from blocking CNS receptors at the chemoreceptor trigger zone
INDICATIONS	Relief of nausea and vomiting, as a tranquilizer
CONTRAINDICATIONS	Hypersensitivity to the drug

PRECAUTIONS	Use cautiously in patients with hypotension and in patients taking other CNS depressants or alcohol.
SIDE EFFECTS	Sedation, hypotension, respiratory depression, extrapyramidal reactions
SIGNIFICANT INTERACTIONS	Droperidol potentiates the CNS depressant effects of opiates or other analgesics.
DOSAGE	2.5 to 7.5 mg IM or 1.25 to 5.0 by slow IV; higher dose up to 10 mg IM may be needed for sedation.
PEDIATRIC DOSAGE	0.08 to 0.165 mg/kg IM or IV
ROUTE	IM or IV
OVERDOSE OR TOXICITY PRESENTATION	Exaggeration of side effects: respiratory depression, sedation, and hypotension
TREATMENT OF OVERDOSE OR OTHER ADVERSE REACTIONS	Give general supportive measures; monitor vitals; administer oxygen and be prepared to assist ventilations; establish IV access. Consider fluid challenge or vasopressors for hypotension.

EPINEPHRINE 1:10,000 (Adrenalin Chloride)

CLASS	Sympathomimetic; bronchodilator
ACTIONS	Stimulates alpha and beta adrenergic receptors, produces bronchodilation, increases heart rate and force of contractions, lowers defibrillation threshold
INDICATIONS	Cardiac arrest, profoundly symptomatic bradycardia, anaphylactic shock
CONTRAINDICATIONS	None when used for life-threatening circumstances
PRECAUTIONS	Protect drug from light
SIDE EFFECTS	In non-cardiac arrest patients, palpitations, angina, arrhythmias, nausea, vomiting, headache, or dizziness possible
SIGNIFICANT INTERACTIONS	Interactions are of no consideration in cases of cardiac arrest; use of epinephrine with other sympathomimetics can cause additive effects.

DOSAGE	**Cardiac arrest:** 1 mg every 3 to 5 minutes or choose one of the following dosing regimens: *Intermediate:* 2 to 5 mg every 3 to 5 minutes *Escalating:* 1 mg, 3 mg, 5 mg every 3 to 5 minutes *High:* 0.1 mg/kg every 3 to 5 minutes **Anaphylaxis:** 0.1 to 0.5 mg (1 to 5 mL) by slow IV infusion; may also be used at a rate of 1 to 4 μg/minute
PEDIATRIC DOSAGE	0.01 mg/kg (0.1 mL/kg)
ROUTES	IV, ET (double dose), IO (pediatric use only)
OVERDOSE OR TOXICITY PRESENTATION	In non-cardiac arrest patients, clinical manifestations of toxicity may include marked increase in blood pressure, arrhythmias, chest pain, respiratory distress, dilated pupils, and severe anxiety.
TREATMENT OF OVERDOSE OR OTHER ADVERSE REACTIONS	Epinephrine is rapidly inactivated in the body, so adverse effects are usually short-lived.

Symptomatic and supportive measures are generally sufficient. Administer oxygen; establish IV access; monitor ABCs; treat lingering arrhythmias and other cardiovascular manifestations per current ACLS guidelines or as directed by medical control.

SPECIAL CONSIDERATIONS

- Monitor vitals and heart rhythms frequently after administration in anaphylaxis.
- Watch for developing arrhythmias.
- If possible, obtain IV access before administration of epinephrine in case complications develop.

EPINEPHRINE 1:1000 (Adrenalin Chloride)

CLASS

Sympathomimetic; bronchodilator

ACTIONS

Stimulates alpha and beta adrenergic receptors, bronchodilation; increases heart rate and force of contractions

INDICATIONS	Anaphylactic shock, severe allergic reactions, acute bronchial asthma, exacerbation of COPD
CONTRAINDICATIONS	None when used for life-threatening circumstances
PRECAUTIONS	In non-life-threatening circumstances, use with caution in elderly patients and patients with cardiac disease, angina, or significant hypertension; protect drug from light.
SIDE EFFECTS	In non-cardiac arrest patients, palpitations, angina, arrhythmias, nausea, vomiting, headache, or dizziness possible
SIGNIFICANT INTERACTIONS	Interactions are of no consideration in cases of life-threatening emergencies.
DOSAGE	0.3 to 0.5 mg SC; for severe anaphylaxis, consider 0.3 to 0.5 mg of a 1:10,000 solution.
PEDIATRIC DOSAGE	0.01 mg/kg (0.1 mL/kg)
ROUTES	SC, IV, ET

OVERDOSE OR TOXICITY PRESENTATION	In non-cardiac arrest patients, clinical manifestations of toxicity may include marked increase in blood pressure, arrhythmias, chest pain, respiratory distress, dilated pupils, and severe anxiety.
TREATMENT OF OVERDOSE OR OTHER ADVERSE REACTIONS	Epinephrine is rapidly inactivated in the body, so adverse effects are usually short-lived. Symptomatic and supportive measures are generally sufficient. Administer oxygen; establish IV access; monitor ABCs, treat lingering arrhythmias and other cardiovascular manifestations per current ACLS guidelines or as directed by medical control.
SPECIAL CONSIDERATIONS	• Monitor vitals and heart rhythms frequently after administration in anaphylaxis. • Watch for developing arrhythmias. • If possible, obtain IV access before

administration of
epinephrine in case
complications develop.

EPINEPHRINE, RACEMIC (Vaponefrin)

CLASS	Adrenergic; bronchodilator
ACTIONS	Stimulates both alpha and beta adrenergic receptors; relaxes bronchial smooth muscle, resulting in bronchodilation
INDICATIONS	Croup (laryngotracheo-bronchitis), bronchial asthma, laryngeal edema associated with anaphylaxis
CONTRAINDICATIONS	Epiglottitis, severe tachyarrhythmias
PRECAUTIONS	Use with caution in elderly patients and those with history of cardiac disease or cardiac arrhythmias.
SIDE EFFECTS	Headache, palpitations, angina, tachycardia; excessive use may result in paradoxical bronchospasm
SIGNIFICANT INTERACTIONS	Use with antihistamines or tricyclic

antidepressants may cause adverse cardiac effects.

DOSAGE

Dilute 0.5 mL of a 2.25% solution of epinephrine (1:1000 solution) in 3 mL of normal saline and administer by nebulizer over 10 to 15 minutes.

PEDIATRIC DOSAGE

Under 20 kg: Dilute 0.25 mL of a 2.25% solution of epinephrine in 2 to 3 mL of normal saline and administer by nebulizer over 10 to 15 minutes.

Over 20 kg: Dilute 0.5 mL of a 2.25% solution of epinephrine in 2 to 3 mL of normal saline and administer by nebulizer over 10 to 15 minutes.

ROUTE

Inhalation, nebulizer

OVERDOSE OR TOXICITY PRESENTATION

Exaggeration of side effects, including palpitations, tachycardia, bronchospasm, and nausea

TREATMENT OF OVERDOSE OR OTHER ADVERSE REACTIONS

Discontinue drug; give general supportive measures; treat lingering problems symptomatically; treat arrhythmias per current ACLS guidelines or as directed by medical control.

SPECIAL CONSIDERATIONS
- Monitor vital signs closely.
- Watch for developing side effects and adverse reactions.

FLUMAZENIL (Romazicon)

CLASS

Benzodiazepine antagonist

ACTIONS

Antagonizes the action of benzodiazepines on the CNS and inhibits activity at benzodiazepine receptor sites

INDICATIONS

Treatment of benzodiazepine overdose/toxicity. Benzodiazepines include the following, among others: alprazolam (Xanax), chlordiazepoxide (Librium), clonazepam (Klonopin), clorazepate (Tranxene), diazepam (Valium), flurazepam (Dalmane), lorazepam (Ativan), midazolam (Versed), oxazepam (Serax), triazolam (Halcion).

CONTRAINDICATIONS	Hypersensitivity to flumazenil or benzodiazepines, patients who have been given a benzodiazepine to control a life-threatening condition such as status epilepticus, patients showing signs of serious tricyclic antidepressant overdose
PRECAUTIONS	Use cautiously in patients with head injury, history of seizures, or panic disorders; may precipitate seizures in patients with mixed drug overdoses
SIDE EFFECTS	Vertigo, nausea, vomiting, flushing, arrhythmias, seizures
SIGNIFICANT INTERACTIONS	Use cautiously in cases of mixed drug overdose; contact medical control for options.
DOSAGE	0.2 mg IV over 30 seconds; follow with additional doses of 0.2 to 0.3 mg at 1-minute intervals until desired effect is achieved. Maximum cumulative dose is 3.0 mg in 1 hour.

PEDIATRIC DOSAGE	Rarely used for children under the age of 12; contact medical control for options.
ROUTES	IV only. Administer through free-flowing IV that is running into a large vein to avoid pain at the injection site.
OVERDOSE OR TOXICITY PRESENTATION	Serious adverse reactions or toxic effects are very rare but when present may include seizures and arrhythmias.
TREATMENT OF OVERDOSE OR OTHER ADVERSE REACTIONS	Monitor ABCs; give general supportive measures; seizures may be repeated with benzodiazepines; treat arrhythmias per current ACLS guidelines or as directed by medical control.
SPECIAL CONSIDERATIONS	Due to short half-life of flumazenil, redosing is often necessary. Be prepared to administer subsequent doses.

FOSPHENYTOIN (Cerebyx)

CLASS	Anticonvulsant
ACTIONS	Anticonvulsant effect believed to result from

	modulation of sodium channels
INDICATIONS	Status epilepticus
CONTRAINDICATIONS	Hypersensitivity to the drug, second- and third-degree heart blocks and bradycardia, Stokes-Adams syndrome
PRECAUTIONS	Use with caution in pregnancy, hypotension, or cardiovascular disease.
SIDE EFFECTS	Dizziness, headache, pruritus, hypotension, ataxia, nystagmus
SIGNIFICANT INTERACTIONS	Avoid use with alcohol, narcotics, depressants, and tricyclic antidepressants.
DOSAGE	15 to 20 mg PE/kg; Cerebyx is prescribed in phenytoin sodium equivalents (PE), and 1 mg PE of Cerebyx equals 1 mg of phenytoin. Do not administer faster than 150 mg PE/minute.
PEDIATRIC DOSAGE	Safety of the drug in children under the age of 12 has not been established.
ROUTE	IV

OVERDOSE OR TOXICITY PRESENTATION	Nystagmus, hypotension, lethargy, vomiting, coma, respiratory depression, arrhythmias
TREATMENT OF OVERDOSE OR OTHER ADVERSE REACTIONS	Discontinue drug if the foregoing symptoms of overdose appear; give general supportive measures; administer oxygen and monitor cardiac rhythms. **Hypotension:** Consider IV fluid challenge and elevate the legs; consider vasopressors. **Arrhythmias:** Treat arrhythmias per current ACLS guidelines or as directed by medical control.
SPECIAL CONSIDERATIONS	Monitor vital signs and heart rhythm continuously during administration of drug.

NOTE: Fosphenytoin (Cerebyx) has replaced IV phenytoin (Dilantin).

FUROSEMIDE (Lasix)
Uritol (Can)

CLASS	Potent loop diuretic
ACTIONS	Inhibits reabsorption of sodium and chloride, promotes rapid diuresis,

reduces venous return to the right atria, helps remove excess fluid in conditions of fluid overload, decreases afterload

INDICATIONS

Congestive heart failure, pulmonary edema

CONTRAINDICATIONS

Dehydration, hypovolemia, and pregnancy; allergy to furosemide

PRECAUTIONS

Use cautiously in patients with renal failure or liver disease; watch for signs of dehydration; protect drug from light; administer slowly.

SIDE EFFECTS

Nausea and vomiting possible, especially if drug is administered too quickly; dehydration; orthostatic hypotension

SIGNIFICANT INTERACTIONS

Increased risk of arrhythmias if patient is taking digitalis preparations, lithium

DOSAGE

20 to 80 mg administered slowly IV

PEDIATRIC DOSAGE

1 mg/kg

ROUTES

IV; also available in oral preparations but not for

	emergency use in the field
OVERDOSE OR TOXICITY PRESENTATION	Severe dehydration, nausea and vomiting, electrolyte imbalance, cardiac arrhythmias, hypotension
TREATMENT OF OVERDOSE OR OTHER ADVERSE REACTIONS	Discontinue drug. Provide supportive care. **Dehydration or hypotension:** Administer fluids. Lactated Ringer's or normal saline is generally recommended. **Cardiac rhythms and arrhythmias:** Monitor rhythm and treat arrhythmias as they develop. **Apparent allergic reaction:** Consider epinephrine 1:1000 (0.3 to 0.5 mg by subcutaneous injection) or diphenhydramine (Benadryl) (25 to 50 mg IV or IM).
SPECIAL CONSIDERATIONS	• Assess lung sounds before and after administration of furosemide. • Be aware that patient may have to urinate shortly after use.

- Peak of action occurs in 30 minutes.

GLUCAGON

CLASS

Antihypoglycemic agent

ACTIONS

Promotes the breakdown of glycogen to glucose in the liver, thereby increasing blood glucose levels; relaxes GI smooth muscle

INDICATIONS

Hypoglycemia; to relax smooth muscle in cases of food obstruction in the esophagus

CONTRAINDICATIONS

Known hypersensitivity to glucagon

PRECAUTIONS

No relevant precautions in the prehospital setting

SIDE EFFECTS

Dizziness, lightheadedness, nausea, vomiting, urticaria

SIGNIFICANT INTERACTIONS

Hyperglycemic effect of glucagon increased and prolonged if used concomitantly with epinephrine; oral anticoagulant agents

DOSAGE

0.5 to 1.0 units; may be repeated in 15 to 20 minutes if needed

PEDIATRIC DOSAGE	Very rarely used in prehospital setting for children; contact medical control for options
ROUTES	IV, IM, SC
OVERDOSE OR TOXICITY PRESENTATION	Serious toxic presentations are rare in the field; if present, they may include vomiting or urticaria.
TREATMENT OF OVERDOSE OR OTHER ADVERSE REACTIONS	Treatment generally consists of nothing more than general supportive measures and symptomatic treatment.
SPECIAL CONSIDERATIONS	• Obtain blood glucose level, if possible, before administration of glucagon. • Obtain pre-glucagon blood sample for hospital use.

HALOPERIDOL (Haldol)

CLASS	Antipsychotic
ACTIONS	Reduces the manifestations of psychotic behavior by blocking CNS dopamine receptors
INDICATIONS	Generally used to treat acute and/or severe

chronic psychotic behavior, as a chemical restraint

CONTRAINDICATIONS   Hypersensitivity to the drug, conditions associated with CNS depression, circulatory collapse or compromise

PRECAUTIONS   Use cautiously in patients with arrhythmias, seizure disorders, Parkinson's, or head injury.

SIDE EFFECTS   Drowsiness, confusion, respiratory depression, hypotension, arrhythmias, nausea, vomiting, extrapyramidal reactions

SIGNIFICANT INTERACTIONS   Additive depressant effects are likely if used with other depressants such as alcohol, narcotics, tranquilizers, or barbiturates; use with antihypertensives may cause significant hypotension.

DOSAGE   2 to 5 mg

PEDIATRIC DOSAGE   Not recommended for pediatric use in the field

ROUTE   IM or IV

OVERDOSE OR TOXICITY PRESENTATION	Unarousable sleep, coma, arrhythmias, seizures, severe hypotension, extrapyramidal reactions
TREATMENT OF OVERDOSE OR OTHER ADVERSE REACTIONS	Give general supportive measures; monitor vitals and cardiac rhythm; administer oxygen at 10 to 15 L/minute; establish IV access. **Arrhythmias:** Treat per current ACLS guidelines, local protocols, or as directed by medical control; consider IV fluid challenge for hypotension; consider diazepam for seizures.
SPECIAL CONSIDERATIONS	Drug is very sensitive to light.

HYDRALAZINE (Apresoline)

CLASS	Peripheral dilator; antihypertensive
ACTIONS	Dilates blood vessels, particularly arteries and arterioles, and lowers blood pressure
INDICATIONS	Hypertensive crisis, sometimes used to treat CHF unresponsive to diuretics

CONTRAINDICATIONS	Hypersensitivity to the drug, mitral valve rheumatic heart disease, coronary artery disease
PRECAUTIONS	Use cautiously in patients with known history of renal disease or CVA.
SIDE EFFECTS	Headache, tachycardia, arrhythmias, hypotension, nausea, vomiting
SIGNIFICANT INTERACTIONS	Use with other antihypertensives or diuretics may produce profound hypotension.
DOSAGE	10 to 40 mg by slow IV bolus, repeat in 10 to 15 minutes as needed.
PEDIATRIC DOSAGE	Rarely used in the field for children under the age of 14
ROUTES	IV route is preferred; may administer IM if IV access is unavailable.
OVERDOSE OR TOXICITY PRESENTATION	Severe hypotension, shock, tachycardia, and other cardiac arrhythmias possible
TREATMENT OF OVERDOSE OR OTHER ADVERSE REACTIONS	Give general supportive measures; monitor vitals and cardiac rhythm; administer oxygen.

Hypotension and shock:
Elevate legs, consider
fluid challenge and
vasopressors, maintain
body heat with blankets.
Arrhythmias: Treat
developing arrhythmias
per current ACLS
guidelines, local
protocols, or as directed
by medical control.

SPECIAL
CONSIDERATIONS

Monitor vitals every 5
minutes after
administration of
hydralazine.

HYDROCORTISONE (Solu-Cortef)

CLASS

Glucocorticoid; anti-
inflammatory

ACTIONS

Suppresses the immune
response in anaphylactic
reactions

INDICATIONS

As an adjunct to
epinephrine in
anaphylaxis, sometimes
used in status
asthmaticus

CONTRAINDICATIONS

No contraindications
when used for life-
threatening emergencies

PRECAUTIONS

Use with caution in
patients with recent

	history of seizures or CHF.
SIDE EFFECTS	Headache, dizziness, euphoria, nausea, vomiting, CHF, edema
SIGNIFICANT INTERACTIONS	Concomitant use with barbiturates or phenytoin (Dilantin) may decrease the effectiveness of hydrocortisone.
DOSAGE	100 to 250 mg by slow IV bolus
PEDIATRIC DOSAGE	0.16 to 1.0 mg/kg
ROUTE	IV preferred but may be given IM if IV access is not available.
OVERDOSE OR TOXICITY PRESENTATION	Acute adverse reactions are rare for one-time emergency use in the field; when present, generally include exaggeration of side effects such as headache, nausea, vomiting, or CHF.
TREATMENT OF OVERDOSE OR OTHER ADVERSE REACTIONS	Discontinue drug; give general supportive measures; provide IV access; administer oxygen; if CHF develops, consider diuretic such as furosemide.

131

SPECIAL
CONSIDERATIONS

- Hydrocortisone
  generally comes in a
  powdered form and
  must be reconstituted.
- Administer slowly to
  avoid adverse
  reactions.
- Monitor patient
  frequently for signs of
  developing CHF.

HYDROMORPHONE (Dilaudid)

CLASS

Opioid; analgesic

ACTIONS

Binds to opiate receptors
in the CNS to produce
an analgesic effect

INDICATIONS

Relief of moderate to
severe pain, sometimes
used when the patient is
allergic to morphine

CONTRAINDICATIONS

Hypersensitivity to the
drug, head trauma,
undiagnosed abdominal
pain

PRECAUTIONS

Use cautiously in elderly
or pregnant patients or
those with a history of
convulsive disorders.

SIDE EFFECTS

Headache, bradycardia,
hypotension, respiratory
depression, nausea,
vomiting

SIGNIFICANT INTERACTIONS	Use with sedatives, tranquilizers, alcohol, antihistamines, or other opioids can result in profound CNS depression.
DOSAGE	• 1.0 mg initial dose by slow IV bolus; follow with additional doses of 0.5 to 1.0 mg every 5 minutes until pain is relieved or respiratory depression occurs. • IM dose is 2 to 4 mg; may not be repeated for at least 3 hours.
PEDIATRIC DOSAGE	Pediatric use not recommended in the field
ROUTES	IV or IM
OVERDOSE OR TOXICITY PRESENTATION	CNS and respiratory depression, miosis (pinpoint pupils), bradycardia, hypotension
TREATMENT OF OVERDOSE OR OTHER ADVERSE REACTIONS	Give general supportive measures; administer oxygen; establish IV access if not yet available; monitor vitals. **Respiratory depression:** Administer naloxone; support ventilations; be prepared to intubate.

Bradycardia: If symptomatic, consider atropine and IV fluids. **Hypotension:** Consider IV fluid challenge, elevation of legs, and/or vasopressors.

SPECIAL CONSIDERATIONS	• Monitor vital signs frequently and watch for signs of respiratory depression. • Have naloxone and intubation equipment available.

INSULIN

CLASS	Hormone
ACTIONS	Promotes the conversion of glucose to glycogen, lowers blood glucose levels
INDICATIONS	Treatment of diabetic ketoacidosis, severely elevated blood glucose levels
CONTRAINDICATIONS	Hypoglycemia, hypersensitivity to the form of insulin available
PRECAUTIONS	Excess dosing can cause hypoglycemia; except in true emergency situations, insulin should

	be administered in the emergency department rather than in the field.
SIDE EFFECTS	Itching, swelling, headache, tachycardia, nausea, hypoglycemia, allergic reactions
SIGNIFICANT INTERACTIONS	Beta blockers may mask certain signs of hypoglycemia such as tachycardia.
DOSAGE	10 to 25 units of regular insulin by IV bolus followed by IV infusion of 0.1 unit/kg/hour; contact medical control for additional dosing options.
PEDIATRIC DOSAGE	Initial IV bolus of 0.1 unit/kg followed by IV infusion of 0.1 unit/kg/hour; contact medical control for additional dosing options.
ROUTE	Generally IV in the field but insulin may also be given by subcutaneous injection; contact medical control for option
OVERDOSE OR TOXICITY PRESENTATION	Usually include signs and symptoms of hypoglycemia: tachycardia, nausea,

135

diaphoresis, anxiety, tremors, and diminished level of consciousness

TREATMENT OF OVERDOSE OR OTHER ADVERSE REACTIONS

Administer oral glucose if patient is conscious; if unconscious, consider IV bolus of D50. Provide general supportive measures including administration of oxygen.

SPECIAL CONSIDERATIONS

- Obtain blood glucose level before administration and recheck in 10 to 15 minutes.
- Monitor patient closely and watch for signs of developing hypoglycemia; have glucose available.
- Insulin can be absorbed in IV tubing; inject at medication port nearest to the skin.
- Insulin must be refrigerated.

IPECAC

CLASS

Emetic agent

ACTIONS

Irritates GI mucosa and causes vomiting

INDICATIONS

Used to induce vomiting in the conscious and alert patient in certain cases of poisoning or drug overdose

CONTRAINDICATIONS

Diminished level of consciousness, absence of gag reflex, seizures, patients who have ingested caustic or petroleum products or strychnine

PRECAUTIONS

- Use with caution in patients with cardiac disease, since ipecac may cause arrhythmias or myocarditis if drug is not vomited; check with medical control before administering during pregnancy.
- Do not confuse syrup of ipecac with concentrated ipecac fluid extract. Administration of fluid extract in dosages appropriate for the syrup can cause severe toxic effects.

SIDE EFFECTS

Arrhythmias, bradycardia, hypotension, depression, diarrhea

SIGNIFICANT INTERACTIONS	Use of ipecac with activated charcoal may render the ipecac ineffective.
DOSAGE	15 to 30 mL of ipecac followed by 2 to 3 glasses of water; may be repeated once in 20 minutes, if necessary. Following vomiting, consider use of activated charcoal.
PEDIATRIC DOSAGE	• Over 1 year of age: 15 mL followed by a glass of water • Under 1 year of age: 5 to 10 mL followed by 100 to 200 mL of water
ROUTE	Oral ingestion only
OVERDOSE OR TOXICITY PRESENTATION	Diarrhea, persistent vomiting (longer than 30 minutes), severe abdominal cramps, cardiac arrhythmias, hypotension, CHF
TREATMENT OF OVERDOSE OR OTHER ADVERSE REACTIONS	Give general supportive measures, including monitoring vitals, administration of oxygen, and use of IV fluids. **Hypotension:** Consider fluid challenge; elevate legs.

Cardiac arrhythmias:
Treat arrhythmias per current ACLS guidelines, local protocols, or as directed by medical control.

CHF: Consider furosemide (Lasix), morphine, and nitroglycerin per local protocols or as directed by medical control.

SPECIAL CONSIDERATIONS	• Ipecac should be used before activated charcoal. • Do not allow patient to drink milk after ipecac. • Save emesis sample for laboratory analysis.

ISOETHARINE (Bronkosol)

CLASS	Adrenergic; bronchodilator
ACTIONS	Relaxes bronchial smooth muscle, resulting in relief of bronchospasm, increased vital capacity, and decreased airway resistance
INDICATIONS	Bronchial asthma, bronchospasm associated with COPD
CONTRAINDICATIONS	Hypersensitivity to the drug

PRECAUTIONS	Use with caution in patients with angina, cardiac disease, hypertension, or cardiac asthma.
SIDE EFFECTS	Headache, dizziness, hypertension, chest pain, arrhythmias, nausea and vomiting
SIGNIFICANT INTERACTIONS	Concomitant with epinephrine or other sympathomimetics may cause adverse cardiovascular effects; beta blockers may inhibit the efficacy of isoetharine.
DOSAGE	**Inhalation:** 1 or 2 inhalations of 340 μg from a metered dose inhaler; repeat in 5 minutes if needed **Nebulizer:** 3 to 7 inhalations of a 0.5% to 1.0% solution
PEDIATRIC DOSAGE	Pediatric use in the field not recommended
ROUTE	Inhalation
OVERDOSE OR TOXICITY PRESENTATION	Exaggeration of side effects, particularly arrhythmias, nausea, vomiting, hypertension

TREATMENT OF OVERDOSE OR OTHER ADVERSE REACTIONS	Discontinue drug; give general supportive measures; administer oxygen; treat arrhythmias per current ACLS guidelines or as directed by medical control.
SPECIAL CONSIDERATIONS	• Monitor vitals continuously. • Watch for developing side effects.

ISOPROTERENOL (Isuprel)

CLASS	Adrenergic; bronchodilator; cardiac stimulant
ACTION	Action on beta 1 adrenergic receptors increases cardiac output, relaxes bronchial smooth muscle
INDICATIONS	Refractory torsade de pointes; symptomatic bradycardia refractory to atropine (heart transplant patients)
CONTRAINDICATIONS	Hypersensitivity to the drug, presence of tachyarrhythmias, in the setting of acute MI
PRECAUTIONS	Use very cautiously in patients who are elderly

	or have a history of cardiac arrhythmias.
SIDE EFFECTS	Headache, arrhythmias, hypertension, nausea, vomiting
SIGNIFICANT INTERACTIONS	Epinephrine and other sympathomimetics
DOSAGE	• 2 to 10 μg/minute; titrate to adequate heart rate and rhythm. • Mix 1 mg of isoproterenol in 500 mL of D_5W or normal saline to obtain concentration of 2 μg/mL.
PEDIATRIC DOSAGE	Not recommended for field use
ROUTE	IV only
OVERDOSE OR TOXICITY PRESENTATION	Cardiac arrhythmias, profound hypotension, vomiting, extreme tremors
TREATMENT OF OVERDOSE OR OTHER ADVERSE REACTIONS	Give general supportive measures; administer oxygen. **Hypotension:** Consider fluid challenge; elevate legs. **Tremors:** Consider barbiturates such as phenobarbital or

anticonvulsant such as diazepam.

Arrhythmias: Treat arrhythmias per current ACLS guidelines or as directed by medical control; consider lidocaine for ventricular ectopy or irritability.

SPECIAL CONSIDERATIONS	Continuously monitor vitals and cardiac rhythm during administration.

LABETALOL (Normodyne, Trandate)

CLASS	Alpha and beta adrenergic blocking agent; antihypertensive agent
ACTIONS	Inhibits peripheral vasoconstriction, promotes vasodilation, and decreases cardiac output, thereby reducing blood pressure
INDICATIONS	Hypertensive crisis, regulation of blood pressure during interfacility transport
CONTRAINDICATIONS	CHF, cardiogenic shock, bronchial asthma, second- or third-degree heart block, and pregnancy

PRECAUTIONS	Use with caution in patients with diabetes, since labetalol can mask tachycardia caused by hypoglycemia.
SIDE EFFECTS	Bradycardia, hypotension, pulmonary edema, bronchospasm, blurred vision, diarrhea
SIGNIFICANT INTERACTIONS	Labetalol may antagonize the bronchodilation effect normally produced by beta adrenergic drugs; use with other antihypertensive drugs may result in additive antihypertensive effect.
DOSAGE	**IV bolus:** 20 mg injected over 2 minutes; additional doses of 20 to 40 mg may be given every 10 minutes until desired blood pressure is achieved or until maximum total dose of 300 mg has been given. **IV infusion:** Add 200 mg of labetalol to 250 mL of D_5W, which creates a concentration of 0.8 mg/mL. Run at rate of 2 mg/minute.
PEDIATRIC DOSAGE	Generally not administered to pediatric patients

TOXICITY PRESENTATION	Severe hypotension, bradycardia, pulmonary edema, bronchospasm
TREATMENT OF OVERDOSE OR OTHER ADVERSE REACTIONS	Give general supportive measures; monitor vitals and heart rate; administer oxygen. **Hypotension:** Elevate legs if not contraindicated. Consider fluid challenge and vasopressors. **Bradycardia:** Consider atropine 0.5 to 1.0 mg IV bolus. **Pulmonary edema:** Consider furosemide (Lasix), morphine, and/or nitroglycerin per local protocol or as directed by medical control.
SPECIAL CONSIDERATIONS	• Closely monitor vital signs and heart rhythm. • Watch for developing CHF, bradycardia, or hypotension.

LIDOCAINE (Xylocaine)

CLASS	Antiarrhythmic; local anesthetic
ACTIONS	Suppresses ventricular ectopic activity, increases ventricular fibrillation

145

	threshold, reduces velocity of electrical impulse through conduction system
INDICATIONS	Ventricular fibrillation, ventricular tachycardia, suppresses PVCs, wide complex tachycardias of uncertain type, wide complex PSVT
CONTRAINDICATIONS	Second- and third-degree heart blocks, PVCs associated with bradycardia, known allergy to drug or other local anesthetics
PRECAUTIONS	Dosage should not exceed 300 mg/hour; consider reducing maintenance dosage in patients with impaired liver function or left ventricular dysfunction.
SIDE EFFECTS	Anxiety, seizures, nausea and vomiting, drowsiness, widening QRS complex
SIGNIFICANT INTERACTIONS	Use of lidocaine with beta blockers, cimetidine, or ranitidine can result in increased lidocaine levels and greater potential for seizures and other adverse effects. Use with

	succinylcholine can prolong apnea.
DOSAGE	**Ventricular fibrillation:** 1.0 to 1.5 mg/kg to be repeated every 3 to 5 minutes with a maximum dose of 3 mg/kg. **Ventricular tachycardia, wide complex tachycardia of uncertain types, PVCs:** 1.0 to 1.5 mg/kg and repeat at 0.5 to 0.75 mg/kg every 5 to 10 minutes with maximum dosage of 3 mg/kg. In either of the above, bolus should be followed by infusion of 1 to 4 mg/minute. Infusion rate should be reduced by 50% in patients over the age of 70.
PEDIATRIC DOSAGE	1.0 mg/kg for bolus; for infusion, give 20 to 50 μg/kg/minute.
ROUTES	IV bolus or IV infusion; in cardiac arrest, may be given via ET if IV access is not available. Give 2 to 2½ times the normal dosage if given by ET and follow with 5 to 10 mL of saline. May administer

via intraosseous route in children (refer to local protocols).

OVERDOSE OR TOXICITY PRESENTATION

Seizures, respiratory depression, and hypotension

TREATMENT OF OVERDOSE OR OTHER ADVERSE REACTIONS

Discontinue drug, support respirations, and monitor cardiac rhythm. **Seizures:** Treat with diazepam (Valium) 5 to 10 mg. **Severe hypotension:** Consider fluid challenge and/or dopamine (5 to 20 μg/kg/minute). **Apparent allergic reaction:** Contact medical control for possible use of epinephrine 1:1000 (0.3 to 0.5 mg) or diphenhydramine (Benadryl) (25 to 50 mg).

SPECIAL CONSIDERATIONS

- Except in cardiac arrest, lidocaine should be administered slowly to avoid seizures, hypotension, or bradycardia
- Patients over the age of 70 may require a reduced dose. Contact medical control for direction.

LORAZEPAM (Ativan)

CLASS	Benzodiazepine; antianxiety agent; sedative-hypnotic
ACTIONS	Depresses the CNS, produces antianxiety effect
INDICATIONS	Status epilepticus, anxiety, alcohol withdrawal
CONTRAINDICATIONS	Known hypersensitivity to benzodiazepines, acute narrow angle glaucoma, alcohol intoxication
PRECAUTIONS	Use cautiously in patients with psychoses, those with Parkinson's, or elderly patients with impaired respiratory function.
SIDE EFFECTS	Bradycardia, hypotension, respiratory depression, drowsiness (especially in the elderly)
SIGNIFICANT INTERACTIONS	Narcotics, depressants, barbiturates, alcohol
DOSAGE	2.0 to 6.0 mg IV (dilute drug in equal volume of sterile water or sodium chloride before administration); 2.0 to 4.0 mg IM

ROUTES	IV, IM
PEDIATRIC DOSAGE	Generally not used in children under the age of 12
OVERDOSE OR TOXICITY PRESENTATION	Coma, depressed or labored breathing, hypotension, bradycardia, slurred speech or confusion
TREATMENT OF OVERDOSE OR OTHER ADVERSE REACTIONS	Monitor ABCs; support blood pressure with fluid challenge and dopamine, if necessary; be prepared to intubate; for serious cases, consider administration of flumazenil, a benzodiazepine antagonist (initial dose of 0.2 mg IV over 30 seconds).
SPECIAL CONSIDERATIONS	Monitor vitals, particularly respiratory status, following administration of lorazepam.

MAGNESIUM SULFATE

CLASS	Electrolyte with anticonvulsant therapeutic properties
ACTION	Acts as a cofactor in numerous enzymatic reactions, essential for

the function of the sodium-potassium adenosine triphosphatase pump, blocks neuromuscular transmission by decreasing acetylcholine in motor nerve terminals

INDICATIONS   Refractory ventricular fibrillation, cardiac arrest associated with torsades de pointes, preeclampsia and eclampsia, life-threatening arrhythmias caused by digitalis toxicity, torsades de pointes

CONTRAINDICATIONS   Heart block, renal disease; no contraindications in cardiac arrest

PRECAUTIONS   Use cautiously in patients on digitalis. Inject slowly to prevent hypotension and/or respiratory depression. Calcium chloride should be available if respiratory depression occurs.

SIDE EFFECTS   Flushing, sweating, mild bradycardia, respiratory depression, drowsiness

SIGNIFICANT INTERACTIONS   Increased CNS depression with barbiturates, general anesthetics, narcotics, and antipsychotics; incompatible with alkalies, alcohol, dobutamine, clindamycin, hydrocortisone, procaine, salicylates

DOSAGE	**Eclampsia:** 1 to 4 mg over 2 to 3 minutes **Ventricular fibrillation:** 1 to 2 g diluted in 100 mL of D_5W and administered over 1 to 2 minutes
PEDIATRIC DOSAGE	Rarely used—not recommended
ROUTES	IV; also, rarely given by IM injection
OVERDOSE OR TOXICITY PRESENTATION	Sharp drop in blood pressure, severe respiratory depression or respiratory paralysis, heart blocks, asystole; may also precipitate ECG changes including increased P-R, QRS, and Q-T intervals
TREATMENT OF OVERDOSE OR OTHER ADVERSE REACTIONS	Establish patent airway and use positive pressure ventilations as needed. Administer one of the following:

Calcium chloride:
500 mg IV

OR

Calcium gluconate: 5 to
10 mEq of a 10% solution
Severe hypotension:
Consider fluid challenge
and/or dopamine (5 to
20 μg/kg/minute) by IV
infusion.
Allergic reaction:
Consider epinephrine
1:1000 (0.3 to 0.5 mg
by SC injection) or
diphenhydramine
(Benadryl) (25 to 50 mg
IV or IM).

SPECIAL
CONSIDERATIONS

Administer slowly to
avoid serious side effects
such as respiratory or
cardiac arrest.

MANNITOL (Osmitrol)

CLASS

Osmotic diuretic

ACTIONS

Inhibits the reabsorption
of water and electrolytes
in the kidneys and thus
promotes diuresis,
reduces intracranial
pressure

INDICATIONS

Treatment of acute
cerebral edema and
intracranial pressure

	resulting from closed head injury
CONTRAINDICATIONS	Pulmonary edema, CHF, severe dehydration
PRECAUTIONS	Use cautiously in patients with known renal disease or tendency to develop CHF; assess lung sounds frequently to monitor for emerging CHF.
SIDE EFFECTS	Headache, tachycardia, CHF, nausea, vomiting, dehydration
SIGNIFICANT INTERACTIONS	Avoid use with CNS depressants.
DOSAGE	1.5 to 2.0 g/kg of a 15% to 25% solution infused over 30 to 60 minutes
PEDIATRIC DOSAGE	Not recommended for children under the age of 12 in the field
ROUTE	IV
OVERDOSE OR TOXICITY PRESENTATION	Severe dehydration, cardiovascular collapse, hypotension, polyuria
TREATMENT OF OVERDOSE OR OTHER ADVERSE REACTIONS	Discontinue infusion and give general supportive measures; monitor ABCs. Any fluid therapy in the presence of hypotension must be done with great

caution. It is advisable to contact medical control for direction in such cases.

SPECIAL
CONSIDERATIONS

Administer mannitol with in-line filter to filter out crystals.

MEPERIDINE HYDROCHLORIDE (Demerol)

CLASS

Narcotic; analgesic

ACTIONS

Depresses pain impulse transmission by acting on opioid receptor sites in the CNS

INDICATIONS

Moderate to severe pain

CONTRAINDICATIONS

Head injury, undiagnosed abdominal pain, hypersensitivity to the drug

PRECAUTIONS

May cause respiratory depression; use with caution in patients with a history of seizure disorders. It is advisable to have naloxone available to reverse any adverse effects.

SIDE EFFECTS

Respiratory depression, lightheadedness, euphoria, nausea, hypotension, bradycardia

SIGNIFICANT INTERACTIONS	Other CNS depressants, antihistamines, barbiturates, benzodiazepines, tricyclics, alcohol, and muscle relaxants can potentiate the CNS effects of meperidine.
DOSAGE	25 to 50 mg IV over 1 to 2 minutes; 50 to 100 mg IM; infusion rate: 15 to 35 mg/hour prn
PEDIATRIC DOSAGE	1.0 to 1.8 mg/kg
ROUTES	IV, IM, SC
OVERDOSE OR TOXICITY PRESENTATION	CNS depression, respiratory depression or apnea, bradycardia, hypotension, cool and clammy skin, pulmonary edema, convulsions
TREATMENT OF OVERDOSE OR OTHER ADVERSE REACTIONS	Monitor ABCs; focus on immediate life threats; administer naloxone (2 mg) and be prepared to administer additional doses due to short half-life. **Cardiac reactions:** Treat per current ACLS guidelines or as directed by medical control; consider atropine (0.5 to 1.0 mg) for symptomatic bradycardia.

Severe respiratory depression or apnea: Be prepared to intubate.
True allergic reactions: Consider epinephrine or diphenhydramine (Benadryl).

SPECIAL
CONSIDERATIONS

- Monitor vital signs, particularly respiratory status, following administration of meperidine.
- Meperidine should not be used in the management of chest pain associated with suspected acute MI unless the patient is allergic to morphine. Meperidine does not produce the same desired hemodynamic effects as morphine.

METHYLPREDNISOLONE (Solu-Medrol)

CLASS

Synthetic steroid; anti-inflammatory; immunosuppressant

ACTIONS

Suppresses the immune system by binding to intracellular corticosteroid receptors

INDICATIONS

Anaphylaxis, status asthmaticus, possible

157

	benefits for certain spinal cord injuries
CONTRAINDICATIONS	Hypersensitivity to adrenocorticoid preparations
PRECAUTIONS	Use with caution in patients with renal disease, hypertension, diabetes, CHF, myasthenia gravis.
SIDE EFFECTS	Depression, headache, hypertension, edema, psychotic behavior
SIGNIFICANT INTERACTIONS	None of significance in presence of severe anaphylaxis
DOSAGE	100 to 250 mg by IV bolus
PEDIATRIC DOSAGE	1 to 2 mg/kg IV bolus
ROUTE	IV
OVERDOSE OR TOXICITY PRESENTATION	Toxicity is rare, but when it occurs it consists of an exaggeration of side effects.
TREATMENT OF OVERDOSE OR OTHER ADVERSE REACTIONS	Treatment consists of general supportive measures; monitor vitals; administer oxygen. Consider furosemide (Lasix) for CHF or edema.

SPECIAL CONSIDERATIONS	Methylprednisolone is supplied in powder form and must be reconstituted before use.

METOPROLOL (Lopressor)

CLASS	Beta adrenergic blocker; antihypertensive
ACTIONS	Decreases heart rate, blood pressure, and cardiac output by blocking adrenergic receptors; reduces the influence of the sympathetic nervous system
INDICATIONS	Field treatment of angina and hypertension, early intervention in acute MI
CONTRAINDICATIONS	Bradycardia, second- and third-degree heart blocks, cardiogenic shock, hypersensitivity to the drug
PRECAUTIONS	Use with caution in patients with diabetes or hepatic dysfunction.
SIDE EFFECTS	Bradycardia, pulmonary edema, CHF, bronchospasm, hypotension

SIGNIFICANT INTERACTIONS	Use with verapamil can cause additive cardiac depressive effects.
DOSAGE	5 mg IV bolus administered slowly; may repeat two more times if necessary at 2- to 3-minute intervals if vital signs remain stable; maximum total dose is 15 mg
PEDIATRIC DOSAGE	Not recommended for children
ROUTE	IV only in the field
OVERDOSE OR TOXICITY PRESENTATION	Exaggeration of side effects including hypotension, bradycardia, bronchospasm, and pulmonary edema
TREATMENT OF OVERDOSE OR OTHER ADVERSE REACTIONS	Give general supportive measures; administer oxygen; monitor heart rhythm and vitals. **Hypotension:** Elevate legs; consider fluid challenge but watch for developing pulmonary edema. **Bradycardia:** If patient is symptomatic, consider atropine but not in presence of an MI. **Pulmonary edema:** High flow oxygen; consider

furosemide or other diuretic.
Bronchospasm: High flow oxygen; consider albuterol.

SPECIAL CONSIDERATIONS	Closely monitor vitals and heart rhythm.

MIDAZOLAM (Versed)

CLASS	Benzodiazepine; tranquilizer; amnesic agent
ACTIONS	Reduces anxiety, provides short-term CNS depressant action, induces amnesia
INDICATIONS	Premedication for endotracheal intubation or synchronized cardioversion, sometimes used as a chemical restraint
CONTRAINDICATIONS	Shock, severe hypotension, narcotic overdose, concomitant use of other CNS depressants or hypersensitivity to benzodiazepines
PRECAUTIONS	Use cautiously in patients with known glaucoma or renal failure and elderly

	patients with history of COPD.
SIDE EFFECTS	Respiratory depression, headache, amnesia, hypotension, cough, nausea
SIGNIFICANT INTERACTIONS	Midazolam potentiates the effects of alcohol, narcotics, tranquilizers, barbiturates, and antidepressants.
DOSAGE	1 to 2.5 mg initially; may be repeated in 1.0 mg increments as needed; total dose should not exceed 0.1 mg/kg.
PEDIATRIC DOSAGE	Generally not recommended for children under age 12
ROUTE	IV; may be administered IM when used as a chemical restraint
OVERDOSE OR TOXICITY PRESENTATION	Severe hypotension, respiratory depression or arrest, coma, confusion
TREATMENT OF OVERDOSE OR OTHER ADVERSE REACTIONS	Give general supportive measures; monitor vitals and heart rhythm; administer oxygen. Consider administration of flumazenil (0.2 mg IV over 30 seconds).

Hypotension: Do IV fluid challenge.
Respiratory depression or arrest: Support ventilations and be prepared to intubate.

SPECIAL CONSIDERATIONS

- Make sure that intubation equipment and oxygen are available before administration.
- Monitor oxygen saturation with pulse oximetry.
- Consider reduction of dosage in the elderly.

MORPHINE SULFATE

CLASS

Narcotic/analgesic

ACTIONS

CNS depressant with analgesic and hemodynamic properties; increases venous capacitance, decreases systemic vascular resistance, relieving pulmonary congestion; causes a reduction in myocardial oxygen requirement; reduces sensitivity to pain

INDICATIONS

Pain and anxiety associated with acute MI, acute pulmonary edema

163

	associated with CHF, severe pain
CONTRAINDICATIONS	Head injury, significant hypotension, undiagnosed abdominal pain, COPD; known hypersensitivity to the drug
PRECAUTIONS	Watch for respiratory depression. Naloxone (Narcan) should be available to reverse possible adverse effects.
SIDE EFFECTS	Dizziness, nausea, vomiting, altered level of consciousness, respiratory depression
SIGNIFICANT INTERACTIONS	Other analgesics, antidepressants, molindone, MAO inhibitors, other narcotics, pentazocine, phenothiazines, phenytoin (Dilantin), sedatives, sleep inducers, tranquilizers
DOSAGE	2 to 5 mg IV administered slowly. Additional 2 mg may be given every 3 to 5 minutes until desired effect is achieved. Do not exceed 15 mg total. Higher total doses may

	be needed during extended transports.
PEDIATRIC DOSAGE	0.1 to 0.2 mg/kg IV
ROUTES	IV or IM; also available in oral form but not for field use
OVERDOSE OR TOXICITY PRESENTATION	Respiratory depression with or without CNS depression, miosis (pinpoint pupils), hypotension, hypothermia, apnea, shock, pulmonary edema, convulsions
TREATMENT OF OVERDOSE OR OTHER ADVERSE REACTIONS	Establish patent airway. Use positive pressure ventilation if significant respiratory depression is present. Be prepared to intubate. Administer 0.4 to 2 mg of naloxone to reverse effect of morphine. Repeat dosage may be necessary, since morphine has a greater duration of action than naloxone. Monitor vitals. If overdose is oral, consider inducing vomiting. Contact medical control for options. **Allergic reaction:** Consider epinephrine

1 : 1000 (0.3 to 0.5 mg) by SQ injection or diphenhydramine (Benadryl) 25 to 50 mg by IV or IM injection. NOTE: Nalmefene (Revex), a narcotic antagonist with a duration of action significantly longer than naloxone, is now available but not yet in use in the prehospital setting.

SPECIAL CONSIDERATIONS

Morphine has a very high potential for addiction.

NALBUPHINE (Nubain)

CLASS

Narcotic agonist-antagonist; analgesic

ACTIONS

Acts as an agonist at opioid receptor sites to produce an analgesic effect

INDICATIONS

Relief of moderate to severe pain

CONTRAINDICATIONS

Hypersensitivity to the drug or known allergy to other opioids such as morphine, codeine, hydrocodone, or hydromorphone; head trauma; undiagnosed abdominal pain

PRECAUTIONS	Use cautiously in pregnancy, patients with known history of bronchial asthma or acute MI when nausea and vomiting are present; consider reduced dosages in elderly patients.
SIDE EFFECTS	Respiratory depression, vertigo, arrhythmias, hypertension, hypotension, palpitations
SIGNIFICANT INTERACTIONS	Use with other narcotics, barbiturates, or sedatives may cause additive CNS depression.
DOSAGE	5 to 20 mg initial dose; if pain is not relieved, administer subsequent doses in 2 to 3 mg increments
PEDIATRIC DOSAGE	Not recommended for pediatric use in the field
ROUTES	IV, IM, or SC; IV is preferred in the field
OVERDOSE OR TOXICITY PRESENTATION	Respiratory depression, apnea, miosis (pinpoint pupils), hypotension, bradycardia
TREATMENT OF OVERDOSE OR OTHER ADVERSE REACTIONS	Give general supportive measures; administer oxygen; obtain IV access if not already available.

167

Respiratory depression or apnea: administer naloxone (Narcan) to reverse the effects of nalbuphine; assist respirations with bag-valve-mask (BVM); be prepared to intubate.
Hypotension: Consider fluid challenge and/or vasopressors; elevate legs.
Bradycardia: Consider atropine if not otherwise contraindicated; give 0.5 to 1.0 mg by IV push.

SPECIAL CONSIDERATIONS

- Administer slowly to avoid adverse reactions.
- Monitor vitals frequently.
- Keep intubation equipment and naloxone readily available.

NALOXONE (Narcan)

CLASS

Narcotic antagonist

ACTION

Reverses the effects of narcotic drugs and certain synthetic analgesics

INDICATIONS

Narcotic overdoses (heroin, morphine, meperidine [Demerol],

methadone, hydromorphone [Dilaudid], fentanyl, percodan, etc.); also used for synthetic analgesics such as Darvocet, Talwin, and Stadol; can be used to rule out narcotic overdose in coma of unknown origin

CONTRAINDICATIONS   None, except known hypersensitivity to the drug

PRECAUTIONS
- Note that the duration of action of naloxone is shorter than that of the drugs it is used to counteract. Patient may lapse back into coma or respiratory depression. Dose often must be repeated.
- Administration to addicted individuals can produce a severe withdrawal syndrome. Consider slow administration until an obvious improvement in respiratory status is observed.
- Ventricular tachycardia and ventricular fibrillation in patients with preexisting cardiac

disease are possible
but uncommon.

SIDE EFFECTS

Nausea and vomiting
possible with high doses
administered rapidly

**SIGNIFICANT
INTERACTIONS**

None of significance in
the prehospital setting

DOSAGE

0.4 to 2.0 mg for narcotic
overdose; may repeat as
needed up to 10 mg.
Higher doses may be
needed for synthetic
narcotics such as fentanyl.

PEDIATRIC DOSAGE

0.01 mg/kg for known or
suspected narcotic-
induced respiratory
depression; may repeat as
necessary.

ROUTES

IV is the route of choice
for fastest action. May
also be administered IM,
SC, or via ET if IV access
is not available. To
administer via ET tube,
double the dose and
follow with 5 to 10 mL
of saline.

**OVERDOSE OR
TOXICITY
PRESENTATION**

Overdoses of naloxone
are extremely rare and of
little significance in the
field.

| **TREATMENT OF OVERDOSE OR OTHER ADVERSE REACTIONS** | Give general supportive measures. Monitor ABCs. |
| **SPECIAL CONSIDERATIONS** | Naloxone has a shorter half-life than most narcotics, making repeat dosing necessary in many cases. |

NIFEDIPINE (Procardia)
Adalat (Can)

CLASS	Calcium channel blocker; antianginal; antihypertensive
ACTIONS	Dilates systemic and coronary arteries; results in reduction in peripheral vascular resistance, blood pressure, and afterload
INDICATIONS	Angina pectoris, hypertensive crisis
CONTRAINDICATIONS	Hypotension or sensitivity to the drug
PRECAUTIONS	Use very cautiously in patients with CHF and those receiving concurrent beta blockers.
SIDE EFFECTS	Hypotension, flushing, dizziness, headache, CHF, nausea and vomiting

SIGNIFICANT INTERACTIONS	Concomitant use with beta blockers may exacerbate angina, CHF, or hypotension.
DOSAGE	10 mg initially; may be followed by second 10 mg or 20 mg dose. Check blood pressure before and after each dose.
PEDIATRIC DOSAGE	Not recommended for pediatric use
ROUTE	PO or sublingual (SL); gel cap may be punctured with a needle and placed under the patient's tongue or bitten open by the patient and dissolved under the tongue or swallowed.
OVERDOSE OR TOXICITY PRESENTATION	Severe hypotension; CHF
TREATMENT OF OVERDOSE OR OTHER ADVERSE REACTIONS	Give general supportive measures; monitor vitals; administer oxygen. • **Hypotension:** Elevate legs; consider IV fluid challenge in absence of signs and symptoms of CHF; consider vasopressor such as dopamine.

- **CHF:** If systolic pressure is 100 mm Hg or more, consider nitroglycerin, furosemide, and/or morphine per current ACLS guidelines, local protocols, or as directed by medical control.

SPECIAL CONSIDERATIONS

Monitor patient's blood pressure before, during, and after administration. NOTE: Nifedipine is now rarely used in the field because of a link between the drug and serious complications.

NITROGLYCERIN (Nitrostat, Nitrol, Tridil)

CLASS

Nitrate; vasodilator; antianginal agent

ACTIONS

Relaxes vascular smooth muscle; causes vasodilation, which results in increased coronary blood flow; reduces preload

INDICATIONS

Ischemic chest pain, CHF

CONTRAINDICATIONS

Hypersensitivity to the drug, hypotension, head trauma, shock, cerebral hemorrhage.

Nitroglycerin should not be administered to any patient who has taken the anti-impotence drug Viagra within the past 24 to 36 hours. Contact medical control for advice.

PRECAUTIONS

Observe for possible rapid decrease in blood pressure.

SIDE EFFECTS

Headache, hypotension, nausea, vomiting, tachycardia

SIGNIFICANT INTERACTIONS

Use with other vasodilators may cause additive hypotensive effects.

DOSAGE

Sublingual: 0.3 to 0.4 mg tablet; repeat up to three times, as necessary, at 5-minute intervals **Sublingual spray:** 0.4 mg spray; repeat up to three times, as necessary, at 5-minute intervals **Ointment:** 1 to 2 inches (15 to 30 mg) on the skin (chest wall)

PEDIATRIC DOSAGE

Not recommended in the field

ROUTES

Sublingual, transdermal, topical, IV; sublingual

tablet or spray is most common in the field

OVERDOSE OR TOXICITY PRESENTATION

Hypotension, bradycardia, heart blocks, reduced respiratory rate

TREATMENT OF OVERDOSE OR OTHER ADVERSE REACTIONS

Give general supportive measures; monitor vitals; administer oxygen; obtain IV access.
Hypotension: Do fluid challenge but use caution in presence of CHF; elevate legs; consider vasopressors.
Arrhythmias: Consider atropine for bradycardia; treat all arrhythmias per current ACLS guidelines or as directed by medical control.

SPECIAL CONSIDERATIONS

- Monitor vitals frequently.
- Nitroglycerin is unstable. If tablet does not taste bitter, efficacy may be compromised. Check expiration date. Store in dark area at room temperature.
- Advise patient that headache is a normal reaction.
- Administer nitroglycerin when patient is sitting or

lying because rapid
hypotensive effect can
occur.

NITROPRUSSIDE (Nipride)

CLASS	Vasodilator; antihypertensive
ACTION	Acts directly on smooth muscle and causes peripheral vasodilation, reduces both preload and afterload and causes a rapid reduction in blood pressure
INDICATIONS	Hypertensive crisis
CONTRAINDICATIONS	Hypersensitivity to the drug; no other contraindications in the presence of life-threatening hypertensive crisis. **Nitroprusside or any other nitrates should not be administered to any patient who has taken the anti-impotence drug Viagra within the past 24 to 36 hours. Contact medical control for advice.**
PRECAUTIONS	Use cautiously in patients with known renal insufficiency.

SIDE EFFECTS	Headache, dizziness, hypotension, palpitations, dyspnea, nausea, vomiting, reflex tachycardia
SIGNIFICANT INTERACTIONS	Use with other antihypertensive agents may cause dangerous additive effects.
DOSAGE	Titrate to blood pressure with an infusion rate of 0.1 to 10 μg/kg/minute; maximum infusion rate is 10 μg/kg/minute for 10 minutes. Consult medical control for desired target blood pressure. Prepare infusion by adding 50 mg of nitroprusside to 250 or 500 mL of D_5W: • 50 mg in 250 mL of D_5W =concentration of 200 μg/mL • 50 mg in 500 mL of D_5W = concentration of 100 μg/mL
PEDIATRIC DOSAGE	Rarely used for children in the field; when used, dosage is same as for adults
ROUTE	IV only
OVERDOSE OR TOXICITY PRESENTATION	Severe hypotension, dyspnea, vomiting

TREATMENT OF OVERDOSE OR OTHER ADVERSE REACTIONS	Give general supportive measures; administer oxygen; monitor vitals frequently; decrease or discontinue drug. **Hypotension:** Consider fluid challenge; elevate legs; consider vasopressors. **Dyspnea:** Elevate head and administer oxygen by nasal cannula or non-rebreather; support ventilations as necessary.
SPECIAL CONSIDERATIONS	• Following preparation of infusion, cover the IV bag with aluminum foil or other opaque material to protect from light. • Monitor vitals every 3 to 5 minutes during administration. • Use minimal dose necessary to achieve desired effect.

NITROUS OXIDE (Nitronox)

CLASS	Analgesic gas; mixture of 50% nitrous oxide and 50% oxygen
ACTIONS	Produces rapid, reversible relief from pain
INDICATIONS	To provide relief from moderate to severe pain from any cause

CONTRAINDICATIONS	Contraindicated in the following cases: • altered level of consciousness • closed head injury • abdominal distention or suspected abdominal trauma • presence of COPD • thoracic trauma • moderate to severe shock • pulmonary edema • suspected pulmonary embolism
PRECAUTIONS	Monitor vitals and level of consciousness closely. Be alert for nausea and vomiting; be prepared to protect the airway. Nitrous oxide should always be patient administered.
SIDE EFFECTS	Lightheadedness, decreased level of consciousness, nausea and vomiting
SIGNIFICANT INTERACTIONS	CNS depressants
DOSAGE	Self-administered by the patient until pain has been relieved; provide oxygen, particularly in cases of cardiac-related

	pain, when nitrous oxide is not being used
PEDIATRIC DOSAGE	Same as for adults
OVERDOSE OR TOXICITY PRESENTATION	When nitrous oxide is patient administered, overdoses or severe adverse reactions are extremely rare and usually consist of exaggeration of side effects such as nausea, vomiting, and decreased level of consciousness.
TREATMENT OF OVERDOSE OR OTHER ADVERSE REACTIONS	Give general supportive measures; monitor vitals and level of consciousness; administer oxygen; protect airway from vomiting.
SPECIAL CONSIDERATIONS	• Be sure that the ambulance is adequately vented to avoid inhalation by EMS personnel. • Follow administration of nitrous oxide with 100% oxygen.

NOREPINEPHRINE (Levophed)

CLASS	Adrenergic; vasopressor
ACTIONS	Directly stimulates alpha adrenergic receptors, which causes peripheral

vasoconstriction; results in increased systolic and diastolic blood pressure; also reduces blood flow to vital organs and for this reason norepinephrine is rarely used in the field

INDICATIONS

Treatment of acute hypotensive states, cardiogenic and neurogenic shock

CONTRAINDICATIONS

Hypotension due to hypovolemia, severe hypoxia

PRECAUTIONS

Use very cautiously in patients suffering from MI or ischemia, since norepinephrine increases myocardial oxygen requirements.

SIDE EFFECTS

Headache, dizziness, bradycardia, arrhythmias, necrosis at the IV site

SIGNIFICANT INTERACTIONS

Use with beta blockers can cause significant increases in hypertension.

DOSAGE

Start infusion at 0.5 to 1.0 μg/minute; increase rate slowly until the desired therapeutic effect (systolic blood pressure of approximately 90 mm Hg)

is achieved. Prepare infusion by adding 4 mg of norepinephrine to 250 mL of D_5W or normal saline, or 8 mg to 500 mL in order to achieve a concentration of 16 μg/mL.

PEDIATRIC DOSAGE

0.1 to 1.0 μg/minute; rarely used in the field for children

ROUTE

IV only

OVERDOSE OR TOXICITY PRESENTATION

Vomiting, convulsions, symptomatic bradycardia, arrhythmias

TREATMENT OF OVERDOSE OR OTHER ADVERSE REACTIONS

Give general supportive measures; administer oxygen; monitor vitals and heart rhythms.
Arrhythmias: Treat as per current ACLS guidelines.
Bradycardia: Consider atropine and transcutaneous pacing.

SPECIAL CONSIDERATIONS

- Ensure patency of IV line because infiltration may cause localized tissue necrosis.
- Monitor blood pressure during administration.

- Protect IV solution
  from light.

OXYGEN

CLASS	Medicinal gas; atmospheric gas
ACTIONS	Oxidizes glucose to produce adenosine triphosphate (ATP), reduces area of infarct in MI; reverses hypoxemia
INDICATIONS	To treat almost all emergency conditions in which hypoxemia is present or may develop, including chest pain, cardiac arrest, cardiac arrhythmias, shock, respiratory distress of any kind, trauma, stroke, head injury, coma from all causes, status epilepticus, inhalation poisoning, syncope
CONTRAINDICATIONS	None in the emergency setting
PRECAUTIONS	Administer cautiously to patients with history of COPD; monitor patient closely and be prepared to assist ventilations; prolonged use in newborn infants may

cause eye damage. Contact medical control for advice regarding concentration to be delivered; avoid use near open flames.

SIDE EFFECTS

In rare cases of COPD, administration may reduce the respiratory drive; long-term use of non-humidified oxygen can cause irritation to nasal mucous membranes.

SIGNIFICANT INTERACTIONS

None

DOSAGE

Usually delivered at a high volume of 10 to 15 L/minute, particularly in cases of chest pain, trauma, respiratory distress, shock, or inhalation poisoning. **Cardiac arrest or carbon monoxide poisoning:** Use concentrations as close to 100% as possible. **COPD:** Give reduced amounts unless a higher concentration is indicated by nature of the patient's emergency condition. Never withhold oxygen from a patient in critical condition.

PEDIATRIC DOSAGE	Same as for adults
ROUTE	Inhalation; nasal cannula, venturi mask, non-rebreather mask; bag-valve-mask (BVM); endotracheal tube; ventilator; mouth-to-mouth or mouth-to-mask
TOXICITY OR OVERDOSE PRESENTATION	Respiratory arrest or insufficiency caused by over-oxygenation of the COPD patient; cyanosis and/or diminished oxygen saturation possible
TREATMENT OF OVERDOSE OR OTHER ADVERSE REACTIONS	Discontinue or reduce concentration; provide ventilatory assist with BVM; consider intubation.
SPECIAL CONSIDERATIONS	Consider use of humidified oxygen for long transports to avoid irritation to the mucous membranes.

OXYTOCIN (Pitocin)

CLASS	Hormonal agent; oxytocic
ACTIONS	Stimulates uterine muscle contraction

INDICATIONS	Generally used in the field to help control postpartum bleeding
CONTRAINDICATIONS	When used to control bleeding, the only contraindication is hypersensitivity to the drug.
PRECAUTIONS	Be sure that the baby or all babies (in the case of multiple births) and the placenta have been delivered before administration of the drug.
SIDE EFFECTS	Nausea, vomiting, hypotension, arrhythmia
SIGNIFICANT INTERACTIONS	Concomitant use with vasoconstrictors such as epinephrine may cause severe hypertension.
DOSAGE	10 to 20 units added to 1000 mL of normal saline or Ringer's lactate and infused according to the severity of the bleeding. Contact medical control for infusion rate. If given IM, the dosage is 5 to 10 units.
PEDIATRIC DOSAGE	Not indicated for pediatric use

ROUTE	IV or IM
OVERDOSE OR TOXICITY PRESENTATION	Severe hypotension, uterine rupture, cardiac arrhythmias, anaphylaxis; since the drug has a very short half-life, toxic effects often resolve spontaneously within a few minutes
TREATMENT OF OVERDOSE OR OTHER ADVERSE REACTIONS	Give general supportive measures; monitor vitals; administer oxygen. **Hypotension:** Elevate legs, consider fluid challenge. Do not use dopamine in the presence of hypovolemia. **Arrhythmias:** Monitor heart rhythm; treat arrhythmias per current ACLS guidelines, local protocols, or as directed by medical control. **Uterine rupture:** Administer high-flow oxygen; place patient in left lateral recumbent position; administer volume-expanding IV fluids to maintain blood pressure; transport rapidly to the hospital.
SPECIAL CONSIDERATIONS	Monitor blood pressure every 5 to 10 minutes after administration.

PANCURONIUM (Pavulon)

CLASS	Non-depolarizing neuromuscular blocking agent; skeletal muscle relaxant
ACTIONS	Prevents acetylcholine from binding to receptors, which results in paralysis of skeletal and respiratory muscles
INDICATIONS	To facilitate intubation
CONTRAINDICATIONS	Hypersensitivity to the drug, neuromuscular disease such as myasthenia gravis
PRECAUTIONS	Use caution in patients with known renal failure and pregnant women receiving magnesium sulfate.
SIDE EFFECTS	Tachycardia, wheezing, residual muscular weakness
SIGNIFICANT INTERACTIONS	Concomitant use with opioid analgesics may increase respiratory depression.
DOSAGE	0.04 to 0.1 mg/kg initial dose; then 0.01 mg/kg

	every 20 to 40 minutes as needed
PEDIATRIC DOSAGE	Same as for adult
ROUTE	IV only
OVERDOSE OR TOXICITY PRESENTATION	Prolonged respiratory depression, apnea, tachycardia
TREATMENT OF OVERDOSE OR OTHER ADVERSE REACTIONS	Give general supportive measures; monitor vitals; maintain airway and assist ventilations until the patient is able to maintain adequate ventilations unassisted. **Tachycardia:** Treat per current ACLS guidelines or as directed by medical control.
SPECIAL CONSIDERATIONS	• Monitor vitals and cardiac rhythm constantly. • Make sure that personnel skilled in intubation and all necessary intubation equipment are readily available. • Precede by administration of a benzodiazepine or narcotic in conscious patients.

PENTAZOCINE (Talwin)

CLASS	Narcotic analgesic
ACTIONS	Binds to receptor sites in the CNS and produces an analgesic effect
INDICATIONS	Relief of moderate to severe pain
CONTRAINDICATIONS	Hypersensitivity to the drug, head injury or undiagnosed abdominal pain
PRECAUTIONS	Use cautiously in older patients who may require a reduced dose and in pregnancy or with history of COPD.
SIDE EFFECTS	Headache, dizziness, hypotension, hypertension, respiratory depression, palpitations, tachycardia, nausea, vomiting
SIGNIFICANT INTERACTIONS	Use with other narcotics, hypnotics, barbiturates, antihistamines, or alcohol can cause additive CNS and respiratory depression.
DOSAGE	30 mg
PEDIATRIC DOSAGE	Not generally used in the field
ROUTE	IV or IM

OVERDOSE OR TOXICITY PRESENTATION	Respiratory depression, tachycardia, severe hypotension, vomiting
TREATMENT OF OVERDOSE OR OTHER ADVERSE REACTIONS	Give general supportive measures; monitor vitals; administer oxygen; obtain IV access. **Respiratory depression:** Protect airway, support ventilations and be prepared to intubate; consider naloxone. **Hypotension:** Do IV fluid challenge; elevate legs and consider vasopressors.
SPECIAL CONSIDERATIONS	• Monitor vitals frequently and be alert for signs of respiratory depression. • Be prepared to support ventilations and have intubation equipment readily available. • Have naloxone on hand.

PHENOBARBITAL (Luminal)

CLASS	Barbiturate; anticonvulsant
ACTIONS	Causes depression of the CNS; suppresses the spread of seizure activity

INDICATIONS	Treatment of grand mal seizures, status epilepticus, and febrile seizures in children
CONTRAINDICATIONS	Hypersensitivity to barbiturates; severe asthma or respiratory distress of any kind because of potential for respiratory depression
PRECAUTIONS	Use with caution in patients with known renal dysfunction or hypotension; administer slowly to avoid cardiovascular side effects.
SIDE EFFECTS	Respiratory depression, drowsiness, vertigo, headache, possible paradoxical excitement, hypotension, bradycardia, nausea, vomiting
SIGNIFICANT INTERACTIONS	May cause significant added CNS depression when used with narcotics, depressants, tranquilizers, sedatives, or alcohol
DOSAGE	100 to 300 mg by slow IV bolus
PEDIATRIC DOSAGE	10 to 20 mg/kg administered slowly by IV bolus

ROUTE	IV
OVERDOSE OR TOXICITY PRESENTATION	Slurred speech, respiratory depression, hypotension
TREATMENT OF OVERDOSE OR OTHER ADVERSE REACTIONS	Monitor vitals; give general supportive measures; administer oxygen. Be prepared to provide ventilatory assist and/or to intubate; monitor cardiac rhythm. Consider IV fluid challenge for hypotension or vasopressors such as dopamine as directed by medical control.
SPECIAL CONSIDERATIONS	Monitor vital signs frequently after administration of phenobarbital; be prepared to provide ventilatory assist.

PHENYTOIN (Dilantin)

CLASS	Anticonvulsant; antiarrhythmic
ACTIONS	Inhibits the spread of seizure activity by decreasing sodium in the neurons of the motor cortex; normalizes sodium influx to the Purkinje fibers, thus

	helping to regulate digitalis-induced arrhythmias
INDICATIONS	Treatment of seizures, occasionally used in the field to treat arrhythmias caused by digitalis toxicity
CONTRAINDICATIONS	Hypersensitivity to the drug, sinus bradycardia, heart blocks, Stokes-Adams syndrome
PRECAUTIONS	Use with extreme caution in pregnancy, hypotension, or cardiovascular disease; do not administer with sugar solutions such as D_5W.
SIDE EFFECTS	Dizziness, headache, hypotension, arrhythmias, nausea, vomiting
SIGNIFICANT INTERACTIONS	Avoid use with depressants, barbiturates, narcotics, alcohol, and tranquilizers; incompatible with dextrose solutions
DOSAGE	**Seizures:** 150 to 250 mg administered slowly **Arrhythmias:** 100 mg administered slowly; may

	be repeated every 5 minutes until the arrhythmia disappears or toxicity occurs; do not exceed total dose of 1000 mg
PEDIATRIC DOSAGE	**Seizures:** 10 to 15 mg/kg administered by slow IV bolus **Arrhythmias:** Very rarely used in the field
ROUTE	IV
OVERDOSE OR TOXICITY PRESENTATION	Drowsiness, vomiting, slurred speech, hypotension, respiratory depression
TREATMENT OF OVERDOSE OR OTHER ADVERSE REACTIONS	Discontinue drug; give general supportive measures; monitor vital signs and cardiac rhythms; administer oxygen; be prepared to assist ventilations and/or intubate. **Hypotension:** Consider IV fluid challenge and/or vasopressors. **Arrhythmias:** Treat arrhythmias per current ACLS guidelines, local protocols, or as directed by medical control.

195

SPECIAL CONSIDERATIONS	Monitor vitals and heart rhythm continuously when administering phenytoin. NOTE: Injectable phenytoin has now been replaced by a new medication known as fosphenytoin sodium. It is available under the trade name of Cerebyx. For more information, refer to fosphenytoin in this chapter.

PHYSOSTIGMINE (Antilirium)

CLASS	Cholinesterase inhibitor; antimuscarinic agent
ACTIONS	Inhibits the destructive effects of cholinesterase, exaggerates the effect of acetylcholine
INDICATIONS	Treatment of tricyclic antidepressant overdose and anticholinergic poisoning
CONTRAINDICATIONS	Should not be used in patients with hypersensitivity to the drug or narrow angle glaucoma
PRECAUTIONS	Administer cautiously in patients with bradycardia,

	hypotension, diabetes, or history of seizures.
SIDE EFFECTS	Dizziness, hallucinations, seizures, bradycardia, hypotension, bronchospasm, vomiting, and diarrhea
SIGNIFICANT INTERACTIONS	Concomitant use with succinylcholine may result in significantly prolonged respiratory depression.
DOSAGE	0.5 to 2.0 mg by slow IV bolus; may repeat in 5 to 10 minutes if necessary
PEDIATRIC DOSAGE	0.02 mg/kg; may repeat in 5 to 10 minutes if necessary
ROUTES	IV preferred but may be administered IM if unable to obtain IV access
OVERDOSE OR TOXICITY PRESENTATION	Vomiting, bronchospasm, hypotension, bradycardia, restlessness, agitation, and diaphoresis possible
TREATMENT OF OVERDOSE OR OTHER ADVERSE REACTIONS	Give general supportive measures; administer oxygen, maintain airway, and support ventilations as necessary; obtain IV access. Consider atropine; contact medical control for dosage.

- Monitor vital signs and neurological status frequently.
- Always have atropine available as an antidote.
- Administer physostigmine at a rate of no more than 1 mg/minute to minimize chances of toxic reactions.

PRALIDOXIME (Protopam Chloride)

CLASS

Antidote

ACTIONS

Reactivates cholinesterase that has been inactivated as a result of organophosphate exposure, reverses respiratory and muscle paralysis caused by organophosphate pesticide poisoning

INDICATIONS

Administered as an adjunct to atropine in acute cases of organophosphate pesticide poisoning

CONTRAINDICATIONS

Hypersensitivity to the drug

PRECAUTIONS	Use very cautiously in patients suffering from myasthenia gravis who are receiving anticholinesterase agents.
SIDE EFFECTS	Headache, dizziness, tachycardia, nausea, vomiting, blurred vision
SIGNIFICANT INTERACTIONS	Avoid use of respiratory depressants such as morphine, aminophylline, succinylcholine, and phenothiazines in patients receiving pralidoxime.
DOSAGE	1 to 2 g by IV infusion over a period of 30 minutes, usually administered after atropine. Prepare infusion by mixing 1 to 2 g of pralidoxime with normal saline (100, 250, or 500 mL—check local protocol).
PEDIATRIC DOSAGE	20 to 40 mg/kg by IV infusion over a period of 30 minutes
ROUTE	IV only
OVERDOSE OR TOXICITY PRESENTATION	Severe headache, vomiting, tachycardia, blurred vision (effects

may also result from the organophosphate pesticide or atropine)

TREATMENT OF OVERDOSE OR OTHER ADVERSE REACTIONS

Give general supportive measures; protect airway; administer oxygen and be prepared to support ventilations; monitor vitals and ECG.

SPECIAL CONSIDERATIONS

- Treatment with pralidoxime should be started within 24 hours to be most effective.
- If administered too rapidly, tachycardia and other side effects are more likely to occur.

PROCAINAMIDE (Pronestyl)

CLASS

Antiarrhythmic

ACTIONS

Decreases myocardial excitability and conduction velocity, increases fibrillation threshold

INDICATIONS

Refractory ventricular fibrillation, ventricular tachycardia with a pulse, wide-complex tachycardia of uncertain type, paroxysmal supraventricular tachycardia

CONTRAINDICATIONS Third-degree heart block, torsades de pointes, prolonged QT interval, patients suffering from digitalis toxicity

PRECAUTIONS Use very cautiously in patients with myasthenia gravis, liver disease, or suspected MI; avoid rapid infusion to reduce the likelihood of adverse effects.

SIDE EFFECTS Confusion, dizziness, hypotension, ventricular arrhythmias, heart blocks, nausea, vomiting

SIGNIFICANT INTERACTIONS Concomitant use with anti-hypertensives may result in severe hypotension.

DOSAGE **Cardiac arrest:** 30 mg/minute, maximum total dose not to exceed 17 mg/kg. In refractory ventricular fibrillation or pulseless ventricular tachycardia, it is acceptable to administer 100 mg IV push every 5 minutes.

Tachycardia: 20 to 30 mg/minute until arrhythmia resolves, hypotension develops, or QRS widens by 50% of its original width; maximum total dose is 17mg/kg.
Maintenance infusion: 1 to 4 mg/minute

PEDIATRIC DOSAGE	Not recommended in the field
ROUTE	IV
OVERDOSE OR TOXICITY PRESENTATION	Severe hypotension, arrhythmias, nausea and vomiting
TREATMENT OF OVERDOSE OR OTHER ADVERSE REACTIONS	Give general supportive measures; monitor vitals and heart rhythm; administer oxygen. **Hypotension:** Do IV fluid challenge, elevate legs, consider vasopressors. **Arrhythmias:** Treat pursuant to current ACLS guidelines or as directed by medical control or local protocols.
SPECIAL CONSIDERATIONS	Monitor patient continuously when administering procainamide.

PROMETHAZINE HYDROCHLORIDE (Phenergan)
Histanil (Can)

CLASS

Antiemetic; antihistamine
(H_1 receptor antagonist)

ACTIONS

Blocks cholinergic
receptors in the vomiting
center, which may
mediate nausea and
vomiting; competes with
histamine for the H_1
receptor site

INDICATIONS

Nausea, vomiting, and
motion sickness; to
potentiate the effects of
analgesics

CONTRAINDICATIONS

Coma, CNS depression,
seizures, severe
dehydration, known
hypersensitivity to
the drug

PRECAUTIONS

Use with caution in
patients (especially
children) with acute or
chronic respiratory
dysfunction because drug
may suppress the cough
reflex; antiemetic action
of promethazine may
mask undiagnosed
disease, poisoning, or
drug overdose. Do not
administer SC as it may
cause local necrosis;

avoid intra-arterial administration as it may cause arteriospasm or gangrene.

SIDE EFFECTS

Dizziness, drowsiness, poor coordination, hypotension, agitation, confusion

SIGNIFICANT INTERACTIONS

Avoid concomitant use with epinephrine as it may result in further hypotension; use with barbiturates, tranquilizers, or alcohol may cause further CNS depression.

DOSAGE

12.5 to 25 mg

PEDIATRIC DOSAGE

0.25 to 0.5 mg/kg

ROUTES

IV, IM

OVERDOSE OR TOXICITY PRESENTATION

May include CNS depression, seizures, flushed skin, dilated pupils

TREATMENT OF OVERDOSE OR OTHER ADVERSE REACTIONS

Monitor ABCs; support respirations as needed; administer oxygen. **Severe hypotension:** Consider vasopressors. **Seizures:** Consider diazepam (Valium). **Allergic reactions:** Consider epinephrine or diphenhydramine (Benadryl).

| SPECIAL CONSIDERATIONS | Promethazine and meperidine (Demerol) may be mixed in the same syringe. |

PROPARACAINE HYDROCHLORIDE (Alcaine)

CLASS	Local anesthetic
ACTIONS	Produces pain relief by preventing transmission of impulses
INDICATIONS	Relief of pain associated with chemical burns of the eye
CONTRAINDICATIONS	Hypersensitivity to the drug
PRECAUTIONS	None of any significance in the field; use for more than 2 hours can result in corneal ulcerations
SIDE EFFECTS	Corneal irritation
SIGNIFICANT INTERACTIONS	None
DOSAGE	1 or 2 drops of a 0.5% solution
PEDIATRIC DOSAGE	1 drop of a 0.5% solution
ROUTE	Eyedrops only
OVERDOSE OR TOXICITY PRESENTATION	Overdose and toxicity are very rare.

TREATMENT OF OVERDOSE OR OTHER ADVERSE REACTIONS	Discontinue medication and treat symptomatically.
SPECIAL CONSIDERATIONS	Administer proparacaine before irrigation of eye with sterile saline or other fluid.

PROPRANOLOL (Inderal)

CLASS	A non-selective beta blocker; antihypertensive; antiarrhythmic; antianginal
ACTIONS	Blocks adrenergic receptors, decreases myocardial oxygen demand, slows heart rate, reduces blood pressure, decreases cardiac output
INDICATIONS	Ventricular tachycardia refractory to other medications, control of rapid atrial fibrillation and atrial flutter, angina, hypertension
CONTRAINDICATIONS	Bradycardia, CHF, second- or third-degree heart block, COPD
PRECAUTIONS	Generally do not use in patients who have received verapamil. Use with caution in patients

206

	with impaired renal or hepatic function.
SIDE EFFECTS	Bradycardia, hypotension, CHF, bronchospasm, wheezing, nausea, vomiting
SIGNIFICANT INTERACTIONS	Use with other antihypertensives may cause severe hypotension. Use with calcium channel blockers, particularly verapamil, may depress myocardial contractility and AV conduction.
DOSAGE	1 to 3 mg by IV bolus administered over 3 to 5 minutes; dose may be repeated in 3 to 5 minutes as needed. To facilitate administration, dilute 3 mg of propranolol in 30 mL of D_5W or normal saline.
PEDIATRIC DOSAGE	0.01 mg/kg by slow IV bolus; rarely used in the field for pediatric patients
ROUTE	IV only in the field
OVERDOSE OR TOXICITY PRESENTATION	Exaggeration of side/adverse effects; bradycardia, hypotension, bronchospasm, CHF, vomiting

TREATMENT OF OVERDOSE OR OTHER ADVERSE REACTIONS	Give general supportive measures; administer oxygen; monitor vitals and heart rhythm.
	Bradycardia: Consider atropine.
	Hypotension: Do fluid challenge, if not otherwise contraindicated; consider vasopressors.
	CHF: Consider diuretics such as furosemide.
	Bronchospasm: Consider bronchodilators.
SPECIAL CONSIDERATIONS	• Monitor vitals frequently.
	• Place patient on cardiac monitor before administration of propranolol.
	• Have atropine readily available in case of overdose or toxicity.

SODIUM BICARBONATE

CLASS	Alkalinizing agent; buffer
ACTIONS	Neutralizes excess buildup of acid caused by severe hypoxic states, helps restore normal pH
INDICATIONS	Used in prolonged cardiac arrest after defibrillation

and cardiac medications, for severe acidotic states, for tricyclic antidepressant overdose

CONTRAINDICATIONS	None when used in cardiac arrest; should not be used in known cases of respiratory or metabolic alkalosis
PRECAUTIONS	Use cautiously in CHF.
SIDE EFFECTS	CHF, alkalosis, cramps
SIGNIFICANT INTERACTIONS	May form a precipitate if mixed with calcium agents
DOSAGE	**Cardiac arrest:** 1 mEq/kg by IV bolus followed by a half dose every 10 minutes thereafter **Other conditions:** As directed by medical control
PEDIATRIC DOSAGE	Same as for adults
ROUTE	IV only
OVERDOSE OR TOXICITY PRESENTATION	Cardiac arrhythmias, CHF, seizures
TREATMENT OF OVERDOSE OR OTHER ADVERSE REACTIONS	Give general supportive measures; monitor vitals and cardiac rhythms. **Arrhythmias:** Treat per current ACLS guidelines

or as directed by medical control.

CHF: Administer oxygen; consider diuretic such as furosemide or bumetanide.

Seizures: Consider diazepam, phenobarbital, or fosphenytoin.

SPECIAL CONSIDERATIONS	• Monitor vitals and cardiac rhythms continuously. • Be alert for signs of developing CHF.

STREPTOKINASE (Streptase)

CLASS	Thrombolytic; plasminogen activator
ACTIONS	Dissolves thrombi or emboli in the setting of acute MI
INDICATIONS	Used to dissolve clots in coronary arteries after acute MI; less frequently used in the prehospital setting to treat pulmonary emboli
CONTRAINDICATIONS	Hypersensitivity to the drug, recent internal bleeding, CVA within 60 days, severe hypertension, active ulcerative colitis, recent history of strep throat

PRECAUTIONS	Use cautiously in patients with recent surgery or trauma. Use with caution in pregnancy or childbirth within the past 30 days.
SIDE EFFECTS	Hypotension, hypertension, reperfusion arrhythmias, spontaneous bleeding, nausea, allergic reactions
SIGNIFICANT INTERACTIONS	Use with anticoagulants may increase the risk of bleeding.
DOSAGE	**For acute MI:** 1,500,000 IU (international units) by IV infusion over 60 minutes **For pulmonary embolism:** Initial dose of 250,000 IU by IV infusion over 30 minutes, followed by sustaining dose of 100,000 IU per hour for 24 to 72 hours
PEDIATRIC DOSAGE	Not recommended for pediatric use in the field
ROUTE	IV only
OVERDOSE OR TOXICITY PRESENTATION	Watch for signs of serious bleeding, including ecchymosis, epistaxis,

hematoma, hypotension, and increasing pulse rate.

TREATMENT OF OVERDOSE OR OTHER ADVERSE REACTIONS

Discontinue drug; give general supportive measures including oxygen and IV fluids. **Arrhythmias:** Treat reperfusion or other arrhythmias per current ACLS guidelines, local protocols, or as directed by medical control.

SPECIAL CONSIDERATIONS

- Drug must be reconstituted.
- Obtain pre-streptokinase blood sample for hospital use.
- Monitor patient before, during, and after administration.

SUCCINYLCHOLINE (Anectine)

CLASS

Depolarizing neuromuscular blocking agent; skeletal muscle relaxant; paralytic

ACTIONS

Depolarizes receptors on skeletal muscle; blocks neuromuscular transmission, resulting in temporary paralysis

INDICATIONS	To facilitate endotracheal intubation
CONTRAINDICATIONS	Hypersensitivity to the drug, narrow angle glaucoma, penetrating eye injury
PRECAUTIONS	Use cautiously in patients with neuromuscular disease such as myasthenia gravis and in severe burns.
SIDE EFFECTS	Hypotension, bradycardia, prolonged respiratory depression, bronchospasm, increased intraocular pressure
SIGNIFICANT INTERACTIONS	Diazepam may shorten duration of action, glycosides such as digoxin may induce arrhythmias.
DOSAGE	1 to 2 mg/kg IV bolus; dose may be repeated once if necessary
PEDIATRIC DOSAGE	1 to 1.5 mg/kg IV bolus; repeat once if necessary
ROUTE	IV only
OVERDOSE OR TOXICITY PRESENTATION	Prolonged apnea, arrhythmias, hypotension

TREATMENT OF OVERDOSE OR OTHER ADVERSE REACTIONS

Give general supportive measures; support ventilations as long as necessary.

Hypotension: Elevate legs and administer fluid challenge unless either is contraindicated by the patient's condition; consider vasopressors in appropriate cases.

Arrhythmias: Treat arrhythmias per current ACLS guidelines, local protocols, or as directed by medical control.

SPECIAL CONSIDERATIONS

- Resulting muscle and respiratory paralysis usually last 2 to 10 minutes. Limit use to personnel who are skilled in intubation; make sure that patient is hooked to a cardiac monitor.
- Often other drugs may be used in conjunction with succinylcholine for intubation, including diazepam, midazolam, and lidocaine. Check local protocols.
- In conscious patients, administer a

benzodiazepine or
narcotic before
succinylcholine.

TERBUTALINE SULFATE (Brethine)

CLASS	Sympathomimetic; bronchodilator; tocolytic (premature labor inhibitor)
ACTIONS	Selective for beta 2 (pulmonary) receptors; effect is to relax bronchial smooth muscle; relaxes uterine smooth muscle and inhibits contractions
INDICATIONS	Moderate to severe asthma, bronchospasm associated with COPD, may also be used in premature labor to inhibit contractions (generally considered second-line drug to magnesium sulfate in premature labor)
CONTRAINDICATIONS	Hypersensitivity to terbutaline or other sympathomimetics
PRECAUTIONS	Use cautiously in patients with cardiovascular disease, particularly when associated with

arrhythmias and hypertension.

SIDE EFFECTS

Anxiety, dizziness, palpitations, arrhythmias, nausea and vomiting, tremors

SIGNIFICANT INTERACTIONS

Use with other sympathomimetics may potentiate adverse cardiovascular effects; when used with beta blockers, bronchodilation may be inhibited.

DOSAGE

0.25 mg SC; may be repeated as needed in 15 to 30 minutes
Metered dose inhaler: 2 inhalations, 1 minute apart
Premature labor: Initial dose of 10 μg/minute by IV infusion, with the maximum dose being 80 μg/min

PEDIATRIC DOSAGE

Same as for adults; not recommended for children under age 12

ROUTES

SC, IV, inhalation

OVERDOSE OR TOXICITY PRESENTATION

Exaggeration of adverse reactions, particularly arrhythmias, seizures, nausea and vomiting

TREATMENT OF OVERDOSE OR OTHER ADVERSE REACTIONS	Give general supportive measures; monitor and support ABCs; administer oxygen. **Arrhythmias:** Treat per current ACLS guidelines or as directed by medical control. **Seizures:** Consider diazepam (5 to 10 mg IV). **Nausea and vomiting:** Consider antiemetic (promethazine) (12.5 to 25 mg).
SPECIAL CONSIDERATIONS	Monitor heart rhythm and vitals continuously.

THIAMINE (Vitamin B$_1$)

CLASS	Vitamin
ACTIONS	Coenzyme necessary for carbohydrate metabolism and the breakdown of glucose
INDICATIONS	Delirium tremens associated with alcohol abuse, coma of unknown origin, vitamin deficiency (rare in the field), sometimes used before D50 in hypoglycemia (particularly in known or suspected alcoholics)

	to avoid consequences of Wernicke's encephalopathy
CONTRAINDICATIONS	None in the emergency setting
PRECAUTIONS	A safe drug in the emergency setting; very rare anaphylactic reactions
SIDE EFFECTS	Hypotension and/or nausea are possible but rare.
SIGNIFICANT INTERACTIONS	None in the field
DOSAGE	100 mg
PEDIATRIC DOSAGE	Rarely given to children in the field; if indicated, consult medical control
ROUTES	IV or IM; administer slowly via IV route
OVERDOSE OR TOXICITY PRESENTATION	Overdoses and toxicity are extremely rare.
TREATMENT OF OVERDOSE OR OTHER ADVERSE REACTIONS	Adverse reactions are treated with supportive therapy; monitor ABCs; administer oxygen. **Hypotension:** Consider fluid challenge.
SPECIAL CONSIDERATIONS	In coma of unknown origin, administer thiamine before D50.

VECURONIUM (Norcuron)

CLASS	Non-depolarizing neuromuscular blocking agent; skeletal muscle relaxant
ACTIONS	Competes for acetylcholine receptor sites, produces muscle paralysis
INDICATIONS	To facilitate endotracheal intubation
CONTRAINDICATIONS	Hypersensitivity to the drug, neuromuscular diseases such as myasthenia gravis
PRECAUTIONS	Use with caution in elderly patients and in pregnant women receiving magnesium sulfate.
SIDE EFFECTS	Prolonged paralysis possible
SIGNIFICANT INTERACTIONS	Concomitant use with other paralytic agents or narcotics may result in prolonged paralysis.
DOSAGE	0.08 to 0.10 mg/kg by IV bolus; may repeat as necessary every 20 to 30 minutes
PEDIATRIC DOSAGE	Rarely used in children under age 10; consult local protocols

ROUTE	IV only
OVERDOSE OR TOXICITY PRESENTATION	Prolonged respiratory paralysis
TREATMENT OF OVERDOSE OR OTHER ADVERSE REACTIONS	Give general supportive measures; maintain airway and assist ventilations until effects of drug wear off.
SPECIAL CONSIDERATIONS	• Be sure that trained personnel and all necessary intubation equipment are available before administration of drug. • Precede use of vecuronium in conscious patients by administration of a benzodiazepine or narcotic. • Monitor vitals frequently.

VERAPAMIL (Calan, Isoptin)

CLASS	Calcium channel blocker; antianginal; antihypertensive; antiarrhythmic
ACTIONS	Inhibits calcium transport across cell membranes, thereby causing dilation of

220

coronary vasculature, decreased vascular resistance, reduction in myocardial oxygen consumption, and decreased SA and AV node conduction

INDICATIONS

Field use generally limited to treatment of symptomatic PSVT not responsive to adenosine and/or vagal maneuvers

CONTRAINDICATIONS

Severe CHF, second- and third-degree heart blocks, sick sinus syndrome, hypotension below 90 mm Hg

PRECAUTIONS

Pregnancy, mild CHF, patients using beta blockers, Wolff-Parkinson-White syndrome

SIDE EFFECTS

Dizziness, headache, CHF, bradycardia, hypotension

SIGNIFICANT INTERACTIONS

Beta blockers, antihypertensives

DOSAGE

2.5 to 5.0 mg over 2 to 5 minutes; may be repeated in 15 to 30 minutes if necessary at double the dose (5.0 to

	10 mg). Maximum dose is 20 mg.
PEDIATRIC DOSAGE	• 0 to 1 year of age: 0.1 to 0.2 mg/kg over 2 minutes • 1 to 15 years of age: 0.1 to 0.3 mg/kg over 2 minutes
ROUTE	IV
OVERDOSE OR TOXICITY PRESENTATION	Hypotension, heart blocks, asystole
TREATMENT OF OVERDOSE OR OTHER ADVERSE REACTIONS	Discontinue drug; monitor vital signs and cardiac rhythms. Administer oxygen and support ventilations as necessary. Be prepared to intubate. **Hypotension:** Consider fluid challenge and any of the following: *Dopamine:* 2 to 5 mg/kg/hour titrated to systolic pressure of 100 mm Hg *Calcium chloride or calcium gluconate:* Contact medical control for dosage. **Bradycardia:** *Atropine:* 0.5 to 1.0 mg IV; may be repeated in 3 to 5 minutes. If unsuccessful, consider cardiac pacing.

Asystole: Start CPR; administer epinephrine and atropine per current ACLS guidelines; consider pacing.

SPECIAL CONSIDERATIONS

Monitor heart rhythm and vitals continuously during administration of verapamil.

CLASS

ACTIONS

INDICATIONS

CONTRAINDICATIONS

PRECAUTIONS

SIDE EFFECTS

SIGNIFICANT
INTERACTIONS

DOSAGE

PEDIATRIC DOSAGE

ROUTES

OVERDOSE OR
TOXICITY
PRESENTATION

TREATMENT OF
OVERDOSE OR OTHER
ADVERSE REACTIONS

SPECIAL
CONSIDERATIONS

CLASS

ACTIONS

INDICATIONS

CONTRAINDICATIONS

PRECAUTIONS

SIDE EFFECTS

SIGNIFICANT
INTERACTIONS

DOSAGE

PEDIATRIC DOSAGE

ROUTES

OVERDOSE OR
TOXICITY
PRESENTATION

TREATMENT OF
OVERDOSE OR OTHER
ADVERSE REACTIONS

SPECIAL
CONSIDERATIONS

CLASS

ACTIONS

INDICATIONS

CONTRAINDICATIONS

PRECAUTIONS

SIDE EFFECTS

SIGNIFICANT
INTERACTIONS

DOSAGE

PEDIATRIC DOSAGE

ROUTES

OVERDOSE OR
TOXICITY
PRESENTATION

TREATMENT OF
OVERDOSE OR OTHER
ADVERSE REACTIONS

SPECIAL
CONSIDERATIONS

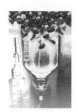

CHAPTER*FOUR*

ADMINISTRATION
OF PREHOSPITAL
MEDICATIONS

Mastering the skills necessary to administer medications in the field under emergency conditions is essential for the prehospital provider. Although medication administration is largely within the paramedic's scope of practice, some jurisdictions now permit intermediate-level personnel to administer certain drugs, and even basic emergency medical technicians, particularly those in states following the National EMT-B curriculum, can assist patients in administering some of their own medications.

There are many routes by which medication may be administered. These routes may be divided into two basic classifications: enteral and parenteral. Enteral simply means by way of the alimentary canal. The alimentary canal consists of the entire digestive tract, from the mouth to the rectum, and includes the stomach and intestines. Routes of administration included within the enteral class are oral, sublingual (under the tongue), buccal (between the cheeks), and rectal. All other routes of administration are classified as parenteral, meaning outside of the alimentary canal. Parenteral routes include subcutaneous (SC), intramuscular (IM), intravenous (IV), transdermal, transtracheal (by endotracheal tube), intraosseous, and inhalation. Each route has its advantages and disadvantages in the field.

The choice of route of administration depends on the nature of the patient's problem, the age of the patient, the drug to be administered, the need for a particular rate of absorption, site availability, and local protocol.

ORAL (PO)

PO medications are swallowed by the patient, and absorption takes place in either the stomach or the intestines. PO medications come in a variety of forms, including tablets, capsules, caplets, lozenges, and liquids.

Advantages
Ease and convenience of administration
Availability of many drugs in oral preparations
No pain or discomfort to the patient

Disadvantages
Requires that patient be conscious and alert
Slow absorption and onset of effect
May cause nausea and vomiting

EXAMPLE A PO medication used in the prehospital setting is aspirin, which is often administered as part of the chest pain protocol.

SUBLINGUAL (SL)

SL medications are administered by placing them under the tongue and allowing them to dissolve and become absorbed through the mucous membranes.

Advantages
Ease and convenience of administration
Rapid absorption

Disadvantages
Very few medications available in SL form
Requires that patient be conscious

Nitroglycerin for chest pain/congestive heart failure is available for SL administration as either a small pill or a spray.

BUCCAL

Buccal medications are intended to be placed between the cheeks and absorbed through the mucous membranes in the mouth.

Advantages
Ease and convenience of administration
Reasonably rapid absorption

Disadvantages
Very few medications available for buccal administration
Requires that patient be conscious

The buccal route is generally not used in the prehospital setting, although nitroglycerin can be administered by this route.

SUBCUTANEOUS (SC)

SC medications are injected into the fatty or connective tissue just below the skin.

Advantages
Relative ease of administration
Patient need not be conscious
Minimal risk to the patient

Disadvantages
Relatively slow absorption rate
Only small volume can be injected (no more than 0.5 mL)

May not be used if patient has poor peripheral circulation

> **EXAMPLE**   Epinephrine 1:1000 for anaphylaxis is typically administered by the SC route.

INTRAMUSCULAR (IM)

IM medication must be injected into the muscle tissue and absorbed through the bloodstream. The most common administration sites are the deltoid muscle in the upper arm and the dorsogluteal muscle in the buttocks. The dorsogluteal area is preferred for larger medication volumes.

Advantages
Patient need not be conscious
Faster absorption rate than SC
Longer duration of action
Availability of many medications
May administer volumes up to 5 mL

Disadvantages
Pain to the patient
Possible complications from poor technique
May not be used if patient has poor peripheral circulation

> **EXAMPLE**   Prehospital medications that may be administered IM include meperidine (Demerol) and glucagon.

ENDOTRACHEAL (ET) OR TRANSTRACHEAL

Administration by the ET route is accomplished by injecting the medication down the ET tube. Absorption takes place through the capillaries of the lungs.

Advantages
Rapid rate of absorption

Disadvantages
Significant skill required to properly place an ET tube
Requires that patient be unconscious
Very few medications administered via this route
Requires 2 to 2½ times the normal dose

EXAMPLE   ET medications include naloxone (Narcan), atropine, epinephrine, and lidocaine. Diazepam (Valium) is no longer recommended for ET administration.

RECTAL

Certain medications may be inserted into the rectum and absorbed through the mucous membranes. The most common form of drug designed for rectal administration is the suppository, but in the emergency setting medication may be injected into the rectum. When injecting medication into the rectum, the needle is generally removed from the syringe and the syringe lubricated to avoid injury. Another approach is to lubricate a short piece of IV tubing (approximately 6 inches), insert it approximately 2 inches into the rectum, and then inject the medication into the tubing. Following injection, the buttocks should be pressed together for 2 to 3 minutes.

Advantages
Absorption is relatively rapid
Patient need not be conscious
Medication not lost if patient vomits

Disadvantages
Few medications available for rectal administration
Inconvenience of accessing the rectum

Diazepam (Valium) is sometimes administered rectally in patients, particularly children, who are having seizures if IV access is not available.

INHALATION

A number of medications are administered by inhalation. Many of these are respiratory inhalers used by patients with asthma, emphysema, or other respiratory conditions. Emergency medical services (EMS) providers also have occasion to administer drugs by this route.

Advantages
Very rapid absorption
Ease and convenience of administration

Disadvantages
Relatively few drugs available for inhalation

Prehospital medications administered by inhalation include albuterol, nitrous oxide, and oxygen.

INTRACARDIAC

The intracardiac route involves injecting medication through the chest wall and into the ventricles of the heart. This route is not used at all in the prehospital environment and is used only rarely in the hospital emergency setting when access is not otherwise attainable.

Advantages
Rapid absorption

Disadvantages
Requires extensive training
Danger of complications

EXAMPLE Epinephrine 1:10,000 may be injected directly into the heart in cardiac arrest in the hospital emergency department setting.

INTRAOSSEOUS (IO)

The IO route is generally used in children under the age of 6 years when IV or other appropriate routes are unavailable in an emergency setting. There has been some recent discussion in the prehospital literature concerning the use of IO infusion in adults. IO administration requires the provider to insert a special needle known as a Jamshidi needle directly into the bone so that fluids and medication may be deposited into the bone marrow cavity. The most common site for IO administration is the anteromedial surface of the tibia, approximately 1 to 3 cm below the tibial tuberosity. Alternate sites are the distal femur and distal tibia.

Advantages
Rapid absorption
Possible to administer almost all drugs by this route

Disadvantages
Requires that patient be unconscious and unresponsive
Requires training
Potential for complications

In the setting of cardiac arrest in children, all IV fluids and advanced cardiac life support (ACLS) medications may be administered by the IO route.

TOPICAL OR TRANSDERMAL

Certain medications may be administered by the topical or transdermal route. Such medications enter the system by absorption through the skin.

Advantages
Ease and convenience of administration
No pain to the patient

Disadvantages
Relatively slow absorption rate
Availability of very few medications for topical use

Commonly seen transdermal medications include nitroglycerin paste and patches and fentanyl (Duragesic) patches.

PREPARING TO ADMINISTER MEDICATION

The preparation needed to administer medication in the field varies to a degree based on the nature and dosage of the medication, the manner in which it is supplied, and the route of administration. However, certain fundamental steps are common to the administration of all medications.

1. Conduct a thorough assessment of the patient, including a history and list of all current medications so that you can be certain that the medication you propose to administer is indicated for the patient's condition.

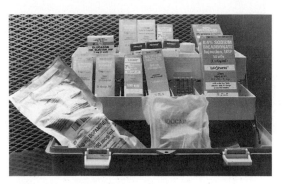

FIGURE 4-1. A typical paramedic drug box.

2. Communicate accurate patient information to the medical control physician so that the physician can order the correct medication in the appropriate dose. In some cases, it will be necessary to ascertain patient body weight for the purposes of dose calculation.

3. Confirm the order with the physician by repeating it back and then write it down. Clarify any questions regarding dosage or route of administration.

4. If administering a medication under standing orders, review the applicable protocol or order to be sure that you are administering the correct medication in the correct dose.

5. If the patient is conscious and competent, confirm that there is no history of allergy to the proposed medication. If the patient cannot be of assistance, check with family members.

6. Obtain the consent of the patient. Explain briefly the purpose of the drug, possible side effects, and consequences of not administering the drug. If

the patient is incompetent, determine whether or not there is a basis to proceed under the doctrine of implied consent. In the case of a minor, obtain parental consent.

7. Check the label on the medication container to be sure that you have selected the right medication in the right concentration. Check the expiration date. If the medication is expired, advise medical control of the expiration date and ask for further orders.
8. Check the medication for usability. Examine the vial, ampule, or Tubex cartridge for clarity and the presence of particles or precipitates.
9. Administer the medication and promptly dispose of needles and other administration equipment.
10. Monitor the patient for responses to the drug, including both therapeutic effect and adverse effects.
11. Document the administration of the drug on your patient care report to include route of administration, dose, patient response, and repeated doses.

Remember the "five patient rights of drug administration." Always be sure that the *right patient* receives the *right dose* of the *right drug* via the *right route* at the *right time.*

PREPARING INJECTABLE MEDICATIONS

The majority of medications used in the field are injected either by IM or SC injection, IV, or down the ET tube. The medications themselves are available in a number of different containers or packages, which vary from system to system. Most commonly seen are vials,

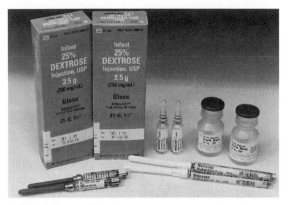

FIGURE 4–2. Injectable medications come in a variety of containers, including pre-loaded syringes, ampules, vials, and Tubex cartridges.

ampules, Tubex cartridges, and pre-filled syringes (Figure 4–2).

DRAWING MEDICATION FROM A VIAL (Figure 4–3)

Vials are small glass bottles containing a quantity of medication for injection. Some vials are single doses, while others may be used for repeated doses. The vial is closed with a rubber stopper and covered with a plastic cap. The procedure is as follows:

1. Confirm the name, dosage, and route of administration of the drug.
2. Check the label for name, concentration, and expiration date.
3. Examine contents for clarity and particles.
4. Select an appropriate syringe and needle based on

237

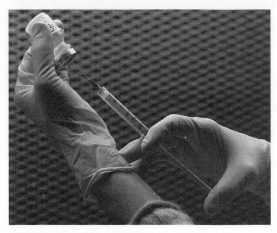

FIGURE 4–3. Drawing medication from a vial.

the quantity of the drug being administered and the route by which it is to be administered. IM injections are usually given with No. 21- to 23-gauge needle, while a No. 25-gauge needle is commonly used for SC administration.

5. Remove the plastic cap from the vial and clean off the rubber stopper with an alcohol prep pad.

6. Remove the cap from the needle and draw air into the syringe in a volume equal to or greater than the volume of the drug that you plan to administer.

7. Hold the vial upside down, insert the needle through the rubber stopper, and inject the air into the vial.

8. Pull back slowly on the plunger until slightly more than the prescribed amount of medication has been drawn into the syringe.

9. Withdraw the needle from the vial and expel any air that may be present, along with any surplus medication.

DRAWING MEDICATION FROM AN AMPULE (Figure 4–4)

Many medications are also available in small glass, single-dose containers known as ampules. When using an ampule, the procedure is as follows:

1. Follow steps 1 to 4 from the previous section on medications contained in vials.
2. Holding the ampule upright, snap your fingers against the stem so that the medication will be directed down into the well of the ampule.
3. Grasp the top of the ampule in your hand, using a gauze pad for protection, and snap it off at the stem. The ampule is usually scored with a colored band where it is to be broken.

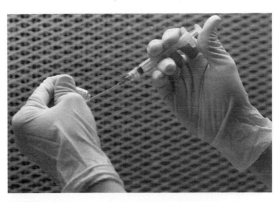

FIGURE 4–4. Drawing medication from an ampule.

4. With the plunger on the syringe pushed all the way forward, insert the needle into the ampule. Do not inject any air into the ampule.
5. Pull slowly back on the plunger until the desired amount of medication has been drawn into the syringe.
6. Withdraw the needle from the ampule, and expel any air and excess drug from the syringe.

PROCEDURE WHEN USING A PRE-FILLED SYRINGE

Many prehospital medications are now available in pre-filled syringes. They are convenient to use and can be administered very rapidly, since there is no need to draw up medication. Pre-filled syringes typically contain a single dose, although there are some exceptions. The procedure is as follows:

1. Follow steps 1 to 4 from the foregoing section on drawing medication from a vial.
2. Pop the plastic caps off of the cartridge containing the medication and the barrel of the syringe, and then carefully twist the medication cartridge into the barrel.
3. Remove the cap from the needle and expel any air that may be present.

PROCEDURE FOR USING A TUBEX SYSTEM

A Tubex system consists of a pre-filled medication cartridge that fits into either a plastic or a metal housing. When using a Tubex, the procedure is as follows:

1. Follow steps 1 to 4 from the foregoing section on drawing medication from a vial.
2. Assemble the Tubex system by inserting the medication cartridge into the housing and screwing it

into place. A number of different housings are available that fit together in slightly different ways. Be sure to become familiar with the systems used in your area.

3. Expel any air from the medication cartridge.

TECHNIQUES FOR INJECTING MEDICATION

As noted earlier, medication may be injected in a number of different ways. In the field, IM, SC, IV, and ET injection routes are the most commonly used. The advanced level prehospital provider must become proficient in these skills.

PROCEDURE FOR INTRAMUSCULAR INJECTION

1. Confirm the order and write it down.
2. Explain what you are going to do to the patient and ask for consent.
3. Ask the patient about possible allergies to the medication.
4. Put on gloves.
5. Assemble all necessary equipment, including a syringe of appropriate size relative to the amount of medication being injected (usually 2 to 5 mL), a needle (21- to 23-gauge), alcohol prep pads, sterile dressing, a bandage, and the medication to be injected.
6. Follow the steps in the previous sections for drawing up medication into a syringe.
7. Select a site for injection. The deltoid muscle in the upper arm and the dorsogluteal muscle in the buttocks are commonly used.
8. Prepare the site by cleaning with an alcohol prep pad.

9. With one hand, pinch together a section of the muscle at the injection site.
10. With the other hand, quickly insert the needle into the muscle at a 90-degree angle (Figure 4–5).
11. Aspirate the syringe to check for blood return. If blood is present, withdraw the needle, place a bandage over the site, and attempt the injection at another site. If blood is not present, inject the medication slowly.
12. Withdraw the needle and gently massage the site to promote absorption.
13. Safely dispose of the syringe.

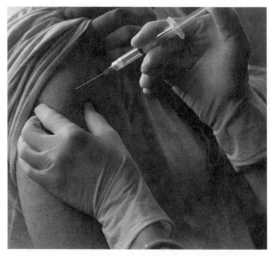

FIGURE 4–5. Administering an intramuscular injection into the deltoid muscle of the upper arm.

14. Document the administration of the drug.
15. Observe the patient for reactions to the drug.

1. Follow steps 1 to 4 from the foregoing section on IM injections.
2. Assemble all necessary equipment, including a syringe (usually a 1-mL syringe), a needle (usually 25 gauge), alcohol prep pads, a bandage, a sterile 4 × 4 dressing, and the medication to be injected.
3. Follow the steps in the previous sections for drawing up the medication unless the medication is in a pre-filled syringe.
4. Select a site for injection. The deltoid muscle in the upper arm is commonly used but other sites include the abdomen and the thighs.
5. Prepare the site by cleaning with an alcohol prep pad.
6. Pinch together a portion of the tissue.
7. With the other hand, insert the needle into the skin at a 45-degree angle (Figure 4–6).
8. Aspirate the syringe slightly to check for blood return. If blood is present, withdraw the needle, place a bandage over the site, and select another site.
9. If blood is not present, inject the medication slowly.
10. Remove the syringe and gently massage the site with a sterile dressing to promote absorption.
11. Safely dispose of the syringe.
12. Document the administration of the drug.
13. Observe the patient for reactions to the medication.

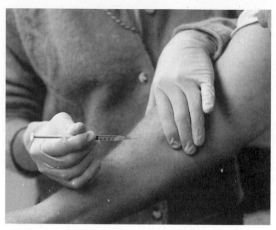

FIGURE 4–6. Administering a subcutaneous injection.

PROCEDURE FOR INJECTION INTO AN INTRAVENOUS LINE

1. Follow steps 1 to 4 from the section on IM injections.
2. Put on gloves.
3. Assemble all necessary equipment, including a syringe of appropriate size, a needle, alcohol prep pads, and the medication to be administered.
4. Follow the steps in the previous section for drawing up the medication unless the medication is in a pre-filled syringe.
5. Clean the medication port on the IV line with an alcohol prep pad.
6. Insert the needle into the medication port and

pinch off the IV tubing between the medication port and the fluid bag.

7. Inject the medication as indicated. Some medications will require slow injection, while others such as adenosine must be injected very quickly.
8. Withdraw the needle and dispose of it safely.
9. Unpinch the line and open the flow regulator wide to allow for the medication to be flushed out of the tubing and into the vein.
10. Readjust the flow rate after 6 to 10 seconds.
11. Document the administration of the drug.
12. Observe the patient for reactions to the drug.

PROCEDURE FOR INJECTION DOWN AN ENDOTRACHEAL TUBE

1. Confirm the order and write it down.
2. Be sure that the medication ordered is one that can be administered via the ET route. ET drugs include atropine, epinephrine, lidocaine, and naloxone. ET administration of diazepam (Valium) is no longer recommended.
3. Put on gloves.
4. Dilute the medication in 5 to 10 mL of sterile water or normal saline. Remember that an ET dose is usually 2 to 2½ times the IV dose.
5. Have the person doing ventilations stop and disconnect the bag-valve-mask from the ET tube.
6. Quickly inject the medication as far down the tube as possible.
7. Reconnect the bag-valve-mask to the ET tube and ventilate briskly for 30 to 60 seconds.
8. Safely dispose of the syringe.
9. Document the administration of the drug.
10. Observe the patient for reactions to the drug.

TECHNIQUE FOR ESTABLISHING INTRAOSSEOUS ACCESS

IO cannulation involves introducing a needle into the intramedullary space of a long bone to provide access for the administration of fluids, blood products, and medication. The procedure is as follows:

1. Obtain an order for the procedure if necessary.
2. Assemble all necessary equipment:
   a. IO needle (Jamshidi needle)
   b. IV fluid and administration set
   c. Alcohol and povidone-iodine prep pads
   d. Sterile gloves
   e. Roller gauze, tape, and sterile dressings
   f. 2 syringes (5 or 10 mL)
3. Locate the site: the preferred site is on the flat portion of the proximal tibia, 2 to 3 cm below the tibial tuberosity.
4. Apply sterile gloves.
5. Clean the site with povidone-iodine and alcohol.
6. Insert the tip of the needle through the skin at a 90-degree angle.
7. Once the needle reaches the bone surface, angulate it slightly toward the foot and advance into the bone using a twisting motion.
8. When you feel a "pop" or "give" you have entered the bone marrow space.
9. Remove the stylet and attach a syringe to the needle. Attempt to aspirate slowly, and check for blood and/or bone marrow. Bone marrow will not always be present.
10. Remove the first syringe and attach a second syringe containing sterile saline. Attempt to flush saline into the site. If the needle is properly placed, the saline should flow easily without resistance.

11. Remove the syringe and attach an IV administration set that is connected to a bag of IV fluid.
12. Administer medication as indicated.
13. Follow the injection of medication with a saline flush of 5 to 10 mL.
14. Stabilize the IO needle in place with gauze and tape.
15. Monitor the site frequently.

IV PIGGYBACK PROCEDURE

On occasion it will be necessary for the paramedic to administer medication using an IV piggyback setup. This procedure can be accomplished as follows:

1. Establish a primary IV line with appropriate fluid.
2. Obtain and confirm the order to administer medication by IV piggyback.
3. Prepare the ordered medication by injecting it into a secondary bag of IV fluid (usually normal saline). Mix the contents by turning the bag several times.
4. Prepare a secondary IV line by attaching an administration set to the bag of fluid containing the medication.
5. Bleed the secondary line of air.
6. Attach a needle to the administration set. An 18-gauge, 1-inch needle is commonly used.
7. Clean the medication port on the primary line with an alcohol prep pad.
8. Insert the needle into the port and secure it with tape.
9. Calculate the proper drip rate in drops per minute.
10. Elevate the secondary IV fluid bag so that it is higher than the primary bag.

11. Adjust the flow rate so that the appropriate amount of medication is being infused.
12. Shut down the primary IV line.
13. Label the secondary bag so that the emergency department will know exactly what you gave the patient.
14. Once the infusion is complete, shut down the secondary line, restart the primary line, and discard the secondary bag, needle, and other equipment.

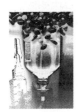

CHAPTER*FIVE*

INTRAVENOUS FLUID ADMINISTRATION

The administration of intravenous (IV) fluids is an integral part of emergency care in the field for two significant reasons: (1) to facilitate fluid replacement in cases of hypovolemia, shock, or dehydration, and (2) to provide access for the administration of medication. Accordingly, IV access should be obtained when the patient has experienced trauma or any medical condition in which the patient may require medication or is dehydrated, unstable, or potentially unstable. Typical indications for IV fluid administration include trauma, any cardiac-related condition, respiratory distress, stroke (cerebrovascular accident [CVA]), poisoning or drug overdose, seizures, diabetic emergencies, childbirth, diminished level of consciousness, dehydration, and burns.

DECISION MAKING IN IV THERAPY

Once the emergency medical services (EMS) provider has decided that it is appropriate to start an IV, several additional decisions must be made. These include the following:

Choice of catheter size
Choice of administration set
Rate of infusion
Choice of IV fluid
Placement of the IV

Selection of a catheter size depends primarily on the purpose for which the IV line is being started. Where the goal of the IV line is to serve as a route for fluid replacement, as in cases of shock or hypovolemia, as large a catheter as possible should be used. Ideally, this will be a 14- or 16-gauge catheter, but in many cases a smaller catheter must be used because of the size and structure of the patient's veins. Many patients, particularly children and the elderly, do not have veins that can accommodate a large catheter, and it may be necessary to use an 18- or 20-gauge catheter. Where fluid replacement is indicated, every effort should be made to obtain access with a larger catheter. Remember, the larger the number, the smaller the diameter of the catheter. Where the IV line is primarily being used as a route for the administration of medication, a smaller catheter, usually an 18- or 20-gauge, will be suitable.

CHOICE OF ADMINISTRATION SET

Administration sets are of two general types: The macrodrip set usually delivers fluid at a rate of 10 to 20 drops per milliliter; the microdrip set delivers fluid at a rate of 50 to 60 drops per milliliter. A macrodrip is used when administering normal saline, lactated Ringer's, or other fluid for volume replacement. The microdrip is generally used when an IV line is being established with D_5W or other fluid to be run at a "to keep open" (TKO) rate for purposes of medication administration. Specialized "blood tubing" may be required when blood products are being used. Local protocols should be checked.

It is now quite acceptable in many jurisdictions, where fluid replacement is not indicated, to use saline or heparin locks instead of connecting a standard administration set and bag of fluid to the IV catheter. These locks allow the EMS provider to administer medication, as needed, by simply injecting the medication into the medication port on the lock and then flushing it with 5 to 10 mL of fluid, generally normal saline. If fluid becomes necessary, it is a simple matter to attach a bag of the appropriate fluid.

RATE OF INFUSION

The rate of infusion depends on the reason that the IV is being established, the patient's condition, local protocols, and the direction of medical control. Where fluid replacement is a high priority, the IV line is sometimes run wide open. When maintaining the IV line solely for the purpose of medication administration, infusion is often set at a TKO rate, also known in some areas as "keep vein open" (KVO). Typically, this will be in the range of 6 to 12 drops (gtt) per minute.

Occasionally the physician or local protocol may direct that a very specific amount of fluid be infused into the patient through the IV line. This will require the provider to calculate the drip rate. To do so, three things must be known:

1. The volume of fluid to be infused
2. The amount of time over which the fluid is to be infused
3. The delivery capabilities of the administration set through which the fluid will be running. This is measured by the number of drops required to deliver 1 mL of fluid. Example: A macrodrip set typically delivers fluid at the rate of 10 gtt/mL. It is also important to know that 1 mL is equal to 1 cubic centimeter (cc).

With the above information, it is possible to calculate the drip rate using the following formula:

$$\dfrac{\text{Volume to be infused} \times \text{gtt/mL of the administration set}}{\text{Infusion time in minutes}} = \text{gtt/minute}$$

EXAMPLE A physician orders an infusion of normal saline at a rate of 200 mL/hr. Your infusion set delivers fluid at a rate of 15 gtt/mL. These numbers are then plugged into the formula as follows:

$$\dfrac{200 \text{ mL} \times 15 \text{ gtt/mL}}{60 \text{ minutes}} = \text{gtt/minute}$$

We multiply 200 times 15 and get a total of 3000. We now have a formula that appears as follows:

$$\dfrac{3000}{60} = \text{gtt/minute}$$

We divide 3000 by 60 and come up with the answer:

$$\dfrac{3000}{60} = 50 \text{ gtt/minute}$$

So, to achieve a volume of 200 mL/hour, we must adjust our administration set to a rate of 50 gtt/minute. This would be slightly slower than 1 drop per second.

CHOICE OF IV FLUID

Fluid selection is usually dictated by the condition of the patient, the types of fluid available, local protocol, and medical control direction. While many different types of fluids are available and in use in hospitals, only a few are commonly used in the prehospital environment. The more common fluids are lactated Ringer's, normal saline, and D_5W. D_5W is used less commonly than it has been in the past.

Before looking at the properties of each of the various IV fluids, it is useful to review the different classifications of fluids and the effect that they have on the body.

IV fluids are divided into two general classifications: colloids and crystalloids. A colloid is a fluid that contains large molecules, usually protein, which remain in the intravascular space for a relatively long period of time. Such fluids are particularly beneficial in maintaining and increasing the patient's intravascular volume. These fluids include dextran, hetastarch (Hespan), and plasma protein fraction (Plasmanate). Colloids are rarely used in the field because they are very expensive, usually have a short half-life, require constant monitoring, and, in certain cases, can interfere with blood cross-matching in the hospital.

Crystalloids are fluids that do not contain protein or other large molecules. They contain water and electrolytes such as potassium, sodium chloride, and calcium chloride. Crystalloids pass through the vascular membrane into the tissue quite rapidly, thus requiring very substantial infusion volumes in cases of hypovolemia or shock. Crystalloids are the most common fluids used in the prehospital environment and include normal saline, lactated Ringer's, and D_5W.

Crystalloids differ from one another based on their relative concentrations of solute molecules to those within the cell. They are hypertonic, hypotonic, or isotonic in nature.

Hypertonic solutions are those which have a concentration of solute molecules higher than the concentration within the cell. This results in a movement of water out of the cell, causing the cells to shrink. An example of a hypertonic crystalloid is $D_{10}W$ (10% dextrose in water).

Hypotonic solutions are those having a solute concentration lower than that within the cell. An infusion of a hypotonic solution causes a movement of fluid from the extracellular space into the cell, causing the cell to swell. One-half normal saline and D_5W are examples of hypotonic solutions.

Isotonic solutions have a solute concentration equal to that within the cell. There is no change in cell size because of fluid transport. Examples of isotonic solutions are lactated Ringer's and normal saline.

PLACEMENT OF THE IV

The actual site of the IV infusion depends on the patient's vasculature and the reason for starting the IV. Arm veins are usually the first choice, and suitable veins can often be found in the forearm, on the back of the hand, and in the antecubital area. Almost any site will be suitable for an IV line that is being used for medication administration, but the larger veins frequently found in the antecubital area are often best when starting an IV line for fluid replacement. The antecubital area is also favored when administering adenosine, a cardiac medication used to treat supraventricular tachycardia. Since adenosine has a very short half-life, it is recommended that it be administered in a vein as close to the heart as possible.

Other possible IV sites include the external jugular vein in the neck and veins in the feet and lower leg. In young children, IO infusion, usually into the tibia, is also an option. IO infusion is used only in true emergencies such as cardiac arrest when the child is unconscious and IV access is not otherwise attainable.

GUIDE TO IV FLUIDS

NORMAL SALINE (0.9% SODIUM CHLORIDE)

CLASS	Isotonic crystalloid solution
ACTION	Normal saline acts as a replacement for water and electrolytes; since the solute concentration is roughly equivalent to that within the cell, there is neither swelling nor shrinking of the cell.
INDICATIONS	Hypovolemia, shock, dehydration, diabetic ketoacidosis, heat stroke, exhaustion
CONTRAINDICATIONS	No true contraindications
PRECAUTIONS	Beware of circulatory overload; use at TKO rate or consider another fluid in patients with congestive heart failure/pulmonary edema.
SIDE EFFECTS	Circulatory overload
SIGNIFICANT INTERACTIONS	None in the context of prehospital care
DOSAGE	Rate of infusion depends on circumstances; IV may be run wide open in cases of shock or hypovolemia, TKO if

being used as an access line for medication, or as directed by local protocol or medical control.

ROUTE   IV only

LACTATED RINGER'S SOLUTION

CLASS   Isotonic crystalloid solution

ACTIONS   Replaces fluid volume depletion, replaces water and electrolytes

INDICATIONS   Primarily used for fluid volume replacement in hypovolemia, shock, and dehydration; may also be used as a TKO line for the administration of medications, if necessary

CONTRAINDICATIONS   Avoid use in patients with renal failure and dialysis patients.

PRECAUTIONS   Beware of circulatory overload; in congestive heart failure or pulmonary edema use very sparingly at TKO rate, use a heparin or saline lock, or consider another fluid.

SIDE EFFECTS   Circulatory overload

SIGNIFICANT INTERACTIONS	None of consequence in the prehospital setting
DOSAGE	Dose depends on circumstances; may be run wide open in cases of hypovolemia or shock; TKO (6 to 10 gtt/minute) when being used as a medication line; or per local protocol or direction of medical control
ROUTE	IV only

½ Normal Saline (0.45% Sodium Chloride)

CLASS	Hypotonic crystalloid solution
ACTION	Acts by slowly replacing water and electrolytes
INDICATIONS	Particularly useful in patients with compromised renal function as a line for medication or for slow rehydration
CONTRAINDICATIONS	Avoid use in shock or hypovolemia where rapid fluid replacement is needed.
PRECAUTIONS	Infusion of large amounts of ½ normal saline can result in electrolyte depletion.

SIDE EFFECTS	None of significance except electrolyte depletion
SIGNIFICANT INTERACTIONS	None of any consequence in the prehospital setting
DOSAGE	Varies depending on the needs of the patient; rate of infusion generally directed by medical control
ROUTE	IV only

5% DEXTROSE IN WATER (D₅W)

CLASS	Hypotonic sugar solution
ACTION	Provides water and dextrose without risk of circulatory overload in patients with congestive heart failure/pulmonary edema
INDICATIONS	Primarily used to establish a medication line; used as a diluent for certain medications to be administered by IV infusion
CONTRAINDICATIONS	Avoid use when rapid fluid replacement is indicated.
PRECAUTIONS	Check patency of IV line because extravasation can

	result in localized tissue necrosis; consider drawing blood sample before infusion of D_5W.
SIDE EFFECTS	None of significance in the field
SIGNIFICANT INTERACTIONS	Incompatible with phenytoin (Dilantin)
DOSAGE	Generally administered TKO
ROUTE	IV only

10% DEXTROSE IN WATER ($D_{10}W$)

CLASS	Hypertonic sugar solution
ACTION	Provides water and dextrose, replaces blood glucose
INDICATIONS	Hypoglycemia, neonatal resuscitation
CONTRAINDICATIONS	Do not use for rapid fluid replacement in hypovolemia, dehydration, or shock.
PRECAUTIONS	Check patency of IV line because $D_{10}W$ can result in local tissue necrosis; draw blood sample before use.
SIDE EFFECTS	None of significance in the field

SIGNIFICANT INTERACTIONS	Phenytoin (Dilantin) is incompatible with $D_{10}W$
DOSAGE	Varies depending on patient status; contact medical control for rate of infusion
ROUTE	IV only

DEXTRAN

CLASS	Synthetic colloid
ACTION	Acts as a plasma volume expander; particularly useful in hypovolemia, since its large molecular size keeps it within the intravascular space for an extended period of time
INDICATIONS	Hypovolemia, hypovolemic shock, severe burns
CONTRAINDICATIONS	Known hypersensitivity to the drug, renal failure, congestive heart failure/pulmonary edema
PRECAUTIONS	Monitor the patient carefully for adverse reactions.
SIDE EFFECTS	Rash, nausea, vomiting, nasal congestion, tightness in the chest

SIGNIFICANT INTERACTIONS	Avoid use with anticoagulants such as heparin or warfarin (Coumadin).
DOSAGE	In hypovolemia, dextran is titrated to the patient's hemodynamic response; for severe burns, follow Consensus Formula (Appendix M) or direction of medical control.
ROUTE	IV only

Plasma Fraction Protein (Plasmanate)

CLASS	Plasma protein; colloid
ACTION	Supplies colloid to the blood, causes fluid shift from the interstitial spaces into the circulation, expands the circulating volume
INDICATIONS	Hypovolemic shock, hypoproteinemia (low protein)
CONTRAINDICATIONS	None in the presence of hypovolemic shock
PRECAUTIONS	Monitor patient status every 5 minutes to determine patient response to Plasmanate; be alert for development

	of pulmonary edema or hypertension.
SIDE EFFECTS	Headaches, hives, nausea, vomiting, chills, flushing
SIGNIFICANT INTERACTIONS	None of significance in the field
DOSAGE	Titrate to hemodynamic response; consult with medical control for infusion rate, which generally should not exceed 10 mL/per minute.
ROUTE	IV only; do not administer through same tubing as other IV fluids

HETASTARCH (HESPAN)

PLASMA	Plasma expander; artificial colloid
ACTION	Increases intravascular volume because of colloidal osmotic effect
INDICATIONS	Hypovolemic shock, severe burns
CONTRAINDICATIONS	Congestive heart failure, bleeding disorders
PRECAUTIONS	Monitor patient response continuously and watch for circulatory overload and pulmonary edema.

SIDE EFFECTS	Headaches, hives, nausea, vomiting, chills, fever
SIGNIFICANT INTERACTIONS	Avoid use in patients using anticoagulants.
DOSAGE	Titrate to patient's hemodynamic response; consult with medical control for infusion rate, which generally should not exceed 1500 mL/day.
ROUTE	IV infusion only

CONVERTING AN INTRAVENOUS INFUSION ORDER INTO A DRIP RATE PER MINUTE

FLUID ORDER IN mL/hour	ADMINISTRATION SET	
	10 gtt/mL	15 gtt/mL
50 mL	8 gtt/minute	12 gtt/minute
100 mL	16–17 gtt/minute	25 gtt/minute
200 mL	33 gtt/minute	50 gtt/minute
300 mL	50 gtt/minute	75 gtt/minute
400 mL	66 gtt/minute	100 gtt/minute
500 mL	83 gtt/minute	125 gtt/minute
600 mL	100 gtt/minute	150 gtt/minute
750 mL	125 gtt/minute	188 gtt/minute
1000 mL	166 gtt/minute	250 gtt/minute

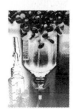

CHAPTER*SIX*

DRUGS
OF
ABUSE

When we hear the term "drugs of abuse" we frequently think of street drugs such as heroin, cocaine, lysergic acid diethylamide (LSD), or marijuana, which are acquired and possessed illegally, used by teenagers and junkies, and have little or no legitimate medical purpose. The term "drug abuse" is defined here as the administration of any medication or drug in a manner that is not consistent with accepted medical practice. Drug abuse is something that spans every age group, even the elderly, and can involve almost any drug. It may include alcohol, prescription medication, or any substance taken improperly for enhanced or mind-altering effect, to achieve a high or euphoria, or even to commit suicide. Drug-related emergencies, especially overdoses, are on the rise, and it is important that the emergency medical services (EMS) provider be prepared to properly assess and treat patients experiencing such problems.

Dealing with drug abuse patients can be difficult and challenging for a variety of reasons:

1. Drug abuse patients are frequently found unconscious, drowsy, and/or exhibiting bizarre and irrational behavior, thus making it nearly impossible to obtain a reliable patient history.
2. Those using illegal drugs may be concerned about the legal consequences of their drug use and often

refuse to provide reliable information for fear of arrest.

3. Many drug-related problems involve multiple drugs or drugs taken in combination with alcohol, making assessment and treatment difficult.

4. Intravenous (IV) drug abusers may be infected with acquired immunodeficiency syndrome (AIDS), hepatitis, and tuberculosis, creating significant health risks for the provider.

The purpose of this chapter is to provide information regarding the assessment and treatment of patients who have overdosed or are suffering toxic reactions related to the abuse of certain drugs. In most cases of overdose, the user intentionally takes the subject drug with the specific intent of attaining a "high," euphoria, or other effect, but accidental overdoses, particularly in the elderly, are also encountered. The classifications of drugs discussed are those most commonly abused, specifically, narcotics, stimulants, barbiturates, hallucinogens, and alcohol. These drugs may be acquired by prescription, by over-the-counter purchase, or through illicit "street trade." Problems associated with other prescription or over-the-counter medications are discussed in Chapter 2; those associated with prehospital medications are addressed in Chapter 4.

ASSESSMENT OF THE SUSPECTED DRUG ABUSER

Assessment of the patient with a suspected drug problem does not differ substantially from assessment of any other patient. Those areas requiring particular attention are as follows:

History. The following information should be obtained, if possible:

1. What did the patient take? If possible, obtain a sample.
2. How much of the drug was taken?
3. When was the drug taken?
4. What was the route of administration? Was it oral, IV, inhaled, etc.?
5. Were other drugs or alcohol taken? If so, how much and when?
6. Has the patient vomited? If so, bring a sample to the hospital.
7. Has anything been done by the patient or by family members or friends to try to assist the patient? If so, what?

Level of Consciousness. This is perhaps the most significant sign and should be observed and recorded at frequent intervals.

Vital Signs. Pulse, blood pressure, and respiratory function should be measured and recorded every few minutes. Observe the quality of the respirations as well as the rate.

Physical Examination. Do the following:
1. Examine the pupils for dilation, miosis (pinpoint pupils), and reaction to light.
2. Check the skin color. Also see if the skin is warm, cool, dry, or moist.
3. Check for unusual odors on the breath.
4. Check the arms and legs for needle marks.

Scene Observation. Check the scene for syringes, pipes, rolling papers, or other drug paraphernalia.

Even if there is strong evidence to suggest drug use, it is always possible that the patient is experiencing another medical problem. For example, finding a comatose patient with needle marks on the arm certainly suggests a narcotic overdose, but you should always conduct a full assessment and consider other possible causes.

TREATMENT

General Principles of Management

Certain general principles of management apply to all drug-related circumstances and should be followed unless otherwise directed by medical control. These include the following:

1. Monitor ABCs (airway, breathing, and circulation).
2. Administer oxygen. If the patient is unconscious, insert an oral or nasal airway and/or be prepared to intubate.
3. Take and record vitals frequently.
4. Start an IV line with lactated Ringer's, normal saline, or other fluid per local protocol. Obtain a sample of the patient's blood.
5. Attach the patient to the cardiac monitor.
6. Contact medical control or the poison center for treatment advice.
7. Contact police if the patient is violent or exhibiting bizarre behavior.
8. Transport rapidly to the hospital.

Specific Classifications of Drugs: Assessment and Treatment

Narcotics

Narcotics or opioids have an extremely high potential for abuse and addiction and are responsible for many deaths each year by accidental overdose. These potent drugs have strong central nervous system (CNS) properties and generally cause death by depression of the respiratory system.

EXAMPLE	Heroin, morphine, meperidine (Demerol), hydromorphone (Dilaudid), codeine, oxycodone (Percodan), methadone, fentanyl, proporyphene (Darvon), "designer" opiates such as "China white" (alpha methyl fentanyl)

SIGNS AND SYMPTOMS	Nausea, vomiting, euphoria, stupor, coma, depressed respirations, miosis (constricted pupils), hypotension. Certain signs such as miosis can be masked if a combination of drugs has been used.
COMMON ROUTES	IV most common but intramuscular (IM), subcutaneous (SC), and oral ingestions are also possible. Some patients also have transdermal patches of fentanyl or other narcotics.
TREATMENT	1. General principles of management as noted above. 2. Consider naloxone (Narcan), 0.4 to 2.0 mg administered IV, IM, SC, or by endotracheal (ET) tube. Significantly higher doses may be needed when treating synthetic narcotics such as fentanyl. May be given as a bolus or titrated

slowly to achieve normal respirations. Check local protocol. For more specific information on naloxone, see page 168. Because of the short half-life of naloxone, redosing may be necessary. Be alert for signs of respiratory depression. If patient has been intubated, be prepared to extubate if there is a response to naloxone.

3. If no response to naloxone, consider the following:

   Thiamine: 100 mg—administered IM or IV

   Dextrose 50%: (D50)—25 g IV

   (For more detailed information regarding thiamine and D50 see pages 217 and 87, respectively.)

NOTE: In some jurisdictions, thiamine and D50 are administered before naloxone in unconscious patients.

4. Continue to monitor vitals and protect airway.
5. Contact medical control for further options and transport rapidly.

Stimulants

Drugs in the stimulant class act by stimulating the CNS. Many stimulants are sympathomimetic agents or mimic the properties of sympathomimetics. As a result, they typically accelerate heart rate and respirations and increase blood pressure.

EXAMPLE Amphetamine (Benzedrine), methamphetamine (Desoxyn, Methedrine), dextroamphetamine (Dexedrine), cocaine, crack cocaine

---

SIGNS AND SYMPTOMS	Agitation, tachycardia, hypertension, sweating, dilated pupils, tachypnea, tremors, increased body temperature, paranoia. In addition, signs and symptoms associated with cocaine or crack use may include chest pain, cardiac arrhythmias, seizures, and stroke.
COMMON ROUTES	IV, ingestion. Some stimulant preparations may also be smoked. Cocaine is usually inhaled through the nasal passages.
TREATMENT	1. General principles of management as noted above. Cocaine is generally inhaled through the nose. 2. If stimulant was ingested, contact medical control for the option of activated

charcoal. Do not induce
vomiting.
3. Treat tachyarrhythmias per
current advanced cardiac
life support (ACLS)
guidelines or as directed
by medical control.
4. Consider *diazepam* or
lorazepam for seizures.

EXAMPLES **Barbiturates:** amobarbital (Amytal),
aprobarbital (Alurate), butabarbital (Butisol), mephobarbital (Mebaral), pentobarbital (Nembutal), phenobarbital (Luminal), secobarbital (Seconal)

Sedatives: alprazolam (Xanax), chlordiazepoxide
(Librium), clonazepam (Klonopin), clorazepate (Tranxene), diazepam (Valium), flurazepam (Dalmane), lorazepam (Ativan), oxazepam (Serax), triazolam (Halcion)

SIGNS AND SYMPTOMS	Drowsiness, lethargy, slurred speech, unsteady gait, respiratory depression, hypotension, shock, coma
COMMON ROUTE	Generally ingested but may be taken IV or IM
TREATMENT	1. General principles of management as noted above. 2. If patient is alert and drug was ingested, consider option of *activated charcoal*. If patient is unconscious and intubated, consider insertion of nasogastric tube

and administer activated charcoal through the tube.

3. Consider flumazenil (Romazicon) 0.2 mg IV for benzodiazepine toxicity. For more information on flumazenil see page 118.

4. Contact medical control for the option of sodium bicarbonate—1 mEq/kg. For more information on sodium bicarbonate, see page 208.

Hallucinogens

EXAMPLE Lysergic acid diethylamide (LSD), phencyclidine (PCP), mescaline, psilocybin, marijuana

SIGNS AND SYMPTOMS	Visual and auditory hallucinations, bizarre behavior, agitation, panic, chills, elevated blood pressure, dilated pupils. In addition, PCP users may demonstrate violent and self-destructive behavior.
COMMON ROUTES	Ingestion, smoking
TREATMENT	Management in the prehospital setting is generally limited to "taking the patient down," supportive care, preventing the patient from harming himself or herself or others, and calming

measures. In certain cases of
violent behavior, consider
contacting medical control for
the option of diazepam or
chlorpromazine.

Acute Alcohol Intoxication
Alcohol is also classified as a potent CNS depressant.

SIGNS AND SYMPTOMS	Decreased level of consciousness, respiratory depression, hypertension or hypotension, bradycardia or tachycardia, agitation, restlessness, arrhythmias, seizures, nausea, vomiting, nystagmus, odor of alcohol on breath, chills. Remember: in assessing these patients, look for signs and symptoms of other conditions such as head injury, hypoglycemia (particularly in children), or mixed drug-alcohol reactions.
COMMON ROUTES	Oral ingestion
TREATMENT	1. General principles of management as noted above.
	2. Start IV of D_5W or normal saline.
	3. Administer thiamine 100 mg by IV.
	4. Administer 25 g of dextrose 50% IV.
	5. Consider naloxone, 0.4 to

2.0 mg IV in cases of
mixed overdose.
6. Consider diazepam 2.5 mg
if seizures develop.

Remember that in all cases of suspected drug overdose, both your local poison control center and on-line
medical control are invaluable resources in helping to
provide effective treatment.

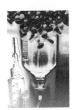

CHAPTER*SEVEN*

PREHOSPITAL TREATMENT OF COMMON EMERGENCIES

Although emergency medical services (EMS) personnel respond to many different types of emergencies, a number occur with great frequency. Among these are cardiac, respiratory, and diabetic emergencies, to name a few. Many of these medical problems can be effectively treated using a variety of medications that are carried by prehospital personnel, primarily paramedics. Since not all EMS services carry the same medications, not all of the medication interventions listed will apply to every reader's practice in the field.

The information is presented in the following manner for each of the selected emergency situations:

1. Common signs and symptoms associated with the condition
2. Treatment objectives
3. Standard treatment interventions
4. A list of possible medications that may be used for the stated condition

The medication indications and dosages are based on standards set forth in nationally recognized references such as the American Heart Association's Guidelines for Advanced Cardiac Life Support (ACLS) and the *Physician's Desk Reference,* among others. The information may differ from the reader's local protocols, which should always be followed.

ANAPHYLACTIC EMERGENCIES

Anaphylaxis is a severe, exaggerated hypersensitivity reaction to an antigen that has been previously encountered. Insect stings, food, and medication are the most common causes of anaphylactic reactions. Anaphylaxis is a true emergency that can easily result in death unless immediate action is taken.

Common Signs and Symptoms. Wheezing, bronchospasm, stridor, accessory muscle use, tachycardia, hypotension, nausea, vomiting, urticaria (hives), pruritus (itching), edema of the face and tongue, tearing of the eyes

Treatment Objectives. To protect and maintain the airway, to reverse respiratory signs and symptoms including laryngeal edema and bronchospasm, to restore hemodynamic stability

Treatment Interventions

1. Assess and constantly monitor the airway; administer high-flow oxygen by face mask. Have intubation and both needle and surgical cricothyrotomy equipment readily available for immediate intervention as necessary. Check local protocols.
2. Monitor vitals.
3. Monitor cardiac rhythm.
4. Establish a large-bore intravenous (IV) line with lactated Ringer's or normal saline and run wide open or as directed by medical control.
5. Place the patient in the shock position.
6. Rapidly transport to the hospital.

Possible Medications. Consult local protocols or medical control for the following options. Dosages may differ.

278

1. **Anaphylaxis kit.** Many patients with known allergies carry their own kits with one or two doses of epinephrine. If the patient has not already done so, consider administering this medication. In many areas, basic level emergency medical technicians (EMTs) are permitted to do so with the approval of medical control.
2. **Epinephrine.** 0.3 to 0.5 mg of a 1:1000 solution administered by subcutaneous (SC) injection *or* 0.1 to 0.5 mg (1–5 mL) of a 1:10,000 solution by slow IV infusion
3. **Epinephrine, racemic.** Nebulize 0.5 mL in 3 mL of normal saline.
4. **Albuterol (Proventil).** Nebulize 2.5 mg in 3 mL of normal saline.
5. **Diphenhydramine (Benadryl).** Administer 25 to 50 mg IV or intramuscularly (IM).
6. **Methylprednisolone (Solu-Medrol).** 100 to 200 mg IV or IM
7. **Hydrocortisone (Solu-Cortef).** 100 to 250 mg IV or IM

Refer to Chapter 3 for further information regarding the foregoing medications, including pediatric dosages.

BEHAVIORAL EMERGENCIES

Behavioral emergencies are common in EMS. Patients who are anxious, agitated, depressed, and/or suicidal are often encountered. The manifestations of these various mental states can be bizarre, combative, dangerous, and irrational behavior that threatens the safety and well-being of the patient, rescue personnel, and other persons in the vicinity. While there are many types of mental disorders, EMS personnel usually respond to those where the patient is extremely anxious, is exhibiting bizarre or irrational behavior, or is believed to be self-destructive or suicidal.

Common Signs and Symptoms. Signs and symptoms vary depending on the type of disorder encountered.

Anxiety attacks: Hyperventilation, dyspnea, chest pain or tightness, palpitations, trembling, sweating, irrational fear that patient is dying

Schizophrenia: Depression or elation, hallucinations, irrational thought, paranoia, unusual posturing, rage, anger, violent behavior

Suicidal behavior: Depression, crying, hopelessness, restlessness, agitation, recent history of a triggering event such as divorce, death of a loved one, termination from employment

It is not the role of the EMS provider to attempt a diagnosis in the field but merely to record the behavior observed and provide effective treatment and transportation. It is also important to remember that what appears to be a case of a mental disorder can often be confused with another medical condition that produces similar signs and symptoms. Such conditions may include drug or alcohol use, head trauma, hypoxia, glucose or magnesium imbalances, cerebrovascular accident (CVA), or an adverse reaction to a prescription medication, among others. EMS personnel must therefore always conduct a complete assessment to the extent permitted by the patient.

Treatment Objectives. To protect the patient and others from harm, to determine whether or not the patient poses a danger to himself or to other persons, to assess the patient for any possible medical or traumatic conditions, to determine whether or not the patient is capable of making rational decisions regarding medical care, to provide effective treatment and transportation to a medical facility, to determine the need for physical or chemical restraints

Treatment Interventions

1. Determine scene safety.
2. Request law enforcement personnel to respond to the scene.
3. Make every effort to obtain the patient's cooperation by using a calm, reassuring, and concerned manner. Never lie to the patient.
4. Conduct an interview of the patient to ascertain information and his or her feelings, medical history, medications, and any physical complaints.
5. Conduct a physical assessment to the extent that it is possible to do so to determine the possible presence of a medical condition or trauma.
6. Provide emergency treatment for any medical conditions or traumatic injuries.
7. If the patient refuses to go the the hospital, contact medical control to determine whether or not the patient should be transported against his or her will and whether physical and/or chemical restraints should be used.
8. Transport to the emergency department.

Possible Medications

1. **Diazepam (Valium):** 2 to 10 mg IV or IM for extreme anxiety
2. **Chlorpromazine (Thorazine):** 25 mg IM for the management of acute psychotic episodes, extreme agitation, or anxiety
3. **Haloperidol (Haldol):** 2 to 5 mg IM or IV for acute psychoses
4. **Lorazepam (Ativan):** 2 to 6 mg IV or IM for anxiety

NOTE: Some of these medications may be used in combination, such as haloperidol and lorazepam.

Contact medical control for further options.

Refer to Chapter 3 for further information regarding the foregoing medications, including pediatric dosages.

CARDIAC ARREST

The EMS provider frequently encounters victims of cardiac arrest from various different causes, including acute myocardial infarction, CVA, poisoning, drug overdose, electric shock, drowning, and trauma.

Common Signs and Symptoms. Absence of pulse and breathing, dilated pupils, and cyanosis. Cardiac monitor shows ventricular fibrillation (VF), ventricular tachycardia (VT) without a pulse, asystole, or pulseless electrical activity (PEA). Late signs include lividity and rigor mortis.

Treatment Objectives. To establish and maintain an effective airway, to provide artificial ventilation and circulation, to correct cardiac arrhythmias

Treatment Interventions

1. Assess airway, breathing, and circulation (ABCs).
2. Initiate cardiopulmonary resuscitation (CPR).
3. Assess cardiac rhythm.
4. Provide electric shock in cases of VF and pulseless VT per ACLS guidelines (see Appendix O).
5. Consider pacing in cases of asystole.
6. Consider causes and treat patients with PEA.

Possible Medications. Consult local protocols or medical control for the following options. Dosages may differ.

1. **Epinephrine 1:10,000.** 1 mg every 3 to 5 minutes or escalating dosage (see page 112)

2. **Lidocaine.** 1 mg/kg in VF or pulseless VT
3. **Bretylium.** 5 mg/kg in VF or pulseless VT
4. **Atropine.** 1 mg every 3 to 5 minutes in asystole or PEA with bradycardia
5. **Magnesium sulfate.** 1 to 2 g in torsades de pointes or refractory VF
6. **Procainamide.** 30 mg/minute in refractory VF
7. **Sodium bicarbonate.** 1 mEq/kg in prolonged cardiac arrest, known preexisting bicarbonate response acidosis, or tricyclic overdose

Refer to Chapter 3 for further information regarding the foregoing medications, including pediatric dosages. See appendices for ACLS algorithms and proper sequence of medication administration.

CARDIAC DYSRHYTHMIAS

A dysrhythmia is described as a cardiac rhythm that is abnormal, disordered, or disturbed. Dysrhythmias may be relatively benign, lethal, or somewhere in-between. In some cases, the presence of a dysrhythmia will be the reason for the request for assistance, whereas in others, the dysrhythmia may be associated with another complaint. It is important to accurately assess and treat dysrhythmias in a manner consistent with current standards. Generally, treatment will follow the American Heart Association's ACLS guidelines

Common Signs and Symptoms. Patients with dysrhythmias are not necessarily symptomatic, and it is not unusual to find a patient with a dysrhythmia who is tolerating the condition surprisingly well. Patients who are symptomatic and unstable commonly present with similar signs and symptoms regardless of whether the dysrhythmia is rapid or slow. Such signs and symptoms include the following: diaphoresis, hypotension, shortness of breath, pulmonary edema, chest pain, decreased level of consciousness, shock. In some cases, a dysrhythmia may be serious even in the absence of symptoms.

Treatment Objectives. To accurately interpret the nature of the dysrhythmia; to restore a normal rhythm, if possible; to restore hemodynamic stability; to assess and treat any associated medical problems; to alleviate pain and other symptoms

Treatment Interventions

1. Assess and monitor ABCs.
2. Monitor vital signs every 5 minutes.
3. Assess lung sounds.
4. Administer oxygen immediately and be prepared to intubate.
5. Monitor oxygen saturation with pulse oximetry.
6. Establish IV access per local protocol.
7. Monitor cardiac rhythm.
8. Perform 12-lead electrocardiogram (ECG) if available.
9. Determine rhythm.
10. Conduct complete assessment and obtain history.
11. Provide such further treatment as indicated.
12. Contact medical control for treatment advice and options.

Possible Medications
For symptomatic bradycardia

1. **Atropine.** 0.5 to 1.0 mg IV push
2. **Dopamine.** 5 to 20 μg/kg/minute titrated to heart rate
3. **Epinephrine 1:10,000.** 2 to 10 μg/minute titrated to heart rate
4. **Isoproterenol (Isuprel).** 2 to 10 μg/minute titrated to heart rate and rhythm; used for bradycardia in

heart transplant patients and in cases of bradycardia refractory to atropine

NOTE: If available, consider transcutaneous pacing.

For symptomatic atrial fibrillation or atrial flutter

5. **Diltiazem (Cardizem).** 0.25 mg/kg slow IV bolus; repeat in 15 minutes with dose of 0.35 mg/kg
6. **Propranolol (Inderal).** 1 to 3 mg IV bolus over 3 to 5 minutes
7. **Verapamil (Calan).** 2.5 mg IV bolus over 1 to 2 minutes
8. **Digoxin (Lanoxin).** 0.25 to 0.50 mg slow IV push over 5 to 8 minutes

For paroxysmal supraventricular tachycardia (PSVT)

9. **Adenosine (Adenocard).** 6 mg rapid IV push; second dose is 12 mg; use adenosine after vagal maneuvers
10. **Verapamil (Calan).** 2.5 to 5.0 mg IV; second dose is 5 to 10 mg after 15 to 30 minutes; use verapamil after adenosine if blood pressure is normal or elevated and the complex remains narrow
11. **Lidocaine.** 1 to 1.5 mg IV push if complex becomes wide

For VT with a pulse

12. **Lidocaine.** 1 to 1.5 mg/kg IV push; repeat in 5 to 10 minutes at half the first dose
13. **Procainamide (Pronestyl).** 20 to 30 mg/minute; maximum dose 17 mg/kg
14. **Bretylium (Bretylol).** 5 to 10 mg/kg IV push over 8 to 10 minutes

Consult medical control for further options.

NOTE: If any tachydysrhythmia becomes unstable at any time, proceed to immediate cardioversion.

For symptomatic or dangerous premature ventricular contractions (PVCs)

15. **Lidocaine.** 1 mg/kg IV push

Consult medical control for further options.

For torsades de pointes

16. **Magnesium sulfate.** 1 to 2 g diluted in 100 mL of D$_5$W given IV over 1 to 2 minutes

Refer to Chapter 3 for further information regarding the foregoing medications, including pediatric dosages.

CHEST PAIN (Acute Myocardial Infarction [MI])

Chest pain calls are very common in EMS. Causes include relatively minor conditions such as bronchitis and costochondritis or far more serious problems such as acute MI. Unfortunately, it is almost impossible to rule out a cardiac problem in the field. Indeed, it can often be difficult in the hospital. Although the EMS provider may suspect a cause other than cardiac, all patients presenting with chest pain must be treated as though they were experiencing an acute MI until proved otherwise.

Common Signs and Symptoms of Acute MI. Chest pain that may radiate to other areas of the body, shortness of breath, nausea, vomiting, diaphoresis, pale skin, weakness, dizziness, palpitations, feeling of impending doom. Remember that an MI may be occurring even in the absence of chest pain.

Treatment Objectives. To maintain ABCs, maintain or restore hemodynamic stability, alleviate pain and anxiety, limit the size of the infarct, prevent or correct serious dysrhythmias; provide rapid transport to emergency department

Treatment Interventions

1. Monitor ABCs and vitals. Check vitals every 5 minutes.
2. Provide immediate oxygen.
3. Monitor oxygen saturation with pulse oximetry.
4. Monitor cardiac rhythm.
5. Establish IV access per local protocol.
6. Perform 12-lead ECG if available.
7. Obtain blood samples per local protocol.
8. Take a detailed history, including risk factors, family history, medications, and prior cardiac problems, if any. Establish possible eligibility for thrombolytic intervention.

Possible Medications. Consult local protocols or medical control for the following options. Dosages may differ.

1. **Nitroglycerin.** 0.3 to 0.4 mg by sublingual tablet or spray; repeat up to three times
2. **Morphine sulfate.** 2 to 5 mg IV
3. **Aspirin.** 160 to 325 mg per local protocol

NOTE: The following beta blockers are sometimes used to help reduce the size of the infarct (not commonly used in the field).

4. **Metoprolol (Lopressor).** 5 mg by slow IV infusion; repeat in 5 minutes
5. **Propranolol (Inderal).** 1 to 3 mg IV every 5 minutes; may be repeated to a maximum dose of 15 mg

If associated with congestive heart failure, consider:

6. **Furosemide (Lasix).** 20 to 80 mg IV
7. **Bumetanide (Bumex).** 0.5 to 1 mg IV bolus
8. **Amrinone (Inocor).** 0.75 mg/kg for congestive heart failure refractory to diuretics
9. **Dobutamine.** 2.5 to 10 μg/kg/minute per medical control

For further options see section in this chapter on congestive heart failure.

If thrombolytic therapy is indicated and available, consider:

10. **Alteplase (tPA).** Contact medical control for dosage.
11. **Streptokinase.** 1,500,000 International Units (IU) IV infusion or as directed by medical control

Contact medical control for further options.

If associated with dysrhythmias or PVCs, refer to the section in this chapter on cardiac dysrhythmias.

Refer to Chapter 3 for further information regarding the foregoing medications, including pediatric dosages.

CONGESTIVE HEART FAILURE (CHF)

CHF is simply defined as the inability of the ventricles to efficiently pump blood out of the heart, causing fluid to back up into the lungs and/or body tissues. CHF may occur very rapidly, as when associated with acute MI, or may develop over time as a result of hypertension, chronic obstructive pulmonary disease, or other causes. In many patients, CHF is a chronic condition and it is only in an acute phase that an ambulance is called. Generally, CHF becomes an emergency when associated with pulmonary edema. In such cases, prompt intervention is necessary because pulmonary edema can quickly lead to death.

CHF may involve either left or right heart failure. In the acute stage, it typically involves both.

Common Signs and Symptoms. Dyspnea, tachycardia, anxiety, restlessness and agitation, diaphoresis, elevated blood pressure, crackles (rales), possible wheezing, cyanosis, and the presence of frothy, pink sputum. In right heart failure, jugular vein distention and peripheral edema, particularly in the feet and ankles, may also be present.

Treatment Objectives. To reduce the workload on the heart, improve respiratory efficiency, decrease anxiety and agitation

Treatment Interventions

1. Transport the patient in a seated, upright position.
2. Administer high-flow oxygen. A non-rebreather device may be sufficient, but be prepared to assist ventilations with a bag-valve-mask or to intubate.
3. Establish an IV at a "keep vein open" (KVO) rate with lactated Ringer's, normal saline, or D_5W (check your local protocols); consider saline or heparin lock.
4. Attach the patient to a cardiac monitor.
5. Monitor pulse oximetry.
6. Provide reassurance.

Possible Medications. Consult local protocols or medical control for the following options. Dosages may differ.

1. **Nitroglycerin.** 0.4 mg sublingually, tablet or spray; repeat as needed every 5 minutes per local protocols
2. **Morphine sulfate.** Usual dosage 2 to 5 mg IV
3. **Furosemide (Lasix).** Usual dosage 20 to 80 mg IV
4. **Bumetanide (Bumex).** 0.5 to 2.0 mg IV bolus over 2 minutes or IM

5. **Amrinone (Inocor).** 0.75 mg/kg IV over 2 to 3 minutes for CHF refractory to diuretics and vasodilators
6. **Hydralazine (Apresoline).** 10 to 40 mg slow IV bolus for CHF refractory to diuretics
7. **Aminophylline.** 5 mg/kg if wheezing is present
8. **Digoxin (Lanoxin).** 0.25 to 0.5 mg IV; sometimes used if atrial fibrillation or other tachyarrhythmias are present
9. **Dobutamine (Dobutrex).** 2.5 to 10 μg/kg/minute IV infusion
10. **Nitroprusside (Nipride).** 0.1 to 5.0 μg/kg/minute by IV infusion to treat associated hypertension

Contact medical control for further options.

Refer to Chapter 3 for further information regarding the foregoing medications, including pediatric dosages.

DIABETIC EMERGENCIES

With approximately 10 million diagnosed and 5 million undiagnosed diabetics in the United States, EMS personnel are frequently called on to provide emergency medical assistance to these individuals for problems related to their diabetic condition. Most such emergencies involve patients experiencing either diabetic ketoacidosis (excessively high blood sugar) or hypoglycemia (low blood sugar). Either of these conditions can be life threatening, and prompt treatment is essential.

Common Signs and Symptoms

Diabetic ketoacidosis: warm, dry skin; tachycardia; nausea and vomiting; Kussmaul's respirations (deep and rapid), polyuria, polydipsia, and polyphagia; fruity odor on the patient's breath

Hypoglycemia: Cool, clammy skin; slurred speech; headache; weakness; agitation; aggressive or irrational behavior; dilated pupils; seizures; diminished level of consciousness; coma

Treatment Objectives. Maintain ABCs, attempt to establish whether the patient is hypoglycemic or in diabetic ketoacidosis, normalize blood sugar levels to the extent possible, provide supportive care

Treatment Interventions

1. Ensure an airway and administer oxygen by mask; be prepared to assist ventilations and/or intubate.
2. Monitor vitals and neurological status every 5 to 10 minutes
3. Establish IV access with normal saline, lactated Ringer's or D$_5$W per local protocol; in suspected cases of ketoacidosis, make every effort to rehydrate the patient with normal saline or lactated Ringer's.
4. Monitor cardiac rhythm continuously.
5. Obtain a thorough history, including medications, dosages, time of last medication, and last meal.
6. Obtain blood glucose level if within scope of local protocol.
7. Monitor oxygen saturation with pulse oximetry.
8. Provide rapid transport to the hospital.

Possible Medications. Consult local protocols or medical control for the following options. Dosages may differ.

1. **Oral glucose (Glucopaste).** As tolerated if patient is conscious and alert for suspected hypoglycemia
2. **Thiamine.** Often given before D50 to prevent Wernicke's encephalopathy; 100 mg by slow IV push; some protocols call for 50 mg IV and 50 mg IM
3. **Dextrose 50%.** 25 g (50 mL) slow IV push for

hypoglycemia or coma of unknown origin; second dose may be necessary

4. **Glucagon.** 0.5 to 1.0 units IV, IM, or subcutaneously (SC) for hypoglycemia; may be repeated in 15 to 20 minutes if needed

5. **Insulin (Humulin, Novolin).** 0.1 units/kg slow IV bolus as directed by medical control for diabetic ketoacidosis

6. **Sodium bicarbonate.** Sometimes administered in the presence of hyperkalemia (very high serum potassium level) as suggested by sharply peaked T waves on the cardiac monitor; check with medical control for dosage.

7. **Naloxone (Narcan).** 0.4 to 2.0 mg by IV bolus; often given if the cause of the patient's coma is uncertain and dextrose is ineffective

Refer to Chapter 3 for further information regarding the foregoing medications, including pediatric dosages.

POISONING AND OVERDOSE EMERGENCIES

A call for an overdose or poisoning emergency can be particularly challenging for the EMS provider. In many cases, it may be impossible to identify the poison or drug involved, making effective treatment difficult. The vast majority of poisonings occur in children, whereas most drug overdoses occur in adults. Prompt and effective treatment is often necessary to save the patient's life.

Common Signs and Symptoms. Signs and symptoms vary greatly depending on the nature of the poison or drug and the manner in which it was introduced into the body. Pupils may be dilated or constricted, respirations may be rapid or depressed, hypotension or hypertension may be present, nausea and vomiting are common; there may be bradycardia or tachycardia, headache, stomach cramps, hallucinations, seizures, decreased level of consciousness or coma, unusual odor on the breath, burns around the mouth, sweating, rash, or muscular weakness.

Treatment Objectives. To protect and maintain the airway; identify the poison or drug involved; provide effective supportive, antidotal, and symptomatic emergency care; transport promptly to an emergency facility

Treatment Interventions

1. Ensure a patent airway and administer oxygen; be prepared to intubate and/or provide ventilatory support.
2. Monitor vitals frequently
3. Establish IV access.
4. Monitor cardiac rhythms.
5. Monitor oxygen saturation with pulse oximetry, if available.
6. Obtain as detailed a history as possible. Identify poison or medication and manner of introduction into the body: ingestion, injection, inhalation, or absorption. Check for needle tracks on the patient's arms.
7. Obtain a sample of the drug or poison involved, as well as a sample of any vomited material.
8. Obtain a blood glucose level if equipment is available.
9. Contact the poison center and medical control for treatment advice.
10. Provide rapid transport to the emergency department.

Possible Medications. Consult local protocols or medical control for the following options. Dosages may differ.

1. **Dextrose 50%.** 25 g if patient is unconscious or blood glucose is low
2. **Naloxone (Narcan).** 0.4 to 2.0 mg in cases of coma of unknown origin or if narcotic drug is suspected
3. **Thiamine.** 50 to 100 mg IV or IM; often given before dextrose 50%
4. **Syrup of ipecac.** 15 to 30 mL by mouth in alert patients to induce vomiting as directed by medical control or the poison center
5. **Activated charcoal.** 1 g/kg as directed by medical control or poison center
6. **Flumazenil (Romazicon).** 0.2 mg to reverse adverse or toxic effects of benzodiazepines
7. **Diazepam (Valium).** 5 mg for seizures
8. **Amyl nitrite.** 1 to 2 ampules for cyanide poisoning
9. **Calcium gluconate.** 5 to 8 mL IV for magnesium sulfate and calcium channel blocker toxicity and black widow bites

For cases of organophosphate poisoning, consider:

10. **Atropine sulfate.** 2 to 3 mg IV
11. **Pralidoxime (Protopam).** 1 to 2 g IV

For cases of tricyclic antidepressant overdose, consider:

12. **Physostigmine (Antilirium).** 0.5 to 2.0 mg IV; also used for anticholinergic toxicity
13. **Sodium bicarbonate.** 1 mEq/kg IV; also used for barbiturate overdose

Contact medical control or the poison center for further options.

Refer to Chapter 3 for further information regarding the foregoing medications, including pediatric dosages.

RESPIRATORY DISTRESS (Asthma/Chronic Obstructive Pulmonary Disease [COPD] Crisis)

Patients with chronic respiratory diseases such as asthma, chronic bronchitis, or emphysema are among the more common users of the EMS system. Typically, these patients take a variety of medications and, in later stages, often use constant oxygen. Though these patients are almost always experiencing some moderate breathing difficulty, requests for EMS assistance usually arise during a period of acute exacerbation. Prompt, effective intervention is necessary in such emergencies.

Common Signs and Symptoms. Though there are clearly distinctions between the different chronic respiratory diseases, the signs and symptoms associated with the acute respiratory crisis phase are very similar. Typical signs and symptoms include wheezing, bronchospasm, tachycardia, cyanosis, rapid but ineffective respirations, diaphoresis, use of accessory muscles, anxiety, and inability to speak.

Treatment Objectives. To decrease airway resistance, increase blood oxygen content, reverse bronchospasm and wheezing, and decrease anxiety

Treatment Interventions

1. Place the patient in an upright position.
2. Assess and monitor vitals.
3. Maintain airway. If patient is unconscious, insert an oropharyngeal airway or consider intubation.
4. Provide immediate oxygen and be prepared to provide ventilatory support.
5. If available, use pulse oximetry to monitor oxygen saturation
6. Monitor cardiac rhythm.

7. Provide reassurance.
8. Provide rapid transport.

Possible Medications. Consult local protocols or medical control for use of the following options. Dosages may differ.

1. **Patient inhaler.** Many patients with asthma or COPD use various inhaled medications. In many areas, EMTs, even at the basic level, may assist patients with the use of their own inhalers if directed to do so by medical control. Common inhalers include albuterol (Proventil), AeroBid, Atrovent, Azmacort, Bronkaid, Beclovent, and Vanceril.

NOTE: Many of the foregoing inhalers are contraindicated in status asthmaticus or severe bronchospasm. Consult medical control for advice.

2. **Albuterol (Proventil).** Nebulize 2.5 mg of drug in 3 mL of sterile saline
3. **Aminophylline.** 250 to 500 mg diluted in D_5W infused over 20 to 30 minutes
4. **Racemic epinephrine.** Nebulize 0.5 mL in 3 mL of sterile saline. Rarely used for adults.
5. **Epinephrine 1:1000.** 0.3 to 0.5 mg by SC injection
6. **Isoetharine (Bronkosol).** 1 or 2 inhalations from a metered dose inhaler (340 μg)
7. **Metaproterenol (Alupent).** 2 to 3 inhalations by metered dose inhaler
8. **Methylprednisolone (Solu-Medrol).** 100 to 250 mg by IV bolus
9. **Terbutaline (Brethine).** 0.25 mg by SC injection *or* 2 inhalations by metered dose inhaler

Refer to Chapter 3 for further information regarding the foregoing medications, including pediatric dosages.

SEIZURES

Seizures are generally the result of abnormal electrical activity in the brain characterized by altered motor behavior and level of consciousness. Among the many causes of seizures are epilepsy, trauma, fever, heat stroke, drug overdose, tumor, stroke, eclampsia, alcohol withdrawal, infection, and hypoglycemia.

Seizures are of several types: grand mal or full body seizures; focal motor seizures, which usually involve a specific part or parts of the body; psychomotor seizures; and petit mal seizures. Status epilepticus is a continuous series of seizures lasting 30 minutes or more. This is a true emergency, since it can result in anoxia, aspiration, and brain damage.

Common Signs and Symptoms. Pre-seizure aura, loss of consciousness, muscle rigidity with alternating relaxation, apnea, incontinence and postictal fatigue and disorientation; seizures resulting from certain conditions such as heat stroke or alcohol withdrawal also have the signs and symptoms associated with other conditions.

Treatment Objectives. Protect the patient from injury, maintain airway and respiration, terminate seizure activity where appropriate, conduct a thorough assessment to determine a possible cause

Treatment Interventions

1. Maintain the safety of the environment to protect the seizing patient from sustaining injury.
2. Maintain and protect the airway. Suction, if necessary, and administer oxygen.
3. Place patient in the coma or Fowler position to avoid aspiration.

4. Obtain IV access with appropriate fluid per local protocol.
5. Monitor cardiac rhythm.

Possible Medications. Consult local protocols or medical control for the following options. Dosages may differ.

1. **Diazepam (Valium).** 2.5 to 10 mg slowly IV if seizures continue
2. **Lorazepam (Ativan).** 2.0 to 6.0 mg by IV bolus
3. **Thiamine.** 50 to 100 mg IV or IM
4. **Naloxone (Narcan).** 0.4 to 2.0 mg IV (if narcotic etiology is suspected)
5. **Dextrose 50%.** 25 g IV if hypoglycemia suspected
6. **Phenytoin (Dilantin).**150 to 250 mg slow IV bolus
7. **Phenobarbital (Luminal).**100 to 300 mg slow IV bolus
8. **Magnesium sulfate.** 2 to 4 g IV for seizures associated with eclampsia

Refer to Chapter 3 for further information regarding the foregoing medications, including pediatric dosages.

ADDITIONAL MEDICATION INTERVENTIONS FOR COMMON EMERGENCIES

Hypertensive Crisis. Contact medical control for the following possible options:

1. **Nitroglycerin (Nitrostat, Nitrol).** 0.3 to 0.4 mg sublingual tablet or spray; may be repeated at 5-minute intervals
2. **Diazoxide (Hyperstat).** 1 to 3 mg/kg by rapid IV push; repeat in 5 to 15 minutes as needed up to a maximum of 150 mg

3. **Hydralazine (Apresoline).** 10 to 40 mg bolus slow IV; may repeat in 10 to 15 minutes
4. **Labetalol (Normodyne).** 20 mg IV bolus over 2 minutes; repeat in 10 minutes; maximum dose 300 mg; may also be infused at 2 mg/minute
5. **Metoprolol (Lopressor).** 5 mg IV; may repeat twice at 5-minute intervals
6. **Nifedipine (Procardia).** 10 mg PO; may repeat once at 10 to 20 mg
7. **Nitroprusside (Nipride).** 0.1 to 10.0 μg/kg/minute IV infusion
8. **Propranolol (Inderal).** 1 to 3 mg IV over 3 to 5 minutes; repeat if needed in 5 minutes

Head Injuries. Contact medical control for the following possible options:

1. **Dexamethasone (Decadron).** 10 mg slow IV bolus for acute cerebral edema
2. **Mannitol (Osmitrol).** 1.5 to 2.0 g/kg by IV infusion over 30 to 60 minutes to relieve intracranial pressure associated with closed head injury

Pain Management. Contact medical control for the following possible options:

1. **Butorphanol (Stadol).** 0.5 to 2.0 mg IV or 1 to 4 mg IM
2. **Hydromorphone (Dilaudid).** 1.0 mg IV or 2 to 4 mg IM
3. **Meperidine (Demerol).** 25 to 50 mg IV or 50 to 100 mg IM
4. **Morphine sulfate.** 2 to 5 mg IV or IM
5. **Nalbuphine (Nubain).** 5 to 20 mg IV, IM, or SC
6. **Nitroglycerin (Nitrostat).** 0.3 to 0.4 mg by sublingual tablet or spray for ischemic chest pain

7. **Nitrous oxide (Nitronox).** Self-administered by the patient
8. **Pentazocine (Talwin).** 30 mg IV or IM

Nausea and Vomiting. Contact medical control for the following possible options:

1. **Dimenhydrinate (Dramamine).** 25 to 100 mg slow IV bolus; may also be given IM
2. **Promethazine (Phenergan).** 12.5 to 25 mg IV or IM

NOTE: These medications may also be used to potentiate the effects of certain analgesics.

Endotracheal Intubation. The following medications may be used to facilitate endotracheal intubation in patients who are conscious or who have a gag reflex. They are often given in various combinations, depending on availability and local protocol. Contact medical control for options:

1. **Diazepam (Valium).** 3 to 5 mg slow IV
2. **Midazolam (Versed).** 1 to 2.5 mg IV; may repeat in 1.0-mg increments
3. **Succinylcholine (Anectine).** 1 to 2 mg/kg by IV bolus; may repeat once if necessary
4. **Vecuronium (Norcuron).** 0.08 to 0.10 mg/kg IV bolus; repeat as necessary every 20 to 30 minutes
5. **Lidocaine (Xylocaine).** 1 to 1.5 mg/kg IV bolus; sometimes administered before intubation to help control intracranial pressure

Refer to Chapter 3 for further information regarding the foregoing medications, including pediatric dosages.

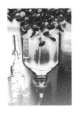

PRESCRIPTION AND OVER-THE-COUNTER MEDICATIONS— GENERIC NAMES

Acarbose (Precose): anti-diabetic agent. Used to treat non-insulin-dependent diabetes mellitus.

Acebutolol (Monitan*, Sectral): beta blocker. Used to treat hypertension (HTN) and to prevent premature ventricular contractions.

Acetaminophen (Feverall): analgesic. Used to treat mild to moderate pain.

Acetazolamide (Diamox): carbonic anhydrase inhibitor. Used to treat glaucoma, petit mal epilepsy, congestive heart failure (CHF), and to prevent and treat high altitude sickness.

Acetohexamide (Dymelor): anti-diabetic agent. Used to treat non-insulin-dependent diabetes mellitus.

Acyclovir (Zovirax): anti-viral agent. Used to treat viral infections.

Albuterol (Proventil, Ventolin): bronchodilator. Used to treat asthma and chronic obstructive pulmonary disease (COPD).

Alclometasone: corticosteroid. Used to treat psoriasis and other dermatoses.

---

* A drug name followed by an asterisk indicates that this is a Canadian trade name.

Allopurinol (Purinol, Zurinol): anti-gout agent. Used to treat gout and prevent gout attacks.

Alprazolam (Xanax): benzodiazepine. Used to treat anxiety, panic attacks, and anxiety associated with depression.

Aluminum hydroxide: antacid. Used to treat gastrointestinal (GI) disorders.

Amantadine (Symadine, Symmetrel): anti-parkinsonism agent, anti-viral agent. Used to treat parkinsonism and respiratory tract infections due to influenza type A virus.

Amikacin (Amikin): antibiotic. Used to treat serious infections.

Amiloride (Midamor, Moduretic): diuretic. Used to treat HTN and excessive fluid retention.

Aminophylline (Phyllocontin, Truphyllin): bronchodilator. Used to treat asthma and COPD.

Amiodarone (Cordarone): anti-arrhythmic agent. Used to treat arrhythmias.

Amitriptyline (Amitril, Elavil): tricyclic antidepressant. Used to treat depression.

Amlodipine (Norvasc): calcium channel blocker. Used to treat HTN and angina.

Amobarbital (Amytal, Tuinal): barbiturate. Used to treat seizure disorders.

Amoxapine (Asendin): tricyclic antidepressant. Used to treat depression.

Amoxicillin (Amoxil, Trimox): antibiotic. Used to treat general infections.

Amphetamine: stimulant. Used to treat attention deficit hyperactive disorder and narcolepsy.

Amphotericin B (Amphotec-F): antibiotic. Used to treat life-threatening infections.

Ampicillin (Omnipen, Polycillin): antibiotic. Used to treat general infections.

Anagrelide (Agrylin): platelet inhibitor. Used to treat essential thrombocythemia.

Aprobarbital (Alurate): barbiturate. Used as a sedative.

Ardeparin (Normiflo): low-molecular-weight heparin. Used to prevent deep vein thrombosis after knee replacement surgery.

Astemizole (Hismanal): antihistamine. Used to treat seasonal allergy symptoms and hives.

Atenolol (Tenoretic, Tenormin): beta blocker. Used to treat exercise-induced angina pectoris and HTN.

Atorvastatin calcium (Lipitor): anti-cholesterol agent. Used to treat high cholesterol.

Atovaquone (Mepron): anti-protozoal agent. Used to treat *Pneumocystis carinii* pneumonia and cerebral toxoplasmosis.

Atropine: antispasmodic. Used to treat spasms of the GI tract.

Auranofin (Ridaura): anti-arthritic agent. Used to treat rheumatoid arthritis in adults.

Azatadine (Optimine, Trinalin): antihistamine. Used to treat allergy symptoms.

Azathioprine: anti-arthritic agent, immunosuppressive. Used to prevent rejection of transplanted organs and to treat severe rheumatoid arthritis.

Azithromycin (Zithromax): antibiotic. Used to treat respiratory tract infections and some skin infections. May be useful in treatment of acquired immunodeficiency syndrome (AIDS)-related infections.

AZT: anti-viral agent. Used to treat human immunodeficiency (HIV) infection.

Bacampicillin (Perglobe*): antibiotic. Used to treat general infections.

Bacitracin (Neosporin): topical antibiotic. Used to treat skin and eye infections.

Becaplermin (Regranex): human-platelet-derived growth factor. Used to treat diabetic ulcers of the lower extremities.

Beclomethasone (Vancenase AQ): corticosteroid. Used in asthma control in patients who do not respond to bronchodilators.

Belladonna (Bellafoline): Used to treat irritable bowel syndrome and ulcers.

Benazepril (Lotensin): acetylcholinesterase (ACE) inhibitor. Used to treat HTN.

Bendroflumethiazide (Rauzide): thiazide diuretic. Used to treat HTN and fluid retention.

Benzonatate (Tessalon): antitussive. Used to treat cough.

Benzphetamine: stimulant. Used to treat obesity.

Benzthiazide (Exna): thiazide diuretic. Used to treat HTN and fluid retention.

Benztropine: anticholinergic. Used to treat Parkinson's disease and parkinsonian reactions to antipsychotic drugs.

Bepridil (Vascor): calcium channel blocker. Used to treat angina and HTN.

Betamethasone (Celestone, Lotrisone): corticosteroid. Used to treat dermatoses.

Betaxolol (Betoptic): beta blocker. Used to treat HTN and glaucoma (eyedrops).

Bethanechol: cholinergic agent. Used to treat urinary retention.

Biperiden (Akineton): anticholinergic. Used to treat Parkinson's disease.

Bisacodyl (Dulcolax): stimulant laxative. Used to treat constipation.

Bisoprolol (Zebeta): beta blocker. Used to treat HTN.

Bitolterol (Tornalate): bronchodilator. Used to treat asthma attacks and to reduce frequency and severity of recurrent asthma attacks.

Bromfenac (Duract): nonsteroidal anti-inflammatory drug (NSAID). Used to treat pain.

Bromocriptine (Parlodel): ergot alkaloid. Used to treat Parkinson's disease.

Bromodiphenhydramine (Ambenyl): antihistamine. Used to treat symptoms of cold and seasonal allergies.

Brompheniramine: antihistamine. Used to treat symptoms of cold and seasonal allergies.

Buclizine (Bucladin-S): antihistamine. Used to treat motion sickness.

Bumetanide (Bumex): diuretic. Used to treat excessive fluid retention due to CHF and liver or kidney disease.

Buprenorphine: narcotic analgesic. Used to treat moderate to severe pain.

Bupropion (Wellbutrin, Zyban): antidepressant. Used to treat depressive disorders and as a smoking cessation aid.

Buspirone (BuSpar): mild tranquilizer. Used to treat anxiety and nervous tension.

Butabarbital (Buticaps): barbiturate. Used as a sedative.

Butalbital: barbiturate. Used to treat tension headaches.

Butorphanol (Stadol): narcotic analgesic. Used to treat postoperative pain.

Calcipotriene (Dovonex): vitamin D_3 analog. Used to treat psoriasis.

Calcitonin (Calcimar): calcium-regulating hormone. Used to treat excessive bone growth (Paget's disease).

Calcium: mineral. Used to treat rickets, tetany, and calcium deficiency.

Capsaicin (Zostrix): plant derivative. Used to treat arthritis pain, neuralgias, and diabetic neuropathy.

Captopril (Capoten, Capozide): ACE inhibitor. Used to treat HTN.

Carbamazepine (Tegretol): anticonvulsant. Used to treat nerve pain, epilepsy, and some psychiatric disorders.

Carbenicillin (Geocillin): antibiotic. Used to treat infections.

Carbidopa: anti-parkinsonian agent. Used to treat Parkinson's disease.

Carisoprodol (Soma): muscle relaxant. Used to treat musculoskeletal disorders.

Carteolol (Cartrol): beta blocker. Used to treat HTN and exercise-induced angina.

Cefaclor (Ceclor): antibiotic. Used to treat infections of the skin, respiratory tract, ear, and urinary tract.

Cefadroxil (Duricef): antibiotic. Used to treat infections of the skin, respiratory tract, ear, and urinary tract.

Cefdinir (Omnicef): antiobiotic. Used to treat general infections.

Cefixime (Suprax): antibiotic. Used to treat infections of the respiratory tract, ear, or urinary tract and gonorrhea.

Cefmetazole (Zefazone): antibiotic. Used to treat wide variety of infections.

Cefotaxime (Claforan): antibiotic. Used to treat a wide variety of infections.

Cefoxitin (Mefoxin): antibiotic. Used to treat general infections.

Cefpodoxime (Vantin): antibiotic. Used to treat general infections.

Cefprozil (Cefzil): antibiotic. Used to treat infections of the respiratory tract and skin.

Ceftazidime (Fortaz): antibiotic. Used to treat a wide variety of infections.

Ceftriaxone (Rocephin): antibiotic. Used to treat general infections.

Cefuroxime (Ceftin): antibiotic. Used to treat ear, skin, respiratory tract, and urinary tract infections.

Cephalexin (Ceporex*, Keflex): antibiotic. Used to treat general infections.

Cephradine (Velosef): antibiotic. Used to treat general infections.

Cerivastatin (Baycol): anti-cholesterol agent. Used to treat high cholesterol.

Cetirizine (Zyrtec): antihistamine. Used to treat seasonal allergy symptoms.

Chloral hydrate: sedative. Used to treat insomnia and postoperative pain.

Chlorambucil (Leukeran): immunosuppressant. Used to treat cancer and to prevent organ transplant rejection.

Chloramphenicol (Chloroptic, Fenicol): antibiotic. Used to treat life-threatening infections.

Chlordiazepoxide (Librax, Libritabs): benzodiazepine. Used to treat anxiety and alcohol withdrawal.

Chlormezanone (Trancopal): sedative. Used to treat anxiety.

Chloroquine (Aralen): anti-protozoal agent. Used to treat and prevent malaria and amebic infection.

Chlorothiazide (Diachlor, Diupres): thiazide diuretic. Used to treat HTN and fluid retention.

Chlorpheniramine: antihistamine. Used to treat symptoms of cold and seasonal allergies.

Chlorpromazine: phenothiazine. Used to treat psychotic disorders and vomiting due to chemotherapy.

Chlorpropamide (Chloronase*, Diabinese): anti-diabetic agent. Used to treat type II, non-insulin-dependent diabetes mellitus.

Chlorprothixene: anti-psychotic agent. Used to treat psychotic disorders.

Chlorthalidone (Hylidone, Regroton): thiazide diuretic. Used to treat HTN and fluid retention.

Chlorzoxazone (Paraflex): muscle relaxant. Used to treat musculoskeletal pain.

Cholestyramine (Questran): anti-cholesterol agent. Used to treat high cholesterol.

Cimetidine (Tagamet): histamine (H_2) blocker. Used to treat and prevent ulcers and esophageal reflux.

Ciprofloxacin (Cipro): antibiotic. Used to treat general infections.

Cisapride (Propulsid): GI stimulant. Used to treat esophageal reflux disease.

Clarithromycin (Biaxin): antibiotic. Used to treat respiratory and skin infections.

Clemastine (Tavist): antihistamine. Used to treat allergy symptoms.

Clidinium (Quarzan): anticholinergic. Used to treat GI disorders.

Clindamycin (Cleocin): antibiotic. Used to treat uncommon infections.

Clofibrate (Artomid-S): anti-cholesterol agent. Used to treat high cholesterol.

Clomipramine (Anafranil): tricyclic antidepressant. Used to treat obsessive-compulsive disorder.

Clonazepam (Klonopin): benzodiazepine. Used to treat epilepsy, panic disorders, and anxiety.

Clonidine (Catapres): anti-hypertensive agent. Used to treat HTN.

Clopidogrel (Plavix): platelet inhibitor. Used to reduce risk of complications of atherosclerosis.

Clorazepate (Tranxene): benzodiazepine. Used to treat anxiety, alcohol withdrawal, and epilepsy.

Clotrimazole (Gyne-Lotrimin): anti-fungal agent. Used to treat yeast and ringworm infections.

Cloxacillin (Cloxapen): antibiotic. Used to treat infections resistant to penicillin.

Clozapine (Clozaril): tranquilizer. Used to treat schizophrenia.

Codeine: narcotic analgesic. Used to treat severe pain and to control cough.

Colchicine (Proben-C): anti-gout agent. Used to treat gout attacks and to prevent gout.

Colestipol (Colestid): anti-cholesterol agent. Used to treat high cholesterol.

Conjugated estrogens: female hormone. Used to treat gynecological disorders.

Cromolyn (Gastrocrom): asthma preventive. Used to prevent allergic reactions and asthma attacks.

Cyanocobalamin: vitamin B_{12}. Used to treat and prevent vitamin B_{12} deficiency.

Cyclacillin: antibiotic. Used to treat general infections.

Cyclandelate (Cyclospasmol): vasodilator. Used to treat vascular disease.

Cyclobenzaprine (Flexeril): muscle relaxant. Used to treat muscle spasm.

Cyclophosphamide (Cytoxan): immunosuppressant. Used to treat cancer and severe rheumatoid arthritis.

Cycloserine (Seromycin): anti-infective agent. Used to treat tuberculosis.

Cyclosporine (Sandimmune): immunosuppressant. Used to prevent organ rejection after transplant surgery.

Cyproheptadine (Periactin): antihistamine. Used to treat cold and allergy symptoms.

Dacliximab (Zenapax): immunosuppressant. Used to prevent organ rejection following transplant surgery.

Dantrolene (Dantrium): muscle relaxant. Used to treat spasticity.

Dapsone (Alvosulfon*): anti-infective agent. Used to treat *Pneumocystis carinii* pneumonia.

Delavirdine (Rescriptor): anti-viral agent. Used to treat HIV-infected patients.

Demecarium (Humorsol): anti-glaucoma agent. Used to treat glaucoma.

Demeclocycline (Declomycin): antibiotic. Used to treat gonorrhea and urinary tract infections (UTIs).

Deserpidine (Harmonyl): alkaloid. Used to treat HTN and psychotic disorders.

Desipramine (Norpramin): tricyclic antidepressant. Used to treat severe depression.

Desmopressin (DDAVP): vasopressin analogue. Used to treat bleeding disorders and diabetes insipidus.

Dexamethasone (Maxidex): corticosteroid. Used to treat allergic and inflammatory conditions.

Dexbrompheniramine: antihistamine. Used to treat cold and seasonal allergy symptoms.

Dexchlorpheniramine: antihistamine. Used to treat cold and seasonal allergy symptoms.

Dextroamphetamine (Dexedrine): amphetamine. Used to treat attention deficit disorder (ADD), narcolepsy, and obesity.

Dextromethorphan: antitussive. Used to treat cough.

Dextrothyroxine (Choloxin): anti-cholesterol agent. Used to treat high cholesterol.

Dezocine (Dalgan): narcotic analgesic. Used to treat moderate to severe pain.

Diazepam (Valium): benzodiazepine. Used to treat anxiety, muscle spasm, epilepsy, and symptoms of alcohol withdrawal.

Diazoxide (Proglycem): vasodilator. Used to treat hypoglycemia.

Dichlorphenamide: anti-glaucoma agent. Used to treat glaucoma.

Diclofenac (Arthrotec, Voltaren): NSAID. Used to treat pain, fever, and inflammation.

Dicloxacillin (Dycill, Dynapen): antibiotic. Used to treat general infections.

Dicyclomine (Bentyl): gastrointestinal anticholinergic. Used to treat GI disorders.

Didanosine (Videx): anti-viral agent. Used to treat HIV infection.

Diethylpropion (Tenuate): anorectic agent. Used to treat obesity.

Difunisal (Dolobid): NSAID. Used to treat pain, fever, and inflammation.

Digitoxin (Crystodigin): digitalis preparation. Used to treat CHF, atrial fibrillation, atrial flutter, and supraventricular tachycardia.

Digoxin: digitalis preparation. Used to treat CHF, atrial fibrillation or flutter, and supraventricular tachycardia.

Dihydrocodeine: narcotic analgesic. Used to treat pain and cough.

Diltiazem (Cardizem): calcium channel blocker. Used to treat angina pectoris and HTN.

Dimenhydrinate (Dramamine): antihistamine. Used to treat motion sickness.

Diphenhydramine (Benadryl): antihistamine. Used to treat motion sickness, vertigo, and allergic reactions.

Diphenidol (Vontrol): anti-emetic agent. Used to treat nausea and vomiting.

Diphenoxylate (Lomotil): anti-diarrheal agent. Used to treat diarrhea.

Dipyridamole (Persantine): platelet inhibitor. Used to prevent post-cardiac surgery thromboembolism and recurrent heart attacks.

Disopyramide (Rhythmodan): anti-arrhythmic agent. Used to treat arrhythmias.

Disulfiram (Antabuse): anti-alcoholism agent. Used to deter the use of alcohol.

Divalproex: anticonvulsant. Used to treat epilepsy and mood disorders.

Docusate (Surfak): laxative. Used to treat constipation.

Dolasetron (Anzemet): anti-emetic agent. Used to prevent chemotherapy-induced nausea and vomiting.

Donepezil (Aricept): anti-dementia agent. Used to treat Alzheimer's disease.

Dornase alpha (Pulmozyme): cystic fibrosis agent. Used to treat cystic fibrosis.

Doxazosin (Cardura): anti-hypertensive agent. Used to treat HTN and benign prostatic hyperplasia (enlarged prostate).

Doxepin (Adapin, Sinequan): tricyclic antidepressant. Used to treat depression.

Doxycycline (Doryx): tetracycline. Used to treat numerous infections.

Dronabinol: anti-emetic agent. Used to treat AIDS-related anorexia and chemotherapy-induced emesis.

Droperidol (Inapsine): anti-emetic agent. Used to treat nausea and vomiting following surgery and as a tranquilizer.

Dyphylline (Dilor): bronchodilator. Used to treat asthma and COPD.

Econazole (Spectazole): anti-fungal agent. Used to treat fungal infections.

Emedastine (Emadine): antihistamine. Used to treat allergic conjunctivitis.

Enalapril (Vasotec): ACE inhibitor. Used to treat HTN, renal artery stenosis, and CHF.

Encainide (Enkaid): anti-arrhythmic agent. Used to treat arrhythmias.

Ephedrine: bronchodilator. Used to treat asthma and COPD.

Epinephrine: sympathomimetic. Used to treat asthma attacks, allergic nasal congestion, glaucoma, and anaphylactic shock.

Eprosartan (Teveten): anti-hypertensive agent. Used to treat hypertension.

Ergoloid mesylate (Hydergine): ergot preparation. Used to treat confusion, depression, and reduced alertness in the elderly.

Ergotamine: ergot preparation. Used to treat migraine headaches and narcolepsy.

Erythrityl tetranitrate (Cardilate): nitrate. Used to treat angina.

Erythromycin (E-Mycin, Ery-Tab): antibiotic. Used to treat general infections.

Estazolam (ProSom): benzodiazepine. Used to treat insomnia.

Estradiol: estrogen. Used to treat gynecological disorders.

Estrogen: female sex hormone. Used to treat gynecological disorders.

Estropipate: estrogen. Used to treat gynecological disorders.

Ethacrynic acid (Edecrin): diuretic. Used to treat fluid retention.

Ethambutol: anti-infective agent. Used to treat pulmonary tuberculosis.

Ethaverine (Ethatab): vasodilator. Used to treat GI tract spasm.

Ethchlorvynol (Placidyl): hypnotic. Used to treat insomnia.

Ethionamide (Trecator-SC): antitubercular agent. Used to treat tuberculosis.

Ethosuximide (Zarontin): anticonvulsant. Used to treat seizure disorders.

Ethotoin: anticonvulsant. Used to treat epilepsy.

Ethylnorepinephrine (Bronkephrine): sympathomimetic. Used to treat hypotension.

Etidronate (Didronel): anti-hypercalcemic agent. Used to treat bone disorders.

Etodolac (Lodine): NSAID. Used to treat pain, fever, and inflammation.

Etretinate (Tegison): anti-flammatory agent. Used to treat psoriasis.

Factor VIII (Monoclate-P): anti-hemophilic agent. Used to treat hemophilia.

Famciclovir (Famvir): anti-viral agent. Used to treat shingles.

Famotidine (Pepcid): histamine (H_2) blocker. Used to treat and prevent ulcers and esophageal reflux.

Felbamate (Felbatol): anticonvulsant. Used to treat seizure disorders.

Felodipine (Plendil): calcium channel blocker. Used to treat angina, CHF, and certain arrhythmias.

Fenoprofen (Nalfon): NSAID. Used to treat pain, fever, and inflammation.

Fentanyl (Sublimaze Duragesic): narcotic analgesic. Used to treat chronic pain.

Ferrous gluconate: iron salt. Used to treat anemia.

Ferrous sulfate: iron salt. Used to treat anemia.

Fexofenadine (Allegra): antihistamine. Used to treat seasonal allergy symptoms.

Finasteride (Proscar, Propecia): androgen hormone inhibitor. Used to treat benign prostatic hyperplasia (enlarged prostate) and male pattern baldness.

Flavoxate (Urispas): antispasmodic. Used to treat muscle spasms of the bladder.

Flecainide (Tambocor): anti-arrhythmic agent. Used to treat arrhythmias.

Fluconazole (Diflucan): anti-fungal agent. Used to treat yeast infection.

Flucytosine (Ancobon): anti-fungal agent. Used to treat endocarditis, osteomyelitis, UTIs, and septicemia. Often used in AIDS-related infections.

Flunisolide (Aerobid): corticosteroid. Used to treat asthma and allergic rhinitis.

Fluocinolone (Lidex): corticosteroid. Used to treat allergic and inflammatory conditions of the skin.

Fluoxetine (Prozac): antidepressant. Used to treat depression and bulimia.

Fluphenazine (Permitil): phenothiazine. Used to treat schizophrenia.

Flurazepam (Dalmane): benzodiazepine. Used to treat insomnia.

Flurbiprofen (Ansaid): NSAID. Used to treat pain, fever, and inflammation.

Flutamide (Evlexin): hormone. Used to treat prostate cancer.

Fluticasone (Cutivate): corticosteroid. Used to treat seasonal allergy symptoms.

Fluvastatin (Lescol): anti-cholesterol agent. Used to treat high cholesterol.

Fluvoxamine (Luvox): antidepressant. Used to treat obsessive-compulsive disorder.

Fosinopril (Monopril): ACE inhibitor. Used to treat HTN and CHF.

Fructose: sugar. Used to treat nausea and vomiting.

Furosemide (Lasix, Uritol): diuretic. Used to treat HTN and fluid retention.

Gabapentin (Neurontin): anticonvulsant. Used to treat epilepsy.

Ganciclovir (Cytovene): anti-viral agent. Used to treat life-threatening infections in immunocompromised patients.

Gemfibrozil (Lopid): anti-cholesterol agent. Used to reduce high cholesterol.

Gentamicin: antibiotic. Used to treat skin infections.

Glimepiride (Amaryl): anti-diabetic agent. Used to treat non-insulin-dependent diabetes mellitus.

Glipizide (Glucotrol): anti-diabetic agent. Used to treat type II diabetes.

Glucagon: sugar. Used to treat hypoglycemia.

Glucose: sugar. Used to treat hypoglycemia.

Glyburide (DiaBeta, Micronase): anti-diabetic agent. Used to treat type II diabetes.

Goserelin (Zoladex): hormone. Used to treat prostate cancer, breast cancer, and endometriosis.

Grepafloxacin (Raxar): antibiotic. Used to treat a variety of infections.

Griseofulvin (Fulvicin): anti-fungal agent. Used to treat ringworm infections.

Guaifenesin: expectorant. Used to treat cough.

Guanabenz (Wytensin): anti-hypertensive agent. Used to treat HTN.

Guanadrel (Hylorel): antihypertensive. Used to treat HTN.

Guanethidine (Esimil): anti-hypertensive agent. Used to treat HTN.

Guanfacine (Tenex): anti-hypertensive agent. Used to treat HTN, heroin withdrawal, and difficult pregnancies.

Halazepam (Paxipam): benzodiazepine. Used to treat anxiety.

Haloperidol (Haldol, Peridol*): anti-psychotic agent. Used to treat schizophrenia, manic-depressive disorder, acute psychosis, and Tourette's syndrome.

Homatropine: anticholinergic. Used to treat eye disorders.

Hydralazine (Alazine): anti-hypertensive agent. Used to treat HTN, CHF, and heart valve insufficiency until surgery.

Hydrochlorothiazide (Aprozide): thiazide diuretic. Used to treat HTN and fluid retention.

Hydrocodone (Hycodan): narcotic analgesic. Used to treat pain and to control cough.

Hydrocortisone (Westcort): corticosteroid. Used to treat allergic and inflammatory conditions of the skin.

Hydroflumethiazide (Salutensin, Saluron): thiazide diuretic. Used to treat HTN and fluid retention.

Hydromorphone (Dilaudid): narcotic analgesic. Used to treat severe pain.

Hydroxychloroquine: anti-inflammatory agent. Used to treat malaria, rheumatoid arthritis, and systemic lupus erythematosus.

Hydroxyzine (Vistaril): antihistamine. Used to treat anxiety, nausea, vomiting, and allergy symptoms.

Hyoscyamine (Cytospaz): belladonna alkaloid. Used to treat GI problems.

Ibuprofen (Motrin, Nuprin): NSAID. Used to treat pain, fever, and inflammation.

Imipramine (Tofranil): tricyclic antidepressant. Used to treat depression.

Indapamide (Lozol): diuretic. Used to treat HTN and CHF.

Indomethacin (Indameth): NSAID. Used to treat pain, fever, and inflammation.

Insulin: anti-diabetic agent. Used to treat insulin-dependent diabetes mellitus and gestational diabetes.

Iodoquinol (Diquinol): anti-infective agent. Used to treat resistant skin infections and asymptomatic carriers of amebic cysts.

Ipratropium (Atrovent): bronchodilator. Used to treat asthma and COPD.

Irbesartan (Avapro): anti-hypertensive agent. Used to treat hypertension.

Isocarboxazid (Marplan): monoamine oxidase (MAO). Used to treat depression and anxiety.

Isoetharine (Bronkometer): bronchodilator. Used to treat asthma, bronchitis, and emphysema.

Isoflurophate (Floropryl): anti-glaucoma agent. Used to treat glaucoma.

Isometheptene: analgesic. Used to treat migraine headache.

Isoniazide: anti-tubercular agent. Used to treat and prevent tuberculosis.

Isoproterenol (Isuprel): sympathomimetic. Used to treat asthma, COPD, and arrhythmias.

Isosorbide dinitrate (Iso-Bid): nitrate. Used to treat and prevent angina attacks.

Isosorbide mononitrate (Imdur, Monoket): nitrate. Used to prevent attacks of angina.

Isotretinoin: anti-acne agent. Used to treat severe acne that has not responded to standard therapy.

Isoxsuprine (Vasodilan): vasodilator. Used to treat vascular disease.

Isradipine (DynaCirc): calcium channel blocker. Used to treat HTN and angina pectoris.

Itraconazole (Sporanox): anti-fungal agent. Used to treat fungal infections.

Kaolin: anti-diarrheal agent. Used to treat diarrhea.

Ketoconazole (Nizoral): anti-fungal agent. Used to treat fungal infections.

Ketoprofen (Orudis): NSAID. Used to treat pain, fever, and inflammation.

Ketorolac: NSAID. Used to treat pain, fever, and inflammation.

Labetalol (Normodyne, Trandate): beta blocker. Used to treat HTN and angina.

Lamotrigine (Lamictal): anti-epileptic agent. Used to treat seizures.

Letrozole (Femara): aromatase inhibitor. Used to treat breast cancer in post-menopausal women.

Levodopa (Larodopa, Sinemet): anti-parkinsonism agent. Used to treat Parkinson's disease.

Levomethadyl (Orlaam): narcotic analgesic. Used to treat opioid dependence.

Levorphanol (Levo-Dromoran): narcotic analgesic. Used to treat moderate to severe pain.

Levothyroxine (Eltroxin, Levothroid, Synthroid): thyroid hormone. Used to treat thyroid disorders.

Lindane (Kwell): anti-parasitic agent. Used to treat scabies and lice.

Liothyronine (Cytomel): thyroid hormone. Used to treat thyroid disorders.

Lisinopril (Prinivil, Zestril): ACE inhibitor. Used to treat HTN and CHF.

Lithium (Carbolith,* Eskalith). tranquilizer. Used to treat manic depression and schizophrenia.

Loperamide (Imodium): anti-diarrheal agent. Used to treat diarrhea.

Loratadine: antihistamine. Used to treat symptoms of seasonal allergies.

Lorazepam (Ativan): benzodiazepine. Used to treat anxiety and insomnia.

Losartan (Cozaar): anti-hypertensive agent. Used to treat HTN.

Lovastatin (Mevacor): anti-cholesterol agent. Used to treat high cholesterol.

Loxapine (Loxitane): anti-psychotic agent. Used to treat schizophrenia and psychotic disorders.

Magaldrate (Riopan): antacid. Used to treat GI disorders.

Magnesium gluconate: magnesium supplement. Used to treat hypomagnesemia and preeclampsia.

Magnesium hydroxide (Magonate): antacid. Used to treat GI disorders.

Magnesium salicylate (Magan): NSAID. Used to treat pain, fever, and inflammation.

Malathion (Ovide): anti-parasitic agent. Used to treat lice and scabies.

Maprotiline (Ludiomil): antidepressant. Used to treat depression, chronic pain, eating disorders, and bedwetting.

Mebendazole (Vermox): anthelmintic agent. Used to treat worm infections—pinworms, roundworms, and hookworms.

Mecamylamine (Inversine): anti-hypertensive agent. Used to treat hypertension.

Meclizine (Antivert): antihistamine. Used to treat motion sickness and dizziness.

Meclofenamate (Meclomen): NSAID. Used to treat pain, fever, and inflammation.

Meclothiazide (Diutensen-R): thiazide diuretic. Used to treat HTN and fluid retention.

Medroxyprogesterone (Curretab, Provera): progestin. Used to treat menstrual disorders and cancer of the breast or uterus.

Mefenamic acid (Ponstel): NSAID. Used to treat pain, fever, and inflammation.

Megestrol: synthetic female hormone. Used to treat breast or uterine cancer.

Meperidine (Demerol, Pethadol): narcotic analgesic. Used to treat pain.

Mephenytoin (Mesantoin): anticonvulsant. Used to treat epilepsy.

Mephobarbital (Mebaral): barbiturate. Used to treat anxiety and seizures.

Meprobamate (Equanil, Miltown): tranquilizer. Used to treat anxiety.

Mesalamine (Asacol): anti-inflammatory agent. Used to treat intestinal inflammatory disorders.

Mesoridazine (Serentil): phenothiazine. Used to treat schizophrenia, behavioral problems, and alcoholism.

Mestranol: oral contraceptive. Used to treat menstrual disorders and to prevent pregnancy.

Metaproterenol (Alupent, Metaprel): bronchodilator. Used to treat asthma and COPD.

Metformin (Glucophage): anti-diabetic agent. Used to treat non-insulin-dependent diabetes mellitus.

Methadone (Dolophine): narcotic analgesic. Used to treat pain and to aid in withdrawal from narcotics.

Methamphetamine: stimulant. Used to treat narcolepsy and ADD.

Methazolamide (Neptazane): anti-glaucoma agent. Used to treat glaucoma.

Methenamine (Mandelamine): antibiotic. Used to treat bladder and kidney infections.

Methocarbamol (Robaxin): muscle relaxant. Used to treat muscle pain and spasm.

Methotrexate (Folex): anti-neoplastic agent. Used to treat acute lymphocytic leukemia, cancer, severe psoriasis, and severe rheumatoid arthritis.

Methscopolamine (Dallergy): anticholinergic. Used to treat peptic ulcer disease.

Methsuximide (Celontin): anti-convulsant agent. Used to treat seizure disorders.

Methyclothiazide: thiazide diuretic. Used to treat HTN and fluid retention.

Methyldopa (Aldomet): anti-hypertensive agent. Used to treat HTN.

Methylergonovine (Methergine): ergot alkaloid. Used to treat breast cancer

Methylphenidate (Ritalin): amphetamine. Used to treat ADD and narcolepsy.

Methylprednisolone (Medrol): corticosteroid. Used to treat allergic and inflammatory symptoms.

Methyltestosterone (Android): male sex hormone. Used to treat breast cancer and primary hypogonadism.

Methysergide (Sansert): serotonin antagonist. Used to treat migraine and cluster headaches.

Metoclopramide (Emex,* Reglan): anti-emetic agent. Used to treat acid reflux and nausea and vomiting due to migraine headaches or cancer-fighting drugs.

Metolazone: thiazide diuretic. Used to treat HTN and fluid retention.

Metoprolol (Lopressor): beta blocker. Used to treat HTN and angina and to prevent recurrent heart attack.

Metronidazole (Femazole, Flagyl): anti-infective agent. Used to treat various infections of the vaginal canal, cervix, male urethra, and intestines.

Metyrosine (Demser): anti-hypertensive agent. Used to treat pheochromocytoma.

Mexiletine (Mexitil): anti-arrhythmic agent. Used to treat cardiac arrhythmias.

Mibefradil (Posicor): calcium channel blocker. Used to treat HTN and angina.

Miconazole: anti-fungal agent. Used to treat fungal vaginal infections.

Midazolam (Versed): benzodiazepine: Used to treat anxiety, insomnia, and psychosis.

Minocycline (Minocin): antibiotic. Used to treat general infections.

Minoxidil (Loniten, Minodyl, Rogaine): anti-hypertensive agent. Used to treat HTN that does not respond to standard therapy. Also used to treat male pattern baldness.

Misoprostol (Cytotec): gastric protectant. Used to prevent drug-induced stomach ulcers. Used in Canada to treat duodenal ulcers.

Molindone (Moban): anti-psychotic agent. Used to treat schizophrenia and depression.

Mometasone (Elocon): corticosteroid. Used to treat skin disorders.

Moricizine (Ethmozine): anti-arrhythmic agent. Used to treat ventricular tachycardia.

Morphine sulfate (MS Contin): narcotic analgesic. Used to treat severe pain.

Nabumetone (Relafen): NSAID. Used to treat pain, fever, and inflammation.

Nadolol (Corgard, Corzide): beta blocker. Used to treat HTN and to prevent exercise-induced angina attacks.

Nafarelin (Synarel): hormone stimulant. Used to treat endometriosis.

Naftifine (Naftin): anti-fungal agent. Used to treat fungal infections.

Nalbuphine (Nubain): narcotic analgesic. Used to treat moderate to severe pain.

Naltrexone (Trexan): narcotic analgesic. Used to treat alcoholism and narcotic addiction.

Naproxen (Aleve, Naprosyn): NSAID. Used to treat pain, fever, and inflammation.

Nefazodone (Serzone): antidepressant. Used to treat depression.

Nelfinavir (Viracept): anti-viral agent. Used to treat HIV infection.

Neomycin: antibiotic. Used to treat infections.

Neostigmine (Prostigmin): anti-myasthenic agent. Used to treat myasthenia gravis and to stimulate bowel function after surgery.

Niacin (Niac, Nicobid): vitamin B_3. Used to treat high cholesterol and vitamin B_3 deficiency.

Nicardipine (Cardene): calcium channel blocker. Used to treat angina and HTN.

Nicotine (Habitrol, Nicoderm): smoking cessation aid. Used to help people quit smoking.

Nifedipine (Adalat, Procardia): calcium channel blocker. Used to treat angina pectoris and HTN.

Nimodipine: calcium channel blocker. Used to treat migraine headaches and the neurological effects of stroke.

Nitrofurantoin (Macrodantin): anti-infective agent. Used to treat urinary tract infections.

Nitroglycerin (Nitrostat, Nitrogard): nitrate. Used to treat angina and CHF.

Nizatidine (Axid): histamine (H_2) blocker. Used to treat and prevent ulcers and reflux.

Norfloxacin (Noroxin): antibiotic. Used to treat genitourinary system infections.

Nortriptyline (Pamelor): tricyclic antidepressant. Used to treat depression and chronic pain.

Nylidrin: vasodilator. Used to treat peripheral vascular disease.

Nystatin (Mycolog-II, Nilstat): anti-fungal agent. Used to treat fungal infections of the mouth, throat, and intestines.

Ofloxacin (Floxin): anti-infective agent. Used to treat infections.

Olsalazine (Dipentum): anti-inflammatory agent. Used to treat inflammatory bowel disease.

Omeprazole (Losec, Prilosec): anti-ulcer agent. Used to treat GI disorders.

Ondansetron (Zofran): anti-emetic agent. Used to treat nausea and vomiting due to cancer treaments.

Opium alkaloid: narcotic analgesic. Used to treat moderate to severe pain.

Orphenadrine (Norflex): muscle relaxant. Used to treat muscle pain.

Oxacillin (Bactocill): antibiotic. Used to treat general infections.

Oxaprozin (Daypro): NSAID. Used to treat pain, fever, and inflammation.

Oxazepam (Serax): benzodiazepine. Used to treat anxiety and alcohol withdrawal.

Oxiconazole (Oxistat): anti-fungal agent. Used to treat dermal fungal infections.

Oxprenolol (Trasicor): beta blocker. Used to treat cardiovascular and CNS disorders.

Oxtriphylline (Choledyl): bronchodilator. Used to treat asthma, COPD.

Oxybutynin (Ditropan): anticholinergic. Used to treat urinary incontinence.

Oxycodone (Percodan, Percocet, Tylox): narcotic analgesic. Used to treat pain.

Oxymetholone (Anadrol-50): testosterone derivative. Used to treat aplastic anemia.

Oxymorphone (Numorphan): narcotic analgesic. Used to treat moderate to severe pain.

Oxytetracycline (Terramycin): antimicrobial. Used to treat skin disorders and infections.

Papaverine (Pavabid): vasodilator. Used to treat peripheral vascular diseases.

Paramethadione (Paradione): anticonvulsant. Used to treat seizure disorders.

Paroxetine (Paxil): antidepressant. Used to treat depression, obsessive-compulsive disorder, and panic disorder.

Pemoline: stimulant. Used to treat ADD.

Penbutolol (Levatol): beta blocker. Used to treat HTN and panic attacks and to prevent recurrent angina or heart attack.

Penicillamine (Cuprimine): chelator. Used to treat copper toxicity, severe rheumatoid arthritis, and excessive cystine in the urine.

Penicillin V (V-Cillin K, Veetids): antibiotic. Used to treat respiratory tract, middle ear, and skin infections.

Pentaerythritol tetranitrate (Duotrate): nitrate. Used to treat angina pectoris.

Pentamidine (Pentam 300, Pneumopent): anti-infective agent. Used to treat *Pneumocystis carinii* pneumonia and to prevent the disease in AIDS patients.

Pentazocine (Talwin): narcotic analgesic. Used to treat pain.

Pentobarbital (Nembutal): barbiturate. Used to treat insomnia.

Pentoxifylline (Trental): bronchodilator. Used to treat peripheral obstructive arterial disease.

Pergolide (Permax): anti-parkinsonism agent. Used to treat Parkinson's disease.

Permethrin (Elimite, Nix): anti-parasitic agent. Used to treat lice and scabies.

Perphenazine (Phenazine, Trilafon): phenothiazine. Used to treat psychotic disorders, agitation, and severe nausea and vomiting.

Phenacemide (Phenurone): anticonvulsant. Used to treat seizure disorders.

Phenazopyridine (Pyridium): analgesic. Used to treat pain and discomfort of UTIs.

Phenelzine (Nardil): MAO inhibitor. Used to treat severe depression.

Phenindamine: antihistamine. Used to treat cold and allergy symptoms.

Phenobarbital (Barbita, Luminal, Solfoton): barbiturate. Used to treat anxiety, nervous tension, insomnia, and epilepsy.

Phenoxybenzamine (Dibenzyline): anti-hypertensive agent. Used to treat pheochromocytoma.

Phensuximide (Milontin): anticonvulsant. Used to treat seizure disorders.

Phenylbutazone (Butazolidin): anti-inflammatory agent. Used to treat gout and arthritis.

Phenylephrine: sympathomimetic. Used to treat symptoms of cold and seasonal allergies.

Phenylpropanolamine: decongestant. Used to treat symptoms of cold and seasonal allergies.

Phenyltoloxamine: antihistamine. Used to treat symptoms of cold, seasonal allergies, and respiratory infections.

Phenytoin (Dilantin, Diphenylan): anticonvulsant. Used to treat epilepsy and to control postoperative seizures.

Pilocarpine (Pilocar, Pilagan): anti-glaucoma agent. Used to treat glaucoma.

Pimozide (Orap): neuroleptic agent. Used to treat Tourette's syndrome.

Pindolol (Visken): beta blocker: Used to treat HTN, to control aggressive behavior, and to prevent migraine headaches.

Pirbuterol (Maxair): bronchodilator. Used to treat asthma and COPD.

Piroxicam (Feldene): NSAID. Used to treat pain, fever, and inflammation.

Polymyxin (Aerosporin): antibiotic. Used to treat eye infections and swelling.

Polythiazide (Renese): thiazide diuretic. Used to treat HTN and fluid retention.

Potassium chloride (K-Dur, Slow-K): electrolyte. Used to treat hypokalemia.

Potassium iodide (SSKI): Used to treat hyperthyroidism.

Pramipexole (Mirapex): anti-parkinsonism agent. Used to treat Parkinson's disease.

Pravastatin (Pravachol): anti-cholesterol agent. Used to treat high cholesterol.

Prazepam (Centrax): benzodiazepine. Used to treat anxiety, psychoneuroses, and tension.

Prazosin (Minipress): anti hypertensive agent. Used to treat HTN and CHF.

Prednisolone (Prelone, Vasocidin): corticosteroid. Used to treat a variety of allergic and inflammatory problems.

Prednisone (Winpred, Orasone): corticosteriod. Used to treat a variety of allergic and inflammatory problems.

Primidone (Sertan,* Mysoline): anticonvulsant. Used to treat grand mal and partial seizures.

Probucol (Lorelco): anti-cholesterol agent. Used to treat high blood levels of cholesterol

Procainamide (Pronestyl): anti-arrhythmic agent. Used to treat and prevent premature ventricle contractions, atrial fibrillation, atrial flutter, and tachycardia.

Prochlorperazine (Stemetil,* Compazine): anti-emetic agent. Used to treat severe nausea and vomiting.

Procyclidine (Kemadrin): anti-parkinsonism agent: Used to treat Parkinson's disease and parkisonism.

Promazine (Sparine): anti-psychotic agent. Used to treat schizophrenia and depression.

Promethazine (Phenergan, Prometh): antihistamine. Used to treat nausea, vomiting, and motion sickness.

Propafenone (Rythmol): anti-arrhythmic agent. Used to treat ventricular arrhythmias.

Propantheline: anticholinergic. Used to treat duodenal ulcer and urinary incontinence.

Propoxyphene (Darvon, Dolene): narcotic analgesic. Used to treat moderate to severe pain.

Propranolol (Detensol,* Inderal): beta blocker. Used to treat angina and HTN and to prevent recurrent heart attack and migraine headaches.

Propylthiouracil: thyroid hormone antagonist. Used to treat hyperthyroidism.

Protriptyline (Triptil, Vivactil): antidepressant. Used to treat depression and bipolar disorders.

Pseudoephedrine: decongestant. Used to treat cold and seasonal allergy symptoms.

Pyrazinamide: anti-infective agent. Used to treat active tuberculosis.

Pyrethrin (RID): anti-parasitic agent. Used to treat lice.

Pyridostigmine (Regonol, Mestinon): anti-myasthenic. Used to treat myasthenia gravis.

Pyrilamine: antihistamine. Used to treat cold and allergy symptoms.

Pyrimethamine (Daraprim): anti-protozoal agent. Used to treat and prevent malaria.

Quazepam (Doral): benzodiazepine. Used to treat insomnia.

Quetiapine (Seroquel): anti-psychotic agent. Used to treat schizophrenia.

Quinethazone (Hydromox): thiazide diuretic. Used to treat HTN and fluid retention.

Quinidine (Quinaglute, Quinate): anti-arrhythmic. Used to treat cardiac arrhythmias.

Quinipril: ACE inhibitor. Used to treat HTN and CHF.

Racepinephrine (Vaponefrine): bronchodilator. Used to treat asthma.

Raloxifene (E-Vista): anti-estrogen agent. Used to prevent osteoporosis in postmenopausal women.

Ramipril (Altace): ACE inhibitor. Used to treat HTN and CHF.

Ranitidine: histamine (H_2) blocker. Used to treat and prevent ulcers and esophageal reflux.

Repaglinide (Prandin): anti-diabetic agent. Used to treat non-insulin-dependent diabetes mellitus.

Reserpine: anti-hypertensive agent. Used to treat HTN and psychiatric disorders.

Ribavirin (Virazole): anti-viral agent. Used to treat respiratory synctial virus (RSV) and pneumonia in AIDS patients.

Rifabutin (Mycobutin): anti-tubercular agent: Used to prevent the spread of a tuberculosis-like infection in HIV-infected patients.

Rifampin (Rifadin, Rofact*): antibiotic. Used to treat active tuberculosis and to prevent tuberculosis in exposed individuals.

Rimantadine (Flumadine): anti-viral agent. Used to treat and prevent influenza A infections.

Risperidone (Risperdal): anti-psychotic agent. Used to treat schizophrenia, aggression, and Tourette's syndrome.

Ritodrine (Yutopar): uterine relaxant. Used to treat premature labor and irritable bowel syndrome.

Rituximab (Rituxan): aromatase inhibitor. Used to treat non-Hodgkin's lymphoma.

Ropinirole (ReQuip): anti-parkinsonism agent. Used to treat Parkinson's disease.

Salicylamide: analgesic. Used to treat pain, anxiety, and fever.

Salmeterol (Serevent): sympathomimetic agent. Used to treat and prevent asthma attacks and to treat exercise-induced bronchospasm.

Salsalate (Salflex, Disalcid): analgesic. Used to treat pain, fever, arthritis, and swelling.

Scopolamine (Seconal): anticholinergic. Used to treat motion sickness.

Secobarbital (Seconal): barbiturate. Used to treat seizure disorders and insomnia.

Selegiline (Eldepryl): MAO inhibitor. Used to treat Parkinson's disease and Alzheimer's disease.

Selenium: anti-fungal agent. Used to treat dandruff and fungal infections of the skin.

Senna fruit extract (Senokot): laxative. Used to treat constipation and irritable bowel syndrome.

Sertraline (Zoloft): antidepressant. Used to treat depression and obsessive-compulsive disorder.

Sibutramine (Meridia): weight loss agent. Used to treat obesity.

Sildenafil (Viagra). Used to treat impotence.

Silver sulfadiazine (Silvadene): topical antibiotic. Used to treat skin infection due to severe burns.

Simethicone: anti-gas agent. Used to treat abdominal retention of gas.

Simvastatin (Zocor): anti-cholesterol agent. Used to treat high blood levels of cholesterol.

Somatrem (Protropin): hormone. Used to treat growth hormone deficiency in children.

Sotalol (Betapace, Sotacor*): beta blocker. Used to treat ventricular arrhythmias.

Spirapril (Renormax): ACE inhibitor. Used to treat CHF, angina pectoris, and atherosclerosis.

Spironolactone (Alatone): diuretic. Used to treat HTN and fluid retention.

Stanozolol (Winstrol): anabolic steroid. Used to treat hereditary angioedema.

Stavudine (Zerit): anti-viral agent. Used to treat HIV-infected patients who cannot tolerate AZT or didanosine.

Strontium chloride-89 (Metastron): radioisotope. Used to treat bone cancer pain.

Sucralfate (Sulcrate,* Carafate): anti-ulcer agent. Used to treat duodenal ulcer disease.

Sulfacetamide: antibiotic. Used to treat eye infections.

Sulfadiazine (Microsulfon): sulfonamide. Used to treat urinary tract infections.

Sulfadoxine (Fansidar): anti-protozoal agent. Used to treat and prevent malaria.

Sulfamethoxazole (Gantanol): antibiotic. Used to treat urinary tract infections.

Sulfasalazine (Azaline, Salazopyrin): antibiotic. Used to treat Crohn's disease and ulcerative colitis.

Sulfinpyrazone: anti-gout agent. Used to treat gout.

Sulfisoxazole (Gantrisin): antibiotic. Used to treat a variety of infections.

Sulindac (Clinoril): NSAID. Used to treat pain, fever, and inflammation.

Sumatriptan (Imitrex): anti-migraine agent. Used to treat migraine and cluster headaches.

Tacrine (THA, Cognex): cholinesterase inhibitor. Used to treat Alzheimer's disease.

Tacrolimus (Prograf): antibiotic. Used to prevent organ transplant rejection.

Tamoxifen (Tamofen,* Nolvadex): Used to treat breast cancer in postmenopausal women.

Tamsulosin (Flomax): Used to treat benign prostatic hyperplasia (enlarged prostate).

Tazarotene (Tazorac): retinoid. Used to treat psoriasis.

Temazepam (Restoril): benzodiazepine. Used to treat insomnia.

Terazosin (Hytrin): anti-hypertensive agent. Used to treat HTN and benign prostatic hyperplasia.

Terbutaline (Brethine): bronchodilator. Used to treat and prevent asthma attacks and to relieve symptoms of chronic bronchitis and emphysema.

Terconazole (Terazol): anti-fungal agent. Used to treat vaginal yeast infections.

Terfenadine (Seldane): antihistamine. Used to treat symptoms of allergic reaction.

Testolactone (Teslac): hormone. Used to treat breast cancer.

Tetracycline (Retet, Sumycin): antibiotic. Used to treat infections.

Theophylline (Respbid, Slo-bid): bronchodilator. Used to treat asthma and COPD.

Thiethylperazine (Torecan): phenothiazine. Used to treat nausea and vomiting.

Thioridazine (Mellaril): phenothiazine. Used to treat depression, agitation, and anxiety.

Thiothixene (Navane): tranquilizer. Used to treat episodes of mania, paranoia, and schizophrenia.

Thyroglobulin (Proloid): hormone. Used to treat hypothyroidism and goiter.

Tiagabine (Gabatril): anticonvulsant. Used to treat partial seizures.

Ticarcillin: antibiotic. Used to treat general infections.

Ticlopidine (Ticlid): platelet inhibitor. Used to treat and prevent stroke.

Tiludronate (Skelid): biphosphonate. Used to treat Paget's disease.

Timolol (Timoptic, Blocadren): beta blocker. Used to treat angina and HTN.

Tincture of opium (Paregoric): narcotic analgesic. Used to treat intestinal cramps and diarrhea.

Tobramycin (Tobrex): antibiotic. Used to treat general infections.

Tocainide (Tonocard): anti-arrhythmic agent. Used to treat ventricular arrhythmias.

Tolazamide (Ronase, Tolinase): anti-diabetic agent. Used to treat type II non-insulin-dependent diabetes mellitus.

Tolbutamide (Orinase): anti-diabetic agent. Used to treat type II non-insulin-dependent diabetes.

Tolmetin (Tolectin): NSAID. Used to treat pain, fever, and inflammation.

Torsemide (Demadex): diuretic. Used to treat HTN and fluid retention.

Tramadol (Ultram): analgesic. Used to treat pain, fever, and inflammation.

Tranylcypromine (Parnate): MAO inhibitor. Used to treat depression.

Trazodone (Trialodine, Desyrel): antidepressant. Used to treat depression and agoraphobia.

Tretinoin (Retin-A): vitamin A. Used to treat acne and other skin conditions.

Triamcinolone (Azmacort, Artisocort): corticosteroid. Used to treat asthma and other inflammatory problems.

Triamterene (Dyrenium): diuretic. Used to treat HTN and fluid retention.

Triazolam (Halcion): benzodiazepine. Used to treat insomnia.

Trichlormethiazide (Trichlorex, Diurese): thiazide diuretic. Used to treat HTN and fluid retention.

Trifluoperazine: phenothiazine. Used to treat psychotic thinking, episodes of mania, paranoia, and schizophrenia.

Triflupromazine (Vesprin): phenothiazine: Used to treat nausea, vomiting and psychotic disorders.

Trihexyphenidyl (Artane): anti-parkinsonism agent. Used to treat Parkinson's disease and parkinsonism.

Trimeprazine: phenothiazine. Used to treat dermatological disorders.

Trimethadione (Tridione): anticonvulsant. Used to treat petit mal seizures.

Trimethobenzamide (Tigan): anti-emetic agent. Used to treat nausea and vomiting.

Trimethoprim (Proloprin, Trimpex): anti-infective agent. Used to treat urinary tract and eye infections.

Trimetrexate (NeuTrexin): Used to treat *Pneumocystis carinii* pneumonia.

Trimipramine (Surmontil): tricyclic antidepressant. Used to treat depression.

Triprolidine: antihistamine. Used to treat cold and allergy symptoms.

Troglitazone (Rezulin): anti-diabetic agent. Used to treat non-insulin-dependent diabetes mellitus.

Trovafloxacin (Trovan): antibiotic. Used to treat general infections.

Ursodiol: anti-cirrhosis agent. Used to treat gallstones.

Valaciclovir (Valtrex): anti-viral agent. Used to treat shingles (herpes zoster).

Valproic acid (Depakote, Epival*): anticonvulsant. Used to treat epilepsy.

Valsartan (Diovan): anti-hypertensive agent. Used to treat HTN.

Vancomycin (Vancocin): anti-infective agent. Used to treat general infections.

Venlafaxine (Effexor): antidepressant. Used to treat depression.

Verapamil (Verelan, Calan): calcium channel blocker. Used to treat angina pectoris, atrial fibrillation, atrial flutter, atrial tachycardia, and HTN.

Warfarin (Coumadin, Sofarin): anticoagulant. Used to treat blood-clotting disorders.

Yohimbine: herbal preparation. Used to treat male impotence.

Zafirlukast (Accolate): antihistamine: Used to treat asthma.

Zalcitabine (Hivid): anti-viral agent. Used to treat advanced HIV infection.

Zidovudine (Retrovir): anti-viral agent. Used to treat HIV-infected patients.

Zolpidem (Ambien): imidazopyridine. Used to treat insomnia.

Zolmitriptan (Zomig): anti-migraine agent. Used to treat migraine headaches.

APPENDIX B

PRESCRIPTION AND OVER-THE-COUNTER DRUGS BY TRADE NAME

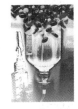

Accolate (zafirlukast): antihistamine. Used to treat asthma.

Accupril (quinapril): acetylcholinesterase (ACE) inhibitor. Used to treat hypertension and CHF.

Accurbron (theophylline): bronchodilator. Used to treat asthma and chronic obstructive pulmonary disease (COPD).

Accutane (isotretinoin): anti-acne agent. Inhibits skin oil production. Used for severe acne.

Acetazolam (acetazolamide): carbonic anhydrase inhibitor. Used to treat glaucoma, petit mal epilepsy, congestive heart failure (CHF), drug-induced edema, and high altitude sickness.

Achromycin (tetracycline): antibiotic. Used to treat severe acne and gum disease.

Actidil (triprolidine): antihistamine. Used to treat cold and allergy symptoms.

Actifed (pseudoephedrine and triprolidine): antihistamine. Used to treat cold and allergy symptoms.

Actigall (ursodiol): gallstone dissolving agent. Used to treat gallstones.

Actisite (tetracycline): antibiotic. Used to treat gum disease (periodontitis).

---

* A drug name followed by an asterisk indicates that this is a Canadian trade name.

Acular (ketorolac): nonsteroidal anti-inflammatory drug (NSAID). Used to treat pain, fever, and inflammation.

Adalat (nifedipine): calcium channel blocker. Used to treat angina and HTN.

Adapin (doxepin): tricyclic antidepressant. Used to treat depression and sleep disorders.

Adrenalin chloride (epinephrine): sympathomimetic. Used to treat asthma, nasal congestion, and anaphylaxis.

Advil (ibuprofen): NSAID. Used to treat pain, fever, and inflammation.

AeroBid (flunisolide): corticosteroid. Used to treat asthma and allergic rhinitis.

Aerolate (theophylline): bronchodilator. Used to treat asthma and COPD.

Aerolone (isoproterenol): sympathomimetic. Used to treat asthma, bronchitis, and emphysema.

Aerosporin (polymyxin): antibiotic. Used to treat infection.

Agrylin (anagrelide): platelet inhibitor. Used to treat essential thrombocythemia.

Akarpine (pilocarpine): anti-glaucoma agent. Used to treat glaucoma.

AK-Chlor (chloramphenicol): antibiotic. Used to treat life-threatening infections.

AK-Cide (prednisolone and sulfacetamide): corticosteroid, antibiotic. Used to treat eye infections.

AK-Dex (dexamethasone): corticosteroid. Used to treat allergic and inflammatory conditions.

Akineton (biperiden): anticholinergic. Used to treat Parkinson's disease.

AK-Pred (prednisolone): corticosteroid. Used to treat a variety of allergic and inflammatory problems.

Ak-Tate (prednisolone): corticosteroid. Used to treat inflammatory problems of the eye.

AK-Zol (acetazolamide): antibiotic. Used to treat glaucoma, petit mal epilepsy, CHF, and high altitude sickness.

Alatone (spironolactone): diuretic. Used to treat HTN and fluid retention.

Alazine (hydralazine): anti-hypertensive agent. Used to treat HTN, CHF, and heart valve insufficiency until surgery.

Aldactazide (hydrochlorothiazide and spironolactone): diuretic. Used to treat HTN and fluid retention.

Aldactone (spironolactone): diuretic. Used to treat HTN and fluid retention.

Aldoclor-150 or -250 (chlorothiazide, methyldopa): diuretic, antihypertensive. Used to treat HTN.

Aldomet (methyldopa): anti-hypertensive agent. Used to treat HTN.

Aldoril (chlorothiazide, methyldopa): diuretic, antihypertensive. Used to treat HTN.

Aleve (naproxen). NSAID. Used to treat pain, fever, and inflammation.

Allegra (fexofenadine): antihistamine. Used to treat seasonal allergy symptoms.

Allerdryl* (diphenhydramine): antihistamine. Used to treat motion sickness and allergic reactions.

Alloprin (allopurinol): anti-gout agent. Used to treat gout.

Almocarpine (pilocarpine): anti-glaucoma agent. Used to treat glaucoma.

Altace (ramipril): ACE inhibitor. Used to treat HTN and CHF.

Alupent (metaproterenol): Used to treat asthma and COPD.

Alurate (aprobarbital): barbiturate. Used as a sedative.

Alvosulfon* (dapsone): anti-infective agent. Used to treat *Pneumocystis carinii* pneumonia.

Amaryl (glimepiride): anti-diabetic agent. Used to treat non-insulin-dependent diabetes mellitus.

Ambenyl cough syrup (codeine, bromodiphenhydramine): narcotic, antihistamine. Used to treat cold symptoms, especially cough.

Ambien (zolpidem): imidazopyridine. Used to treat insomnia.

Amcill (ampicillin): antibiotic. Used to treat general infections, septicemia, and meningitis.

Amen (medroxyprogesterone): progestin. Used to treat menstrual disorders and cancer of the breast.

Amersol* (ibuprofen): NSAID. Used to treat pain, fever, and inflammation.

Amesec (ephedrine, aminophylline): sympathomimetic, bronchodilator, barbiturate. Used to treat asthma and COPD.

Amikin (amikacin): antibiotic. Used to treat serious infections.

Aminophyllin (aminophylline): bronchodilator. Used to treat asthma and COPD.

Amitril (amitriptyline): tricyclic antidepressant. Used to treat depression.

Amoxil (amoxicillin): antibiotic. Used to treat general infections.

Ampicin* (ampicillin): antibiotic. Used to treat general infections, septicemia, and meningitis.

Ampicin PRB* (ampicillin, probenecid): antibiotic, antigout agent. Used to treat gout.

Amytal sodium (amobarbital): barbiturate. Used to treat seizure disorders.

Anacin (aspirin and caffeine): analgesic. Used to treat mild pain.

Anacin with codeine (aspirin, caffeine, codeine): narcotic analgesic. Used to treat moderate to severe pain.

Anadrol-50 (oxymetholone): testosterone derivative. Used to treat aplastic anemia.

Anafranil (clomipramine): antidepressant. Used to treat obsessive-compulsive disorder.

Anaprox (naproxen): NSAID. Used to treat pain, fever, and inflammation.

Anaprox DS (naproxen): NSAID. Used to treat pain, fever, and inflammation.

Ancasal* (aspirin): analgesic. Used to treat mild pain.

Ancobon (flucytosine): anti-fungal agent. Used to treat endocarditis, osteomyelitis, pneumonia, and AIDS-related infections.

Ancotil (flucytosine): anti-fungal agent. Used to treat endocarditis, osteomyelitis, pneumonia, and acquired immunodeficiency syndrome (AIDS)-related infections.

Android-10 or -25 (methyltestosterone): male sex hormone. Used to treat breast cancer and primary hypogonadism.

Anexsia (hydrocodone, acetaminophen): narcotic analgesic. Used to treat moderate to severe pain.

Ansaid (flurbiprofen): NSAID. Used to treat pain, fever, and inflammation.

Antabuse (disulfiram): anti-alcoholism agent. Used to deter the use of alcohol.

Antispasmodic (atropine, hyoscyamine, phenobarbital, scopolamine): antispasmodic. Used to treat spasms and pain due to urinary tract infections (UTIs).

Antivert (meclizine): antihistamine. Used to treat motion sickness and dizziness.

Anturane (sulfinpyrazone): anti-gout agent. Used to treat gout.

Anzemet (dolasetron): anti-emetic agent. Used to prevent chemotherapy-induced nausea and vomiting.

Apo-Allopurinol* (allopurinol): anti-gout agent. Used to treat gout and prevent gout attacks.

Apo-Amitriptyline* (amitriptyline): tricyclic antidepressant. Used to treat depression.

Apo-Amoxi* (amoxicillin): antibiotic. Used to treat general infections.

341

Apo-Ampi* (ampicillin): antibiotic. Used to treat general infections.

Apo-Benztropine* (benztropine): anticholinergic. Used to treat parkinsonism.

Apo-Carbamazepine* (carbamazepine): anticonvulsant. Used to treat nerve pain, epilepsy, and some psychiatric disorders.

Apo-Chlorpropamide* (chlorpropamide): anti-diabetic agent. Used to treat type II diabetes mellitus.

Apo-Chlorthalidone* (chlorthalidone): thiazide diuretic. Used to treat HTN and fluid retention.

Apo-Cimetidine* (cimetidine): histamine (H_2) blocker. Used to treat and prevent ulcers and esophageal reflux.

Apo-Cloxi* (cloxacillin): antibiotic. Used to treat infections resistant to forms of penicillin.

Apo-Diazepam* (diazepam): benzodiazepine. Used to treat anxiety, muscle spasm, epilepsy, insomnia, and symptoms of alcohol withdrawal.

Apo-Dipyridamole* (dipyridamole): platelet inhibitor. Used to prevent post-cardiac surgery thromboembolism and recurrent heart attacks.

Apo-Erythro Base* (erythromycin): antibiotic. Used to treat general infections.

Apo-Erythro-ES* (erythromycin): antibiotic. Used to treat general infections.

Apo-Erythro-S* (erythromycin): antibiotic. Used to treat general infections.

Apo-Fluphenazine* (fluphenazine): phenothiazine. Used to treat schizophrenia.

Apo-Flurazepam* (flurazepam): benzodiazepine. Used to treat insomnia.

Apo-Furosemide* (furosemide): Used to treat HTN and fluid retention.

Apo-Haloperidol* (haloperidol): anti-psychotic agent.

Used to treat schizophrenia, manic-depressive disorder, acute psychosis, and Tourette's syndrome.

Apo-Hydro* (hydrochlorothiazide): thiazide diuretic. Used to treat HTN and fluid retention.

Apo-Ibuprofen* (ibuprofen): NSAID. Used to treat pain, fever, and inflammation.

Apo-Indomethacin* (indomethacin): NSAID. Used to treat pain, fever, and inflammation.

Apo-ISDN* (isosorbide dinitrate): nitrate. Used to treat angina attacks.

Apo-Lorazepam* (lorazepam): benzodiazepine. Used to treat anxiety and insomnia.

Apo-Methazide* (hydrochlorothiazide, methyldopa): diuretic, anti-hypertensive agent. Used to treat HTN.

Apo-Mctoclop* (metoclopramide): anti-emetic agent. Used to treat nausea and vomiting due to migraine headaches or cancer-fighting drugs.

Apo-Metoprolol* (metoprolol): beta-blocker. Used to treat HTN and angina.

Apo-Nadol* (nadolol): beta blocker. Used to treat HTN and to prevent exercise-induced angina attacks.

Apo-Naproxen* (naproxen): NSAID. Used to treat pain, fever, and inflammation.

Apo-Nifed* (nifedipine): calcium channel blocker. Used to treat angina pectoris and HTN.

Apo-Nitrofurantoin* (nitrofurantoin): anti-infective agent. Used to treat urinary tract infections.

Apo-Oxtriphylline* (oxtriphylline): bronchodilator. Used to treat asthma and COPD.

Apo-Penicillin VK* (penicillin V): antibiotic. Used to treat respiratory, ear, and skin infections.

Apo-Perphenazine* (perphenazine): phenothiazine. Used to treat acute and chronic psychotic disorders, as well as severe nausea and vomiting, and to calm agitation.

Apo-Piroxicam* (piroxicam): NSAID: Used to treat pain, fever, and inflammation.

Apo-Prazo* (prazosin): anti-hypertensive agent. Used to treat HTN and CHF.

Apo-Prednisone* (prednisone): corticosteroid. Used to treat allergic and inflammatory problems, including asthma, bursitis, tendonitis, and arthritis.

Apo-Primidone* (primidone): anticonvulsant. Used to treat grand mal and partial seizures.

Apo-Procainamide* (procainamide): anti-arrhythmic agent. Used to treat and prevent premature arrhythmias.

Apo-Propranolol* (propranolol): beta blocker. Used to treat angina, HTN, and migraine headaches.

Apo-Quinidine* (quinidine): anti-arrhythmic agent. Used to treat arrhythmias.

Apo-Ranitidine* (ranitidine): histamine (H_2) blocker. Used to treat and prevent ulcers and esophageal reflux.

Apo-Sulfamethoxazole* (sulfamethoxazole): antibiotic. Used to treat UTIs.

Apo-Sulfatrim* (sulfamethoxazole, trimethoprim): antibiotic. Used to treat UTIs.

Apo-Tetra* (tetracycline): antibiotic. Used to treat severe acne and gum disease.

Apo-Thioridazine* (thioridazine): phenothiazine. Used to treat depression, agitation, and anxiety.

Apo-Timolol* (timolol): beta blocker. Used to treat angina and HTN.

Apo-Tolbutamide* (tolbutamide): anti-diabetic agent. Used to treat non-insulin-dependent diabetes.

Apo-Triazide* (hydrochlorothiazide, trimethoprim): diuretic, potassium-sparing diuretic. Used to treat HTN and fluid retention.

Apo-Trifluoperazine* (trifluoperazine): phenothiazine. Used to treat psychotic thinking, episodes of mania, paranoia, and schizophrenia.

Apresazide (hydralazine, hydrochlorothiazide): anti-hypertensive agent, diuretic. Used to treat HTN and fluid retention.

Apresoline (hydralazine): anti-hypertensive agent. Used to treat HTN, CHF, and heart valve insufficiency.

Apresoline-Esidrix (hydralazine, hydrochlorothiazide): anti-hypertensive agent, diuretic. Used to treat HTN and fluid retention.

Aquatensen (methyclothiazide): thiazide diuretic. Used to treat CHF, HTN, drug-induced fluid retention, and certain liver and kidney disorders.

Aralen (chloroquine): anti-malarial agent. Used to treat malaria, amebic infection, arthritis, and lupus erythematosus.

Aricept (donepezil): cholinesterase. Used to treat Alzheimer's disease.

Aristocort (triamcinolone): corticosteroid. Used to treat asthma and other inflammatory problems.

Arm-a-Med (metaproterenol): beta agonist. Used to treat asthma and COPD.

Artane (trihexyphenidyl): anti-parkinsonism agent. Used to treat Parkinson's disease.

Arthrotec (diclofenac, misoprostol): buffered NSAID. Used to treat rheumatoid arthritis and osteoarthritis.

Asacol (mesalamine): anti-inflammatory agent. Used to treat intestinal inflammatory disorders.

Asantine (aspirin, dipyridamole): anticoagulant. Used to prevent formation of blood clots after cardiac surgery and to help prevent stroke and heart attack.

Asendin (amoxapine): tricyclic antidepressant. Used to treat depression.

Aspergum (aspirin): analgesic. Used to treat mild pain.

Astramorph PF (morphine): narcotic analgesic. Used to treat severe pain.

Astrin (aspirin): analgesic. Used to treat mild pain.

Atabrine hydrochloride (quinacrine): anti-protozoal agent. Used to treat tapeworm, malaria, and lupus erythematosus.

Atarax (hydroxyzine): antihistamine. Used to treat anxiety, nausea, vomiting, and allergy symptoms.

Ativan (lorazepam): benzodiazepine. Used to treat anxiety and insomnia.

Atromid-S (clofibrate): anti-hypertensive agent, diuretic. Used to treat HTN and fluid retention.

Atrovent (ipratropium): bronchodilator. Used to treat asthma and COPD.

Augmentin (amoxicillin, clavulanate): antibiotic. Used to treat general infections.

Avapro (irbesartan): anti-hypertensive agent. Used to treat hypertension.

Aventyl (nortriptyline): tricyclic antidepressant. Used to treat depression and chronic pain.

Axid (nizatidine): histamine (H_2) blocker. Used to treat and prevent ulcers, reflux.

Axotal (aspirin, butalbital): analgesic, barbiturate. Used to treat pain and tension headaches.

Azaline (sulfasalazine): antibiotic. Used to treat Crohn's disease and ulcerative colitis.

Azdone (aspirin, hydrocodone): narcotic analgesic. Used to treat moderate and severe pain.

Azmacort (triamcinolone): corticosteroid. Used to treat asthma and other inflammatory problems.

Azo Gantanol (phenazopyridine, sulfamethoxazole): analgesic, antibiotic. Used to treat UTIs.

Azo Gantrisin (phenazopyridine, sulfisoxazole): analgesic, antibiotic. Used to treat UTIs.

AZT (zidovudine): Used to treat HIV infection.

Azulfidine (sulfasalazine): antibiotic. Used to treat Crohn's disease and ulcerative colitis.

Bactocill (oxacillin): antibiotic. Used to treat general infections.

Bactrim (sulfamethoxazole, trimethoprim): antibiotic. Used to treat UTIs.

Bancap HC (hydrocodone, acetaminophen): narcotic analgesic. Used to treat moderate and severe pain.

Barbita (phenobarbital): barbiturate. Used to treat anxiety, nervous tension, insomnia, and epilepsy.

Baycol (cerivastatin): anti-cholesterol agent: Used to treat high cholesterol.

Bayer Aspirin (aspirin): analgesic. Used to treat mild pain.

Beclovent (beclomethasone): corticosteroid. Used to treat asthma and COPD.

Beconase AQ (beclomethasone): corticosteroid. Used to treat asthma.

Beepen-VK (penicillin V): antibiotic. Used to treat respiratory tract, middle ear, and skin infections.

Belladenal (belladonna, phenobarbital): barbiturate. Used to treat irritable bowel syndrome.

Bellergal (ergotamine, phenobarbital): ergot preparation. Used to treat migraine headaches.

Benadryl (diphenhydramine): antihistamine. Used to treat motion sickness, Parkinson's disease, and allergic reactions.

Benemid (probenecid): anti-gout agent. Used to treat gout.

Bensylate* (benztropine): anticholinergic. Used to treat parkinsonism and parkinsonian reactions.

Bentyl (dicyclomine): Used to treat gastrointestinal (GI) disorders.

Benuryl (probenecid): anti-gout agent. Used to treat gout.

Benylin (diphenhydramine): antihistamine. Used to treat motion sickness and allergic reactions.

Benzamycin (erythromycin, benzoyl peroxide): topical antibiotic. Used to treat acne.

Bepadin (bepridil): calcium channel blocker. Used to treat angina.

347

Betaloc* (metoprolol): beta blocker. Used to treat HTN and angina and to prevent recurrent heart attack.

Betapace (sotalol): beta blocker. Used to treat ventricular arrhythmias.

Betapen-VK (penicillin): antibiotic. Used to treat respiratory tract, middle ear, and skin infections.

Bethaprim (sulfamethoxazole, trimethoprim): antibiotic. Used to treat urinary tract infections.

Betoptic (betaxolol): beta blocker. Used to treat HTN and glaucoma (eye drops).

Biaxin (clarithromycin): antibiotic. Used to treat respiratory tract and skin infections.

Bicillin C-R (penicillin): antibiotic. Used to treat respiratory tract, middle ear, and skin infections.

Biohisdex DHC (diphenylpyraline, hydrocodone, phenylephrine): narcotic analgesic. Used to treat pain and to control cough.

Biohisdine DHC (diphenylpyraline, hydrocodone, phenylephrine): narcotic analgesic. Used to treat pain and to control cough.

Biphetamine (dextroamphetamine, amphetamine): stimulant. Used to treat attention deficit hyperactive disorder and narcolepsy.

Biquin Durules (quinidine): antiarrhythmic. Used to treat cardiac arrhythmias.

Blephamide (prednisolone): corticosteroid. Used to treat a variety of allergic and inflammatory problems.

Blocadren (timolol): beta blocker. Used to treat angina and HTN.

Brethaire (terbutaline): bronchodilator. Used to treat and prevent asthma attacks and COPD.

Brethine (terbutaline): bronchodilator. Used to treat and prevent asthma attacks and COPD.

Brevicon (norethindrone): oral contraceptive. Used to treat menstrual disorder and to prevent pregnancy.

348

Bricanyl (terbutaline): bronchodilator. Used to treat and prevent asthma and COPD.

Bronalide (flunisolide): corticosteroid. Used to treat asthma and allergic rhinitis.

Brondecon (guaifenesin, oxtriphylline): bronchodilator. Used to treat asthma COPD.

Bronitin Mist (epinephrine): sympathomimetic. Used to treat asthma and allergic nasal congestion.

Bronkaid Mist (epinephrine): sympathomimetic. Used to treat asthma attacks, allergic nasal congestion, glaucoma, and anaphylactic shock.

Bronkephrine (ethylnorepinephrine): sympathomimetic. Used to treat hypotension.

Bronkodyl (theophylline): bronchodilator. Used to treat and prevent asthma and COPD.

Bronkometer (isoetharine): bronchodilator. Used to treat asthma, bronchitis, and emphysema.

Bronkosol (isoetharine): bronchodilator. Used to treat asthma, bronchitis, and emphysema.

Bucladin-S (buclizine): antihistamine. Used to treat and prevent symptoms of motion sickness.

Bumex (bumetanide): diuretic. Used to treat excessive fluid retention due to CHF or disease.

Buprenex (buprenophine): narcotic analgesic. Used to treat moderate to severe pain.

BuSpar (buspirone): mild tranquilizer. Used to treat anxiety, nervous tension, and panic disorders.

Butazolidin (phenylbutazone): anti-inflammatory agent. Used to treat gout and arthritis.

Buticaps (butabarbital): barbiturate. Used as a sedative.

Butisol Sodium (butabarbital): barbiturate. Used as a sedative.

Cafergot (caffeine, ergotamine): ergot preparation. Used to treat migraine headaches and narcolepsy.

Cafergot PB (atropine, caffeine, ergotamine, phenobarbital): ergot preparation. Used to treat migraine headaches and narcolepsy.

Caladryl (calamine, diphenhydramine): antihistamine. Used to treat dermal allergies.

Calan (verapamil): calcium channel blocker. Used to treat angina, HTN, and arrhythmias.

Calcimar (calcitonin): calcium-regulating hormone. Used to treat excessive bone growth (Paget's disease).

Canesten* (clotrimazole): anti-fungal agent. Used to treat yeast and ringworm infections.

Capital with codeine (acetaminophen, codeine): analgesic. Used to treat moderate to severe pain.

Capoten (captopril): ACE inhibitor. Used to treat HTN.

Capozide (captopril, hydrochlorothiazide): ACE inhibitor, diuretic. Used to treat HTN.

Carafate (sucralfate): anti-ulcer agent. Used to treat duodenal ulcer disease.

Carbolith* (lithium): tranquilizer. Used to treat manic depression and schizophrenia.

Cardene (nicardipine): calcium channel blocker. Used to treat angina and HTN.

Cardioquin (quinidine): anti-arrhythmic agent. Used to treat arrhythmias.

Cardizem (diltiazem): calcium channel blocker. Used to treat angina pectoris and HTN.

Cardura (doxazosin): anti-hypertensive agent. Used to treat HTN and enlarged prostate.

Carfin (warfarin): anticoagulant. Used to treat blood-clotting disorders.

Cartrol (carteolol): beta blocker. Used to treat HTN and exercise-induced angina.

Cataflam (diclofenac): NSAID. Used to treat pain, fever, and inflammation.

Catapres (clonidine): anti-hypertensive agent. Used to treat HTN.

350

Ceclor (cefaclor): antibiotic. Used to treat infections of the skin, respiratory tract, ear, and urinary tract.

Ceftin (cefuroxime): antibiotic. Used to treat infections of the ear, skin, respiratory tract, and urinary tract.

Cefzil (cefprozil): antibiotic. Used to treat infections of the respiratory tract and skin.

Celestone (betamethasone): corticosteroid. Used to treat inflammation.

Celontin (methsuximide): anticonvulsant. Used to treat seizure disorders.

Centrax (prazepam): benzodiazepine. Used to treat anxiety and agitation.

Cephanex (cephalexin): antibiotic. Used to treat a variety of infections.

Ceporex (cephalexin): antibiotic. Used to treat a variety of infections.

Chardonna-2 (belladonna, phenobarbital): barbiturate. Used to treat anxiety, nervous tension, insomnia, and epilepsy.

Chloromycetin (chloramphenicol): antibiotic. Used to treat life-threatening infections.

Chloronase* (chlorpropamide): anti-diabetic agent. Used to treat non-insulin-dependent diabetes mellitus.

Chloroptic (chloramphenicol): antibiotic. Used to treat life-threatening infections.

Chlorpromanyl* (chlorpromazine): phenothiazine. Used to treat psychotic disorders and vomiting due to toxic chemotherapy.

Chlor-Trimeton (chlorpheniramine): antihistamine. Used to treat symptoms of cold and allergies.

Choledyl* (oxtriphylline): bronchodilator. Used to treat asthma and COPD.

Choloxin (dextrothyroxine): anti-cholesterol agent. Used to treat high cholesterol.

Cholybar (cholestyramine): anti-cholesterol agent. Used to treat high blood levels of low-density lipoprotein (LDL) cholesterol and itching due to partial biliary obstruction.

Cibalith-S (lithium): tranquilizer. Used to treat manic depression and schizophrenia.

Cin-Quin* (quinidine): anti-arrhythmic agent. Used to treat arrhythmias.

Cipro (ciprofloxacin): antibiotic. Used to treat general infections.

Claforan (cefotaxime): antibiotic. Used to treat a wide variety of infections.

Claritin (loratidine): antihistamine. Used to treat symptoms of seasonal allergies.

Claritin-D: antihistamine. Used to treat symptoms of seasonal allergies.

Clavulin* (amoxicillin, clavulanate): antibiotic. Used to treat general infections.

Cleocin (clindamycin): antibiotic. Used to treat uncommon infections.

Clinoril (sulindac): NSAID. Used to treat pain, fever, and inflammation.

Cloxapen (cloxacillin): antibiotic. Used to treat infections resistant to original forms of penicillin.

Clozaril (clozapine): tranquilizer. Used to treat schizophrenia.

Co-Advil (ibuprofen, pseudoephedrine): analgesic, decongestant. Used to treat colds and allergies.

Co-Betaloc (hydrochlorothiazide, metoprolol): diuretic, beta blocker. Used to treat HTN and angina.

Codiclear DH (guaifenesin, hydrocodone): narcotic analgesic. Used to treat pain and to control cough.

Codimal DH (hydrocodone, phenylephrine, pyrilamine): narcotic analgesic. Used to treat pain and to control cough.

Codimal DM (dextromethorphan, phenylephrine, pyrilamine): antitussive, sympathomimetic. Used to treat symptoms of cold and seasonal allergies.

Codimal-L.A. (chlorpheniramine, pseudoephedrine): antihistamine, decongestant. Used to treat symptoms of cold and seasonal allergies.

Codimal PH (codeine, phenylephrine, pyrilamine): narcotic analgesic. Used to treat pain and to control cough.

Cogentin (benztropine): anticholinergic. Used to treat parkinsonism and parkinsonian reactions.

Co-Gesic (acetaminophen, codeine): narcotic analgesic. Used to treat pain and to control cough.

Cognex (tacrine): cholinesterase inhibitor. Used to treat Alzheimer's disease.

Colace (docusate): laxative. Used to treat constipation

ColBenemid (colchicine, probenecid): anti-gout agent. Used to treat gout.

Colestid (colestipol): anti-cholesterol agent. Used to treat high blood cholesterol.

Combipres (chlorthalidone, clonidine): diuretic, anti-hypertensive agent. Used to treat HTN.

Combivent (albuterol, ipratropium): bronchodilator. Used to treat COPD.

Comoxol (sulfamethoxazole): antibiotic. Used to treat urinary tract infections.

Compazine (prochlorperazine): anti-emetic agent. Used to treat severe nausea and vomiting.

Compoz (diphenhydramine): antihistamine. Used to treat motion sickness and allergic reactions.

Congess JR/SR (guaifenesin, pseudoephedrine): expectorant, decongestant. Used to treat symptoms of cold and seasonal allergy.

Constant-T (theophylline): bronchodilator. Used to treat asthma and COPD.

Coptin (sulfadiazine, trimethoprim): antibiotic. Used to treat UTIs.

Cordarone (amiodarone): anti-arrhythmic agent. Used to treat arrhythmias.

Corgard (nadolol): beta blocker. Used to treat HTN and to prevent exercise-induced angina attacks.

Coronex (isosorbide dinitrate): nitrate. Used to treat angina attacks.

Corzide (nadolol, bendroflumethiazide): beta blocker, thiazide diuretic. Used to treat HTN.

Cotrim (sulfamethoxazole, trimethoprim): antibiotic. Used to treat UTIs.

Coumadin (warfarin): anticoagulant. Used to treat blood-clotting disorders.

Cozaar (losartan): anti-hypertensive agent. Used to treat HTN.

Crystodigin (digitoxin): digitalis preparation. Used to treat CHF and cardiac arrhythmias.

Cuprimine (penicillamine): chelator. Used to treat copper toxicity and severe rheumatoid arthritis.

Curretab (medroxyprogesterone): progestin. Used to treat menstrual disorders and cancer of the breast or uterus; a contraceptive.

Cutivate (fluticasone): corticosteroid. Used to treat symptoms of seasonal allergies.

Cyclopar (tetracycline): antibiotic. Used to treat severe acne and gum disease.

Cyclospasmol (cylandelate): vasodilator. Used to treat vascular disease.

Cycrin (medroxyprogesterone): progestin. Used to treat menstrual disorders and cancer of the breast or uterus. Also used as contraceptive.

Cylert (pemoline): stimulant. Used to treat attention deficit disorder.

Cystospaz (hyoscyamine): belladonna alkaloid. Used to treat GI problems.

Cytomel (liothyronine): thyroid hormone. Used to treat thyroid disorders.

Cytotec (misoprostol): anti-ulcer agent. Used to prevent drug-induced stomach ulcers.

Cytovene (ganciclovir): anti-viral agent. Used to treat life-threatening infections.

Cytoxan (cyclophosphamide): immunosuppressant. Used to treat cancer and severe rheumatoid arthritis.

Dalacin C (clindamycin): antibiotic. Used to treat uncommon infections.

Dalgan (dezocine): narcotic analgesic. Used to treat moderate to severe pain.

Dallergy (chlorpheniramine, methscopolamine, phenylephrine): antihistamine. Used to treat allergy symptoms.

Dalmane (flurazepam): benzodiazepine. Used to treat insomnia.

Damason-P (aspirin, hydrocodone): narcotic analgestic. Used to treat moderate to severe pain.

Dantrium (dantrolene): muscle relaxant. Used to treat spasticity.

Daranide (dichlorphenamide): anti-glaucoma agent. Used to treat glaucoma.

Daraprim (pyrimethamine): anti-protozoal agent. Used to treat and prevent malaria.

Darvocet-N (acetaminophen, propoxyphene): narcotic analgesic. Used to treat moderate to severe pain.

Darvon (propoxyphene): narcotic analgesic. Used to treat moderate to severe pain.

Darvon with aspirin (aspirin, propoxyphene): narcotic analgesic. Used to treat moderate to severe pain.

Daypro (oxaprozin): NSAID. Used to treat pain, fever, and inflammation.

Dazamide (acetazolamide): carbonic anhydrase inhibitor. Used to treat glaucoma, CHF, and high altitude sickness.

DDAVP (desmopressin): vasopressin analogue. Used to treat bleeding disorders and diabetes insipidus.

Decaderm (dexamethasone): corticosteroid. Used to treat allergic and inflammatory conditions.

Decadron (dexamethasone): corticosteroid. Used to treat allergic and inflammatory conditions.

Decadron with xylocaine (dexamethasone, lidocaine): corticosteroid, analgesic. Used to treat allergic and inflammatory conditions.

Decaspray (dexamethasone): corticosteroid. Used to treat allergic and inflammatory conditions.

Declomycin (demeclocycline): antibiotic. Used to treat gonorrhea and UTIs.

Deconamine (chlorpheniramine, pseudoephedrine): antihistamine, decongestant. Used to treat symptoms of cold and allergies.

Delestrogen (estradiol): female sex hormone. Used to treat gynecological disorders.

Delsym (dextromethorphan): antitussive. Used to treat cough.

Delta-Cortef (prednisolone): corticosteroid. Used to treat a variety of allergic and inflammatory problems.

Deltasone (prednisone): corticosteroid. Used to treat a variety of allergic and inflammatory problems.

Demadex (torsemide): diuretic. Used to treat HTN, CHF, and fluid retention.

Demerol (meperidine): narcotic analgesic. Used to treat pain.

Demi-Regroton (chlorthalidone, reserpine): diuretic, anti-hypertensive agent. Used to treat HTN.

Demser (metyrosine): Used to treat pheochromocytoma.

Demulen (ethynodiol): oral contraceptive: used to treat menstrual disorders and to prevent pregnancy.

Depa (valproic acid): anticonvulsant. Used to treat epilepsy.

Depakene (valproic acid): anticonvulsant. Used to treat epilepsy.

Depakote (divaproex): anticonvulsant. Used to treat epilepsy.

Depen (penicillamine): chelator. Used to treat copper toxicity and severe rheumatoid arthritis.

Depo Provera (medroxyprogesterone): progestin. Used to treat menstrual disorders and cancer of the breast or uterus. Also used as a contraceptive.

Deponit (nitroglycerin): nitrate. Used to treat angina and CHF.

Deproic* (valproic acid): anticonvulsant. Used to treat epilepsy.

Deronil (dexamethasone): corticosteroid. Used to treat allergic and inflammatory conditions.

Desoxyn (methamphetamine): stimulant. Used to treat narcolepsy and ADD.

Desyrel (trazodone): antidepressant. Used to treat depression.

Detensol* (propranolol): beta blocker. Used to treat angina, HTN, and migraine headaches.

Dexadrine (dextroamphetamine): amphetamine. Used to treat ADD, narcolepsy, and obesity.

Dexasone (dexamethasone): corticosteroid. Used to treat allergic and inflammatory conditions.

Dexone (dexamethasone): corticosteroid. Used to treat allergic and inflammatory conditions.

DiaBeta (glyburide): anti-diabetic agent. Used to treat type II non-insulin-dependent diabetes mellitus.

Diabinese (chlorpropamide): anti-diabetic agent. Used to treat type II non-insulin-dependent diabetes mellitus.

Diachlor (chlorothiazide): thiazide diuretic. Used to treat HTN and fluid retention.

Dialose (docusate): laxative. Used to treat constipation.

Diamox (acetazolamide): carbonic anhydrase inhibitor. Used to treat glaucoma and CHF, and to prevent and treat acute high altitude sickness.

Diazemuls (diazepam): benzodiazepine. Used to treat anxiety, muscle spasm, and epilepsy.

Diazepam Intensol (diazepam): benzodiazepine. Used to treat anxiety, muscle spasm, epilepsy, insomnia, and symptoms of alcohol withdrawal.

Dibenzyline (phenoxybenzamine): antihypertensive agent. Used to treat pheochromocytoma.

Dicumarol (bishydroxycoumarin): anticoagulant. Used to treat blood-clotting disorders.

Didrex (benzphetamine): stimulant. Used to treat obesity.

Didronel (etidronate): anti-hypercalcemic agent. Used to treat bone disorders.

Diflucan (fluconazole): anti-fungal agent. Used to treat yeast infections.

Dilacor XR (diltiazem): calcium channel blocker. Used to treat angina pectoris and HTN.

Dilantin (phenytoin): anticonvulsant. Used to treat epilepsy and to control postoperative seizures.

Dilatrate-SR (isosorbide dinitrate): nitrate. Used to treat angina attacks.

Dilaudid (hydromorphone): narcotic analgestic. Used to treat severe pain.

Dilor (dyphylline): bronchodilator. Used to treat asthma and COPD.

Dilor-G (dyphylline, guaifenesin): bronchodilator, expectorant. Used to treat asthma and COPD.

Dimetane-DC Cough (brompheniramine, codeine, phenylpropanolamine): narcotic analgesic. Used to treat cold symptoms, especially cough.

Dimetane Expectorant-DC (brompheniramine, hydrocodone, phenylpropanolamine): antihistamine, narcotic analgesic, decongestant. Used to treat cold symptoms, especially cough.

Dimetapp-C (brompheniramine, codeine): narcotic analgesic. Used to treat cold symptoms, especially cough.

Diovan (valsartan): anti-hypertensive agent. Used to treat HTN.

Dipentum (olsalazine): anti-inflammatory. Used to treat inflammatory bowel disease.

Diphenhist (diphenhydramine): antihistamine. Used to treat motion sickness and allergic reactions.

Diphenylan sodium (phenytoin): anticonvulsant. Used to treat epilepsy and to control postoperative seizures

Disalcid (salsalate): analgesic. Used to treat pain, fever, and inflammation.

Ditropan (oxybutynin): anticholinergic. Used to treat urinary incontinence.

Diucardin (hydroflumethiazide): thiazide diuretic. Used to treat HTN and fluid retention.

Diuchlor-H* (hydrochlorothiazide): thiazide diuretic. Used to treat HTN and fluid retention.

Diulo (metolazone): thiazide diuretic. Used to treat HTN and fluid retention.

Diupres (chlorothiazide): thiazide diuretic. Used to treat HTN and fluid retention.

Diurese (trichlormethiazide): thiazide diuretic. Used to treat HTN and fluid retention.

Diurigen (chlorothiazide): thiazide diuretic. Used to treat HTN and fluid retention.

Diuril (chlorothiazide): thiazide diuretic. Used to treat HTN and fluid retention.

Diutensen (cryptenamine, methyclothiazide): diuretic. Used to treat HTN and fluid retention.

Diutensen-R (methyclothiazide, reserpine): thiazide diuretic, anti-hypertensive agent. Used to treat HTN.

Dixarit (clonidine): anti-hypertensive agent. Used to treat HTN.

Dizac (diazepam): benzodiazepine. Used to treat anxiety, muscle spasm, and epilepsy.

Dolene (propoxyphene): narcotic analgesic. Used to treat moderate to severe pain.

Dolobid (diflunisal): NSAID. Used to treat pain, fever, and inflammation.

Dolophine hydrochloride (methadone): narcotic analgesic. Used to treat pain and to aid in withdrawal from heroin or other narcotics.

Dopar (levodoapa): anti-parkinsonism agent. Used to treat Parkinson's disease.

Doral (quazepam): benzodiazepine. Used to treat insomnia.

Doryx (doxycycline): tetracycline. Used to treat numerous infections.

Dovonex (calcipotriene): vitamin D_3 analog. Used to treat psoriasis.

Doxidan (docusate): stimulant laxative. Used to treat constipation.

Doxychel (doxycycline hyclate): tetracycline. Used to treat numerous infections.

Dramamine (dimenhydrinate): antihistamine. Used to treat motion sickness.

Drixoral (dexbrompheniramine): antihistamine. Used to treat cold and seasonal allergy symptoms.

Dulcolax (bisacodyl): stimulant laxative. Used to treat constipation.

Duocet (acetaminophen, hydrocodone): narcotic analgesic. Used to treat moderate and severe pain.

Duo-Medihaler (isoproterenol, phenylephrine): sympathomimetic. Used to treat symptoms of cold and allergies.

Duotrate (pentaerythritol tetranitrate): nitrate. Used to treat angina pectoris.

Duract (bromfenac): NSAID. Used to treat pain.

Duradyne (acetaminophen, hydrocodone): narcotic analgesic. Used to treat moderate and severe pain.

Duragesic (fentanyl): narcotic analgesic. Used to treat chronic pain.

Duralith (lithium): tranquilizer. Used to treat manic depression and schizophrenia.

Duramorph (morphine): narcotic analgesic. Used to treat severe pain.

Durapam (flurazepam): benzodiazepine. Used to treat insomnia.

Duraquin (quinidine): anti-arrhythmic agent. Used to treat cardiac arrhythmias.

Duratuss (guaifenesin, hydrocodone, pseudoephedrine); expectorant, narcotic analgesic, decongestant. Used to treat cold symptoms, especially cough.

Duretic (methyclothiazide): anti-hypertensive agent. Used to treat HTN and edema.

Duricef (cefadroxil): antibiotic. Used to treat a variety of infections.

DV (dienestrol): female sex hormone. Used to treat gynecological disorders.

Dyazide (hydrochlorothiazide, triamterene): diuretic. Used to treat HTN and fluid retention.

Dycill (dicloxacillin): antibiotic. Used to treat general infections.

Dymelor (acetohexamide): anti-diabetic agent. Used to treat non-insulin-dependent diabetes mellitus.

DynaCirc (isradipine): calcium channel blocker. Used to treat HTN and angina pectoris.

Dynapen (dicloxacillin): antibiotic. Used to treat general infections.

Dyrenium (triamterene): diuretic. Used to treat HTN and fluid retention.

Dysne-Inhal* (epinephrine): sympathomimetic. Used to treat asthma attacks, allergic nasal congestion, glaucoma, and anaphylactic shock.

E-Mycin (erythromycin): antibiotic. Used to treat general infections.

Easprin (aspirin): analgesic. Used to treat mild pain.

Econopred (prednisolone): corticosteroid. Used to treat

361

a variety of allergic and inflammatory problems of the eye.

Ecotrin (aspirin): analgesic. Used to treat mild pain.

Edecrin (ethacrynic acid): diuretic. Used to treat fluid retention.

E.E.S. (erythromycin): antibiotic. Used to treat general infections.

Effexor (venlafaxine): antidepressant. Used to treat depression.

Elavil (amitriptyline): tricyclic antidepressant. Used to treat depression and some pain syndromes.

Eldepryl (selegiline): monoamine oxidase (MAO) inhibitor. Used to treat Parkinson's disease and Alzheimer's disease.

Elimite (permethrin): anti-parasitic agent. Used to treat lice and scabies.

Elixomin (theophylline): bronchodilator. Used to treat asthma and COPD.

Elixophyllin (theophylline): bronchodilator. Used to treat asthma and COPD.

Elocon (mometasone): corticosteroid. Used to treat skin disorders.

Eltroxin* (levothyroxine): thyroid hormone. Used to treat thyroid disorders.

Emadine (emedastine): antihistamine. Used to treat allergic conjunctivitis.

Emex* (metoclopramide): anti-emetic agent. Used to treat acid reflux and nausea and vomiting due to migraine headaches or cancer-fighting drugs.

Emitrip (amitriptyline): tricyclic antidepressant. Used to treat depression and some pain syndromes.

Emla (lidocaine, prilocaine): topical anesthetic. Used to treat skin irritation.

Empirin (aspirin): analgesic. Used to treat mild pain.

Empirin with codeine (aspirin, codeine): narcotic analgesic. Used to treat moderate to severe pain.

Empracet (acetaminophen, codeine): narcotic analgesic. Used to treat moderate to severe pain.

Emtec (acetaminophen, codeine): narcotic analgesic. Used to treat moderate to severe pain.

Endep (amitriptyline): tricyclic antidepressant. Used to treat depression and some pain syndromes.

Endocet* (acetaminophen, oxycodone): narcotic analgesic. Used to treat moderate to severe pain.

Endodan (aspirin, oxycodone): narcotic analgesic. Used to treat moderate to severe pain.

Enduron (methyclothiazide): thiazide diuretic, rauwolfia alkaloid. Used to treat HTN.

Enduronyl (methyclothiazide, deserpidine): thiazide diuretic, alkaloid. Used to treat HTN.

Enovid (mestranol, norethynodrel): oral contraceptive. Used to treat menstrual disorders and to prevent pregnancy.

Entex LA (phenylpropanolamine, guaifenesin): decongestant, expectorant. Used to treat symptoms of cold and seasonal allergies.

Entrophen (aspirin): analgesic. Used to treat mild pain.

E-Pam* (diazepam): benzodiazepine. Used to treat anxiety, muscle spasm, epilepsy, insomnia, and symptoms of alcohol withdrawal.

Ephed II (ephedrine): bronchodilator. Used to treat asthma and COPD.

Epifrin (epinephrine): sympathomimetic. Used to treat asthma attacks, allergic nasal congestion, glaucoma, and anaphylactic shock.

Epimorph* (morphine): narcotic analgesic. Used to treat severe pain.

Epipen (epinephrine): sympathomimetic. Used to treat anaphylactic shock.

Epitol (carbamazepine): anticonvulsant. Used to treat nerve pain, epilepsy, and some psychoses.

Epitrate (epinephrine): sympathomimetic. Used to treat

asthma attacks, allergic nasal congestion, glaucoma, and anaphylactic shock.

Epival* (valproic acid): anticonvulsant. Used to treat epilepsy.

Equagesic (aspirin, meprobamate): analgesic, tranquilizer. Used to treat anxiety, tension, and insomnia.

Equanil (meprobamate): tranquilizer. Used to treat anxiety.

Ercaf (caffeine, ergotamine): ergot preparation. Used to treat migraine headaches and narcolepsy.

Ergomar (ergotamine): ergot preparation. Used to treat migraine headaches and narcolepsy.

Ergostat (ergotamine): ergot preparation. Used to treat migraine headaches and narcolepsy.

ERYC (erythromycin): antibiotic. Used to treat general infections.

EryDerm (erythromycin): antibiotic. Used to treat general infections.

Erygel (erythromycin): antibiotic. Used to treat general infections.

Erypar (erythromycin): antibiotic. Used to treat general infections.

EryPed (erythromycin): antibiotic. Used to treat general infections.

Ery-Tab (erythromycin): antibiotic. Used to treat general infections.

Erythrocin stearate (erythromycin): antibiotic. Used to treat general infections.

Erythromid (erythromycin): antibiotic. Used to treat general infections.

Eryzole (erythromycin, sulfisoxazole): antibiotic. Used to treat a variety of infections.

Esgic (acetaminophen, butalbital, caffeine): analgesic, barbiturate. Used to treat pain and tension headaches.

Esgic with codeine (acetaminophen, butalbital, caffeine, codeine): narcotic analgesic, barbiturate. Used to treat pain and tension headaches.

Esidrix (hydrochlorothiazide): thiazide diuretic. Used to treat HTN and fluid retention.

Esimil (guanethidine, hydrochlorothiazide): anti-hypertensive agent, thiazide diuretic. Used to treat HTN.

Eskalith (lithium): tranquilizer. Used to treat manic depression and schizophrenia.

Estinyl (estrogen): female sex hormone. Used to treat gynecological disorders.

Estrace (estrogen): female sex hormone. Used to treat gynecological disorders.

Estraderm (estrogen): female sex hormone. Used to treat gynecological disorders.

Estraguard (estrogen): female sex hormone. Used to treat gynecological disorders.

Estratab (estrogen): female sex hormone. Used to treat gynecological disorders.

Estrovis (estrogen): female sex hormone. Used to treat gynecological disorders.

Ethatab (ethaverine): vasodilator. Used to treat GI tract spasm.

Ethmozine (moricizine): anti-arrhythmic agent. Used to treat ventricular tachycardia.

Etrafon (amitriptyline, perphenazine): antidepressant, tranquilizer. Used to treat nausea, vomiting, and depression.

Euflex Used to treat prostate cancer.

Euglucon (glyburide): anti-diabetic agent. Used to treat type II non-insulin-dependent diabetes mellitus.

Eulexin (flutamide): Used to treat prostate cancer.

Euthroid (levothyroxine, liothyronine): thyroid hormone. Used to treat thyroid disorders.

Evista (raloxifene): estrogen receptor modulator. Used to prevent osteoporosis in post-menopausal women.

Excedrin (acetaminophen, aspirin, caffeine): analgesic. Used to treat mild pain.

Excedrin P.M. (acetaminophen, diphenhydramine): analgesic, antihistamine. Used to treat mild pain.

Exdol (acetaminophen, caffeine, codeine): narcotic analgesic. Used to treat moderate to severe pain.

Exna (benzthiazide): thiazide diuretic. Used to treat HTN and fluid retention.

Famvir (famciclovir): anti-viral agent. Used to treat shingles (acute herpes zoster).

Fansidar (pyrimethamine, sulfadoxine): anti-protozoal agent. Used to treat and prevent malaria.

Felbatol (felbamate): anticonvulsant. Used to treat seizure disorders.

Feldene (piroxicam): NSAID. Used to treat pain, fever, and inflammation.

Femara (letrozole): aromatase inhibitor. Used to treat breast cancer in post-menopausal women.

Femazole (metronidazole): anti-infective agent. Used to treat various infections of the vaginal canal, cervix, male urethra, and intestines.

Femcet (acetaminophen, butalbital, caffeine): analgesic, barbiturate. Used to treat pain and tension headaches.

Feminone (estrogen): female sex hormone. Used to treat gynecological disorders.

Femogen (estrogen): female sex hormone. Used to treat gynecological disorders and osteoporosis.

Femogex (estrogen): female sex hormone. Used to treat gynecological disorders.

Fenicol* (chloramphenicol): antibiotic. Used to treat life-threatening infections.

Feosol (ferrous sulfate): iron salt. Used to treat anemia.

Fergon (ferrous sulfate): iron salt. Used to treat anemia.

Fevernol (acetaminophen): analgesic. Used to treat mild to moderate pain.

Fioricet (acetaminophen, butalbital, caffeine): analgesic, barbiturate. Used to treat pain and tension headaches.

Fiorinal (aspirin, butalbital, caffeine): analgesic, barbiturate. Used to treat pain and tension headaches.

Fiorinal with codeine (acetaminophen, butalbital, caffeine, codeine): narcotic analgesic, barbiturate. Used to treat pain and tension headaches.

Flagyl (metronidazole): anti-infective agent. Used to treat various infections of the vaginal canal, cervix, male urethra, and intestines.

Flexeril (cyclobenzaprine): muscle relaxant. Used to treat muscle spasm.

Flomax (tamsulosin): adrenergic blocker. Used to treat benign prostatic hyperplasia (enlarged prostate).

Floropryl (isoflurophate): anti-glaucoma agent. Used to treat glaucoma.

Floxin (ofloxacin): anti-infective agent. Used to treat general infections.

Flumadine (rimantadine): anti-viral agent. Used to treat and prevent influenza A infections.

Folex (methotrexate): antineoplastic agent. Used to treat acute lymphocytic leukemia, cancer, severe psoriasis, and severe rheumatoid arthritis.

Fortaz (ceftazidime): antibiotic. Used to treat a wide variety of infections.

Fulvicin (griseofulvin): anti-fungal agent. Used to treat ringworm (tinea) infections.

Furadantin (nitrofurantoin): anti-infective agent. Used to treat UTIs.

Furalan (nitrofurantoin): antibiotic. Used to treat UTIs.

Furanite (nitrofurantoin): antibiotic. Used to treat UTIs.

Furoside (furosemide): diuretic. Used to treat HTN and fluid retention.

Gabitril (tiagabine): anticonvulsant. Used to treat partial seizures.

Gantanol (sulfamethoxazole): antibiotic. Used to treat UTIs.

Gantrisin (sulfisoxazole): antibiotic. Used to treat a variety of infections.

Gardenal (phenobarbital): barbiturate. Used to treat anxiety, nervous tension, insomnia, and epilepsy.

Gastrocrom (cromolyn): asthma preventive. Used to prevent allergic reactions and asthma attacks.

Gemnisyn (acetaminophen, aspirin): analgesic. Used to treat mild to moderate pain.

Genahist (diphenhydramine): antihistamine. Used to treat motion sickness and allergic reactions.

Genora (norethindrone, mestranol): oral contraceptive. Used to treat menstrual disorders and to prevent pregnancy.

Geocillin (carbenicillin): antibiotic. Used to treat infections.

Glaucon (epinephrine): sympathomimetic. Used to treat asthma attacks, allergic nasal congestion, glaucoma, and anaphylactic shock.

Glucophage (metformin): anti-diabetic agent. Used to treat non-insulin-dependent diabetes mellitus.

Glucotrol (glipizide): anti-diabetic agent. Used to treat type II non-insulin-dependent diabetes mellitus.

Glynase (glyburide): anti-diabetic agent. Used to treat type II non-insulin-dependent diabetes mellitus.

Grifulvin V (griseofulvin): anti-fungal agent. Used to treat ringworm (tinea) infections.

Grisactin (griseofulvin): anti-fungal agent. Used to treat ringworm (tinea) infections.

Grisovin FP (griseofulvin): anti-fungal agent. Used to treat ringworm (tinea) infections.

Grisp-PEG (griseofulvin): anti-fungal agent. Used to treat ringworm (tinea) infections.

Guaifed (guaifenesin, pseudoephedrine): expectorant, decongestant. Used to treat cold and seasonal allergy symptoms.

Gyne-Lotrimin (clotrimazole): anti fungal agent. Used to treat vaginal yeast infections.

Gynergen* (ergotamine): ergot preparation. Used to treat migraine headaches and narcolepsy.

Habitrol (nicotine): smoking cessation aid. Used to help people quit smoking.

Halcion (triazolam): benzodiazepine. Used to treat insomnia.

Haldol (haloperidol): anti-psychotic agent. Used to treat schizophrenia, acute psychosis, and Tourette's syndrome.

Halfprin (aspirin): analgestic. Used to treat mild pain.

Halperon (haloperidol): anti-psychotic agent. Used to treat schizophrenia, acute psychosis, and Tourette's syndrome.

Haltran (ibuprofen): NSAID. Used to treat pain, fever, and inflammation.

Hexadrol (dexamethasone): corticosteroid. Used to treat allergic and inflammatory conditions.

Hismanal (astemizole): antihistamine. Used to treat seasonal allergy symptoms and hives.

HIVID (zalcitabine): anti-viral agent. Used to treat advanced HIV infection.

Humorsol (demecarium): anti-glaucoma agent. Used to treat glaucoma.

Humulin (insulin): anti-diabetic agent. Used to treat insulin-dependent diabetes mellitus

Hycodan (homatropine, hydrocodone): narcotic analgesic. Used to treat cold symptoms, especially cough.

Hycomine Compound (acetaminophen, caffeine, chlorpheniramine, hydrocodone, phenylephrine): narcotic analgesic. Used to treat pain and to control cough.

Hycomine-S (ammonium chloride, hydrocodone,

phenylephrine, pyrilamine): narcotic analgesic. Used to treat cold symptoms, especially cough.

Hycomine syrup (hydrocodone, phenylpropanolamine): narcotic analgesic, decongestant. Used to treat cold symptoms, especially cough.

Hycotuss expectorant (guaifenesin, hydrocodone): expectorant, narcotic analgesic. Used to treat cold symptoms, especially cough.

Hydergine (ergoloid mesylate): ergot preparation. Used to treat confusion, depression, and reduced alertness in the elderly.

Hydrex (benzthiazide): thiazide diuretic. Used to treat HTN and fluid retention.

Hydrocet (acetaminophen, hydrocodone): narcotic analgesic. Used to treat moderate to severe pain.

Hydro-Chlor (hydrochlorothiazide): thiazide diuretic. Used to treat HTN and fluid retention.

HydroDIURIL (hydrochlorothiazide): thiazide diuretic. Used to treat HTN and fluid retention.

Hydromox (quinethazone): thiazide diuretic. Used to treat HTN and fluid retention.

Hydromox R (quinethazone, reserpine): thiazide diuretic, antihypertensive. Used to treat HTN.

Hydropres (hydrochlorothiazide, reserpine): thiazide diuretic, antihypertensive. Used to treat HTN.

Hydro Z (hydrochlorothiazide): thiazide diuretic. Used to treat HTN and fluid retention.

Hygroton (chlorthalidone): thiazide diuretic. Used to treat HTN and fluid retention.

Hylidone (chlorthalidone): thiazide diuretic. Used to treat HTN and fluid retention.

Hylorel (guanadrel): anti-hypertensive agent. Used to treat HTN.

Hytrin (terazosin): anti-hypertensive agent. Used to treat HTN and benign prostatic hyperplasia.

Hyzaar (hydrochlorothiazide, losartan): thiazide diuretic, anti-hypertensive agent. Used to treat HTN.

Ibuprohm (ibuprofen): NSAID. Used to treat pain, fever, and inflammation.

Ibu-Tab (ibuprofen): NSAID. Used to treat pain, fever, and inflammation.

Iletin II NPH (insulin): anti-diabetic agent. Used to treat insulin-dependent diabetes mellitus and gestational diabetes.

Ilosone (erythromycin): antibiotic. Used to treat general infections.

Ilotycin (erythromycin): antibiotic. Used to treat general infections.

Imdur (isosorbide mononitrate): nitrate. Used to prevent attacks of angina pectoris.

Imitrex (sumatriptan): anti-migraine agent. Used to treat migraine and cluster headaches.

Imodium (loperamide): anti-diarrheal agent. Used to treat diarrhea.

Imodium A-D (loperamide): anti-diarrheal agent. Used to treat diarrhea.

Imuran (azathioprine): anti-arthritic agent, immunosuppressant. Used to prevent rejection of transplanted organs and to treat severe rheumatoid arthritis.

Inapsine (droperidol): anti-emetic agent; tranquilizer. Used to treat nausea and vomiting and for chemical restraint.

Indameth* (indomethacin): NSAID. Used to treat pain, fever, and inflammation.

Inderal (propranolol): beta blocker. Used to treat angina, HTN, and migraine headaches.

Inderide (hydrochlorothiazide, propranolol): thiazide diuretic, beta blocker. Used to treat HTN.

Indochron E-R (indomethacin): NSAID. Used to treat pain, fever, and inflammation.

Indocid (indomethacin): NSAID. Used to treat pain, fever, and inflammation.

Indocin (indomethacin): NSAID. Used to treat pain, fever, and inflammation.

Infergen (interferon alfacon-1): interferon. Used to treat hepatitis C.

Inflamase (prednisolone): corticosteroid. Used to treat a variety of allergic and inflammatory problems.

Initard (insulin): anti-diabetic agent. Used to treat insulin-dependent diabetes mellitus and gestational diabetes.

Insomnal (diphenhydramine): antihistamine. Used to treat motion sickness and allergic reactions.

Insulatard NPH (insulin): anti-diabetic agent. Used to treat insulin-dependent diabetes mellitus.

Intal (cromolyn): asthma preventive. Used to prevent allergic reactions and asthma attacks.

Inversine (mecamylamine): anti-hypertensive agent. Used to treat hypertension.

Ipran (propranolol): beta blocker. Used to treat angina, HTN, and migraine headaches.

Ismelin (gaunethidine): anti-hypertensive agent. Used to treat HTN.

Ismelin-Esidrix (guanethidine, hydrochlorothiazide): anti-hypertensive agent, thiazide diuretic. Used to treat HTN.

Ismo (isosorbide mononitrate): nitrate. Used to prevent attacks of angina pectoris.

Iso-Bid (isosorbide dinitrate): nitrate. Used to treat angina and to prevent future attacks.

Isoclor expectorant (codeine, guaifenesin, pseudo-ephedrine, alcohol): narcotic, expectorant. Used to treat cold symptoms, especially cough.

Isodil (isosorbide dinitrate): nitrate. Used to treat angina and to prevent future attacks.

Isonate (isosorbide dinitrate): nitrate. Used to treat angina and to prevent future attacks.

Isoptin (verapamil): calcium channel blocker. Used to treat angina, arrhythmias, and HTN.

Isopto Carpine (pilocarpine): anti-glaucoma agent. Used to treat glaucoma.

Isopto Fenicol (chloramphenicol): antibiotic. Used to treat life-threatening infections.

Isordil (isosorbide dinitrate): nitrate. Used to treat angina and to prevent future attacks.

Isordil Tembids (isosorbide dinitrate): nitrate. Used to treat angina and to prevent future attacks.

Isordil Titradose (isosorbide dinitrate): nitrate. Used to treat angina and to prevent future attacks.

Isotamine (isoniazid): anti-tubercular agent. Used to treat and prevent tuberculosis.

Isuprel (isoproterenol): sympathomimetic. Used to treat asthma and COPD.

K-Dur (potassium chloride): potassium supplement. Used to treat hypokalemia.

K-Lor (potassium chloride): potassium supplement. Used to treat hypokalemia.

K-Lyte (potassium chloride): potassium supplement. Used to treat hypokalemia.

K-Norm (potassium): potassium supplement. Used to treat hypokalemia.

K-Tab (potassium chloride): potassium supplement. Used to treat hypokalemia.

Kaon-CI (potassium chloride): potassium supplement. Used to treat hypokalemia.

Kaopectate (kaolin, pectin): anti-diarrhea agent. Used to treat diarrhea.

Kay Ciel (potassium chloride): potassium supplement. Used to treat hypokalemia.

Keflet (cephalexin): antibiotic. Used to treat a variety of infections.

Keflex (cephalexin): antibiotic. Used to treat a variety of infections.

Keftab (cephalexin): antibiotic. Used to treat infections.

Kefurox (cefuroxime): antibiotic. Used to treat infections of the ear, skin, respiratory tract, and urinary tract.

Kemadrin (procyclidine): anti-parkinsonism agent. Used to treat Parkinson's disease.

Kenacort (triamcinolone): corticosteroid. Used to treat asthma and other inflammatory problems.

Kenalog (triamcinolone): corticosteroid. Used to treat asthma and other inflammatory problems.

Kerlone (betaxolol): beta blocker. Used to treat HTN and glaucoma (eye drops).

Kinesed (atropine, phenobarbital): barbiturate. Used to treat anxiety, nervous tension, insomnia, and epilepsy.

Klonopin (clonazepam): benzodiazepine. Used to treat epilepsy, panic disorders, and anxiety.

Klor-Con (potassium chloride): potassium supplement. Used to treat hypokalemia.

Klotrix (potassium chloride): potassium supplement. Used to treat hypokalemia.

Kolyum (potassium chloride): potassium supplement. Used to treat hypokalemia.

Korvess (potassium chloride): potassium supplement. Used to treat hypokalemia.

Kwell (lindane): anti-parasitic agent. Used to treat scabies and lice.

Lamictal (lamotrigine): anti-epileptic agent. Used to treat seizures.

Laniazide (isoniazid): anti-tubercular agent. Used to treat and prevent tuberculosis.

Lanoxicaps (digoxin): digitalis preparation. Used to treat CHF and arrhythmias.

Lanoxin (digoxin): digitalis preparation. Used to treat CHF and arrhythmias.

Larodopa (levodopa): anti-parkinsonism agent. Used to treat Parkinson's disease.

Larotid (amoxicillin): antibiotic. Used to treat general infections.

Lasix (furosemide): diuretic. Used to treat HTN and fluid retention.

Ledercilin VK (penicillin V): antibiotic. Used to treat respiratory tract, middle ear, and skin infections.

Lenoltec with codeine (acetaminophen, caffeine, codeine): narcotic analgesic. Used to treat moderate to severe pain.

Lente Iletin I (insulin): anti-diabetic agent. Used to treat insulin-dependent diabetes mellitus.

Lente Iletin II (beef) (insulin): anti-diabetic agent. Used to treat insulin-dependent diabetes.

Lente Iletin III (pork) (insulin): anti-diabetic agent. Used to treat insulin-dependent diabetes.

Lente Insulin (insulin): anti-diabetic agent. Used to treat insulin-dependent diabetes.

Lescol (fluvastatin): anti-cholesterol agent. Used to treat high cholesterol.

Leukeran (chlorambucil): immunosuppressant. Used to treat cancer and to prevent organ transplant rejection.

Levate* (amitriptyline): tricyclic antidepressant. Used to treat depression and some pain syndromes.

Levatol (penbutolol): beta blocker. Used to treat HTN and panic attacks and to prevent recurrent angina.

Levlen (estrogen): oral contraceptive. Used to treat menstrual disorders and to prevent pregnancy.

Levo-Dromoran (levorphanol): narcotic analgesic. Used to treat moderate to severe pain.

Levorphan (levorphanol): narcotic analgesic. Used to treat moderate to severe pain.

Levothroid (levothyroxine): thyroid hormone. Used to treat thyroid disorders.

Levoxine (levothyroxine): thyroid hormone. Used to treat thyroid disorders.

Levsin (hyoscyamine): belladonna alkaloid. Used to treat GI problems.

Librax (chlordiazepoxide, clidinium): benzodiazepine, anticholinergic. Used to treat tension, nervousness, and spasms of the GI or genitourinary tract.

Libritabs (chlordiazepoxide): benzodiazepine. Used to treat anxiety and alcohol withdrawal.

Librium (chlordiazepoxide): benzodiazepine. Used to treat anxiety and alcohol withdrawal.

Lidex (fluocinolone): corticosteroid. Used to treat allergic and inflammatory conditions of the skin.

Limbitrol (amitriptyline, chlordiazepoxide): tricyclic antidepressant, benzodiazepine. Used to treat depression and anxiety.

Lipitor (atorvastatin calcium): anti-cholesterol agent. Used to treat high cholesterol.

Lithane (lithium): tranquilizer. Used to treat manic depression and schizophrenia.

Lithizine* (lithium): tranquilizer. Used to treat manic depression and schizophrenia.

Lithobid (lithium): tranquilizer. Used to treat manic depression and schizophrenia.

Lithonate (lithium): tranquilizer. Used to treat manic depression and schizophrenia.

Lithotabs (lithium): tranquilizer. Used to treat manic depression and schizophrenia.

Lodine (etodolac): NSAID. Used to treat pain, fever, arthritis, and inflammation.

Lodrane (theophylline): bronchodilator. Used to treat asthma and COPD.

Loestrin: oral contraceptive. Used to treat menstrual disorders and to prevent pregnancy.

Loestrin Fe: iron, oral contraceptive. Used to treat menstrual disorders and to prevent pregnancy.

Lomotil (atropine, diphenoxylate): anti-diarrheal. Used to treat diarrhea and intestinal cramps.

Loniten (minoxidil): anti-hypertensive agent. Used to treat HTN that does not respond to standard therapy. Also used to treat male-pattern baldness.

Lo/Ovral (estrogen): oral contraceptive. Used to treat menstrual disorders and to prevent pregnancy.

Lopid (gemfibrozil): anti-cholesterol agent. Used to reduce high cholesterol.

Lopressor (metoprolol): beta blocker. Used to treat HTN and angina pectoris.

Lopressor HCT (hydrochlorothiazide, metoprolol): diuretic, beta blocker. Used to treat HTN and angina.

Lopurin* (allopurinol): anti-gout agent. Used to treat gout and prevent gout attacks.

Lorazepam Intensol (lorazepam): benzodiazepine. Used to treat anxiety and insomnia.

Lorcet (acetaminophen, hydrocodone): analgesic. Used to treat moderate to severe pain.

Lorelco (probucol): anti-cholesterol agent. Used to treat high blood levels of cholesterol.

Lortab (acetaminophen, hydrocodone): narcotic analgesic. Used to treat moderate to severe pain.

Lortab ASA (aspirin, hydrocodone): narcotic analgesic. Used to treat moderate to severe pain.

Losec (omeprazole): anti-ulcer agent. Used to treat GI disorders.

Lotensin (benazepril): ACE inhibitor. Used to treat HTN.

Lotrel (benazepril, amlodipine): ACE inhibitor, calcium channel blocker. Used to treat HTN.

Lotrimin (clotrimazole): anti-fungal agent. Used to treat yeast and ringworm infections.

Lotrisone (betamethasone, clotrimazole): corticosteroid, antifungal. Used to treat yeast and ringworm infections.

Loxitane (loxapine): anti-psychotic agent. Used to treat schizophrenia and psychotic disorders.

Lozol (indapamide): diuretic. Used to treat HTN and CHF.

Ludiomil (maprotiline): antidepressant. Used to treat depression, eating disorders, and bed-wetting.

Lufyllin (dyphylline): brochodilator. Used to treat asthma and COPD.

Luminal (phenobarbital): barbiturate. Used to treat anxiety, nervous tension, insomnia, and epilepsy.

Luvox (fluvoxamine): antidepressant. Used to treat obsessive-compulsive disorder.

Macrobid (nitrofurantoin): anti-infective agent. Used to treat UTIs.

Macrodantin (nitrofurantoin): anti-infective agent. Used to treat UTIs.

Magan (magnesium salicylate): NSAID. Used to treat pain, fever, and inflammation.

Magonate (magnesium gluconate): magnesium supplement. Used to treat hypomagnesemia and preeclampsia.

Mandelamine (methenamine): antibiotic. Used to treat bladder and kidney infections.

Marax (ephedrine, hydroxyzine, theophylline): sympathomimetic, antihistamine, bronchodilator. Used to treat asthma and COPD.

Marinol (dronabinol): anti-emetic agent. Used to treat AIDS-related anorexia and chemotherapy-induced emesis.

Marplan (isocarboxazid): MAO inhibitor. Used to treat depression and anxiety.

Maxair (pirbuterol): bronchodilator. Used to treat asthma and COPD.

Maxidex (dexamethasone): corticosteroid. Used to treat allergic and inflammatory conditions.

Maxolon (metoclopramide): anti-emetic agent. Used to treat nausea and vomiting due to migraine headaches or cancer-fighting drugs.

Maxzide (hydrochlorothiazide, triamterene): diuretic. Used to treat HTN and fluid retention.

Mazepine (carbamazepine): anticonvulsant. Used to treat nerve pain and epilepsy.

Measurin (aspirin): analgesic. Used to treat pain.

Mebaral (mephobarbital): barbiturate. Used to treat anxiety and seizures.

Meclodium (meclofenamate): NSAID. Used to treat pain, fever, and inflammation.

Meclomen (meclofenamate): NSAID. Used to treat pain, fever, and inflammation.

Medicycline (tetracycline): antibiotic. Used to treat a variety of infections.

Medihaler-Epi (epinephrine): sympathomimetic. Used to treat asthma attacks and allergies.

Medipren (ibuprofen): NSAID. Used to treat pain, fever, and inflammation.

Medrol (methylprednisolone): corticosteroid. Used to treat a variety of allergic and inflammatory problems.

Mefoxin (cefoxitin): antibiotic. Used to treat general infections.

Megace (megestrol): synthetic female hormone. Used to treat breast or uterine cancer.

Mellaril (thioridazine): phenothiazine. Used to treat depression, agitation, and anxiety.

Menest (estrogen): female sex hormone. Used to treat gynecological disorders.

Menrium (chlordiazepoxide, estrogen): female sex hormone. Used to treat gynecological disorders.

Mepergan (meperidine, promethazine): narcotic analgesic, anti-emetic agent. Used to treat moderate to severe pain and to control nausea and vomiting.

Mepron (atovaquone): anti-protozoal agent. Used to treat *Pneumocystis carinii* pneumonia and toxoplasmosis.

Meprospan (meprobamate): tranquilizer. Used to treat anxiety.

Meridia (sibutramine): weight loss agent. Used to treat obesity.

Mesantoin (mephenytoin): anticonvulsant. Used to treat epilepsy.

Mestinon (pyridostigmine): anti-myasthenic agent. Used to treat myasthenia gravis.

Metahydrin (trichlormethiazide): thiazide diuretic. Used to treat HTN and fluid retention.

Metaprel (metaproterenol): beta blocker. Used to treat asthma and COPD.

Metastron (strontium): radioisotope. Used to treat bone cancer pain.

Metatensin (reserpine, trichlormethiazide): thiazide diuretic, anti-hypertensive agent. Used to treat HTN.

Methergine (methylergonovine): ergot alkaloid. Used to treat breast cancer and primary hypogonadism.

Meticorten (prednisone): corticosteroid. Used to treat allergic and inflammatory problems, including asthma, colitis, bursitis, tendonitis, and arthritis.

Metizol (metronidazole): anti-infective agent. Used to treat various infections of the vaginal canal, cervix, male urethra, and intestines.

MetroGel (metronidazole): anti-infective agent. Used to treat various infections of the vaginal canal, cervix, male urethra, and intestines.

Metryl (metronidazole): anti-infective agent. Used to treat various infections of the vaginal canal, cervix, male urethra, and intestines.

Mevacor (lovastatin): anti-cholesterol agent. Used to treat high blood levels of cholesterol.

Meval (diazepam): benzodiazepine. Used to treat anxiety, muscle spasm, epilepsy, insomnia, and symptoms of alcohol withdrawal.

Mexate (methotrexate): antineoplastic agent. Used to treat acute lymphocytic leukemia and cancer.

Mexitil (mexiletine): anti-arrhythmic agent. Used to treat cardiac arrhythmias.

Micro-K (potassium chloride): potassium supplement. Used to treat hypokalemia.

Micronase (glyburide): anti-diabetic agent. Used to treat type II non-insulin-dependent diabetes .

Micronor oral contraceptive. Used to treat menstrual disorders and to prevent pregnancy.

Microsulfon (sulfadiazine): antibiotic. Used to treat urinary tract infections.

Midamor (amiloride): diuretic. Used to treat HTN and excessive fluid retention.

Midol (aspirin, caffeine): analgesic. Used to treat mild pain.

Midol PMS (acetaminophen, pamabrom, pyrilamine): analgesic, antihistamine. Used to treat moderate pain.

Midol 200 (ibuprofen): NSAID. Used to treat pain, fever, and inflammation.

Millazine (thioridazine): phenothiazine. Used to treat depression, agitation, and anxiety.

Milontin (phensuximide): anticonvulsant. Used to treat seizure disorders.

Miltown (meprobamate): tranquilizer. Used to treat anxiety.

Minestrin: oral contraceptive. Used to treat menstrual disorders and to prevent pregnancy.

Minims* (pilocarpine): anti-glaucoma agent. Used to treat glaucoma.

Minipress (prazosin): anti-hypertensive agent. Used to treat HTN and CHF.

Minitran (nitroglycerin): nitrate. Used to treat or prevent angina.

Minizide (polythiazide, prazosin): thiazide diuretic, anti-hypertensive agent. Used to treat HTN.

Minocin (minocycline): antibiotic. Used to treat general infections.

Minodyl (minoxidil): anti-hypertensive agent. Used to treat HTN and male-pattern baldness.

Miocarpine* (pilocarpine): anti-glaucoma agent. Used to treat glaucoma.

Mirapex (pramipexole): anti-parkinsonism agent. Used to treat Parkinson's disease.

Mixtard (insulin): anti-diabetic agent. Used to treat insulin-dependent diabetes mellitus.

Moban (molindone): anti-psychotic agent. Used to treat schizophrenia and depression.

Mobenol* (tolbutamide): anti-diabetic agent. Used to treat type II non-insulin-dependent diabetes mellitus.

Modecate* (fluphenazine): phenothiazine. Used to treat schizophrenia.

Modicon (estrogen, progestin): oral contraceptive. Used to treat menstrual disorders and to prevent pregnancy.

Moditen* (fluphenazine): phenothiazine. Used to treat schizophrenia.

Moduret (amiloride, hydrochlorothiazide): diuretic. Used to treat HTN and excessive fluid retention.

Moduretic (amiloride, hydrochlorothiazide): diuretic. Used to treat HTN and fluid retention.

Monistat 7 (miconazole): antifungal agent. Used to treat vaginal fungal infections.

Monitan* (acebutolol): Used to treat HTN and to prevent premature ventricular contractions.

Mono-Gesic (salsalate): analgesic. Used to treat pain, fever, and inflammation.

Monoclate-P (factor VIII): anti-hemophilic agent. Used to treat hemophilia.

Monoket (isosorbide mononitrate): nitrate. Used to prevent attacks of angina pectoris.

Monopril (fosinopril): ACE inhibitor. Used to treat HTN and CHF.

Morphine HP (morphine): narcotic analgesic. Used to treat severe pain.

Morphitec* (morphine): narcotic analgesic. Used to treat severe pain.

M.O.S.* (morphine): narcotic analgesic. Used to treat severe pain.

Motofen (atropine, difenoxin): anti-diarrheal agent. Used to treat severe diarrhea.

Motrin (ibuprofen): NSAID. Used to treat pain, fever, and inflammation.

MS Contin (morphine): narcotic analgesic. Used to treat severe pain.

MSIR (morphine): narcotic analgesic. Used to treat severe pain.

Mudrane GG Elixir (ephedrine, phenobarbital, theophylline, quafenesin): expectorant, bronchodilator. Used to treat asthma and COPD.

Mudrane GG Tablets (aminophylline, ephedrine, phenobarbital, quafenesin): bronchodilator, sympathomimetic, barbiturate. Used to treat asthma and COPD.

Myambutol (ethambutol): anti-infective agent. Used to treat pulmonary tuberculosis.

Mycelex (clotrimazole): anti-fungal agent. Used to treat vaginal yeast infections.

Myclo* (clotrimazole): anti fungal agent. Used to treat yeast and ringworm infections.

Mycobutin (rifabutin): anti-tubercular agent. Used to prevent the spread of a tuberculosis-like infection in HIV-infected patients.

Mycolog II (nystatin, triamcinolone): anti-fungal agent, corticosteroid. Used to treat fungal infections.

Mycostatin (nystatin): anti-fungal agent. Used to treat fungal infections of the mouth, throat, and intestines.

Myidone (primidone): anticonvulsant. Used to treat grand mal and partial seizures.

Mykrox (metolazone): thiazide diuretic. Used to treat HTN and fluid retention.

Mysoline (primidone): anticonvulsant. Used to treat grand mal and partial seizures.

Nadopen-V (penicillin): antibiotic. Used to treat respiratory tract, middle ear, and skin infections.

Naftin (naftidine): anti-fungal. Used to treat fungal infections.

Nalcrom (cromolyn): asthma preventive. Used to prevent allergic reactions and asthma attacks.

Naldecon CX (codeine, guaifenesin, phenylpropanolamine): cold remedy. Used to treat cold symptoms, especially cough.

Nalfon (fenoprofen): NSAID. Used to treat pain, fever, and inflammation.

Napamide (disopyramide): anti-arrhythmic agent. Used to treat cardiac arrhythmias.

Naprosyn (naproxen): NSAID. Used to treat pain, fever, and inflammation.

Naqua (trichlormethiazide): thiazide diuretic. Used to treat HTN and fluid retention.

Naquival (reserpine, trichlormethiazide): anti-hypertensive agent, diuretic. Used to treat HTN.

Nardil (phenelzine): MAO inhibitor. Used to treat severe depression.

Nasacort (triamcinolone): corticosteroid. Used to treat asthma and other inflammatory problems.

Nasalcrom (cromolyn): asthma preventive. Used to prevent allergic reactions and asthma attacks.

Nasalide (flunisolide): corticosteroid. Used to treat asthma and allergic rhinitis.

Natrimax* (hydrochlorothiazide): thiazide diuretic. Used to treat HTN and fluid retention.

Naturetin (bendroflumethiazide): thiazide diuretic. Used to treat HTN and fluid retention.

Navane (thiothixene): tranquilizer. Used to treat agitation, psychosis, and schizophrenia.

Naxen* (naproxen): NSAID. Used to treat pain, fever, and inflammation.

NebuPent (pentamidine): anti-infective agent. Used to treat and prevent *Pneumocystis carinii* pneumonia.

Nelova (estrogen and progestin) oral contraceptives. Used to treat menstrual disorders and to prevent pregnancy.

Nembutal (pentobarbital): barbiturate. Used to treat insomnia.

Neo-Codema* (hydrochlorothiazide): thiazide diuretic. Used to treat HTN and fluid retention.

Neosar (cyclophosphamide): immunosuppressant. Used to treat cancer and severe rheumatoid arthritis.

Neosporin ointment (bacitracin, neomycin, polymyxin): topical antibiotic. Used to treat skin and eye infections.

Neo-Tetrine* (tetracycline): antibiotic. Used to treat severe acne and gum disease.

Neothylline-GG (dyphylline, guaifenesin): bronchodilator, expectorant. Used to treat asthma and COPD.

Nephronex* (nitrofurantoin): anti-infective agent. Used to treat UTIs.

Neptazane (methazolamide): anti-glaucoma agent. Used to treat glaucoma.

Neumega (oprelvekin): Used to treat chemotherapy-induced thrombocytopenia.

Neurontin (gabapentin): anticonvulsant. Used to treat epilepsy.

Neuro-Spasex (homatropine, phenobarbital): barbiturate. Used to treat anxiety, nervous tension, insomnia, and epilepsy.

NeuTrexin (trimetrexate): Used to treat *Pneumocystis carinii* pneumonia.

Nia-Bid (niacin): vitamin B_3. Used to treat high blood levels of cholesterol and vitamin B_3 deficiency.

Niac (niacin): vitamin B_3. Used to treat high blood levels of cholesterol and vitamin B_3 deficiency.

Niacels (niacin): vitamin B_3. Used to treat high blood levels of cholesterol and vitamin B_3 deficiency.

Nicobid (niacin): vitamin B_3. Used to treat high blood levels of cholesterol and vitamin B_3 deficiency.

Nicoderm (nicotine): smoking cessation aid. Used to help people quit smoking.

Nico-400 (niacin): vitamin B_3. Used to treat high blood levels of cholesterol and vitamin B_3 deficiency.

Nicolar (niacin): vitamin B_3. Used to treat high blood levels of cholesterol and vitamin B_3 deficiency.

Nicorette (nicotine): smoking cessation aid. Used to help people quit smoking.

Nicotinex (niacin): vitamin B_3. Used to treat high blood levels of cholesterol and vitamin B_3 deficiency.

Nicotrol (nicotine): smoking cessation aid. Used to help people quit smoking.

Nilstat (nystatin): anti-fungal agent. Used to treat fungal infections of the mouth, throat, and intestines.

Nimotop (nimodipine): calcium channel blocker. Used to treat migraines and the neurological effects of stroke.

Nisentil (alphaprodine): analgesic. Used to provide short-term analgesia.

Nitro-Bid (nitroglycerin): nitrate. Used to treat angina and CHF.

Nitrocap (nitroglycerin): nitrate. Used to treat angina and CHF.

Nitrocine (nitroglycerin): nitrate. Used to treat angina pectoris and CHF.

Nitrodisc (nitroglycerin): nitrate. Used to treat angina pectoris and CHF.

Nitro-Dur (nitroglycerin): nitrate. Used to treat angina pectoris and CHF.

Nitrogard (nitroglycerin): nitrate. Used to treat angina pectoris and CHF.

Nitroglyn (nitroglycerin): nitrate. Used to treat angina pectoris and CHF.

Nitrol (nitroglycerin): nitrate. Used to treat angina pectoris and CHF.

Nitrolingual Spray (nitroglycerin): nitrate. Used to treat angina pectoris and CHF.

Nitrong (nitroglycerin): nitrate. Used to treat angina pectoris and CHF.

Nitrospan (nitroglycerin): nitrate. Used to treat angina pectoris and CHF.

Nitrostabilin (nitroglycerin): nitrate. Used to treat angina pectoris and CHF.

Nitrostat (nitroglycerin): nitrate. Used to treat angina pectoris and CHF.

Nix (permethrin): anti-parasitic agent. Used to treat lice and scabies.

Nizoral (ketoconazole): anti-fungal agent. Used to treat fungal infections.

Nolamine (chlorpheniramine, phenindamine, phenylpropanolamine): antihistamine, decongestant. Used to treat cold and allergy symptoms.

Nolvadex (tamoxifen): antineoplastic. Used to treat breast cancer in post-menopausal women and to stimulate ovulation.

Norcept-E: 1/35 oral contraceptive. Used to treat menstrual disorders and to prevent pregnancy.

Norcet (acetaminophen, hydrocodone): narcotic analgesic. Used to treat moderate and severe pain.

Nordette (estrogen and progestin): oral contraceptive. Used to treat menstrual disorders and to prevent pregnancy.

Norflex (orphenadrine): muscle relaxant. Used to treat muscle pain.

Norgesic (aspirin, caffeine): analgesic. Used to treat mild pain.

Norinyl (estrogen and progestin): oral contraceptive. Used to treat menstrual disorders and to prevent pregnancy.

Norisodrine Aerotrol (isoproterenol): sympathomimetic. Used to treat asthma, bronchitis, and emphysema.

Norlestrin (estrogen and progestin): oral contraceptive. Used to treat menstrual disorders and to prevent pregnancy.

Normiflo (ardeparin): low molecular weight heparin. Used to prevent deep vein thrombosis after surgery.

Normodyne (labetalol): beta blocker. Used to treat HTN and angina.

Normozide (hydrochlorothiazide, labetalol): thiazide diuretic, beta blocker. Used to treat HTN and angina.

Noroxin (norfloxacin): antibiotic. Used to treat genitourinary system infections.

Norpace (disopyramide): anti-arrhythmic agent. Used to treat cardiac arrhythmias.

Norpramin (desipramine): tricyclic antidepressant. Used to treat severe depression.

Nor-Q.D. (progestogen): Used to treat menstrual disorders.

Nor-Tet (tetracycline): antibiotic. Used to treat severe acne and gum disease.

Norvasc (amlodipine): calcium channel blocker. Used to treat HTN and angina pectoris.

Novahistex C (codeine, phenylephrine): narcotic, decongestant. Used to treat cold symptoms, especially cough.

Novahistex DH (diphenylpyraline, hydrocodone, phenylephrine): narcotic analgesic. Used to treat cold symptoms, especially cough.

Novahistine DH (chlorpheniramine, codeine, pseudoephedrine): antihistamine, narcotic, decongestant. Used to treat cold symptoms, especially cough.

Novahistine Expectorant (codeine, guaifenesin, pseudoephedrine): narcotic, expectorant, decongestant. Used to treat cold symptoms, especially cough.

Novamoxin* (amoxicillin): antibiotic. Used to treat general infections.

Novasen* (aspirin): analgesic. Used to treat mild pain.

Novo-Ampicillin* (ampicillin): antibiotic. Used to treat general infections and certain types of septicemia and meningitis.

Novoanaprox* (naproxen): NSAID. Used to treat pain, fever, and inflammation.

Novobutamide* (tolbutamide): anti-diabetic agent. Used to treat non-insulin-dependent diabetes.

Novochlorpromazine* (chlorpromazine): phenothiazine. Used to treat psychotic disorders and vomiting due to toxic chemotherapy.

Novocimetine* (cimetidine): histamine (H_2) blocker. Used to treat and prevent ulcers and esophageal reflux.

Novocloxin* (cloxacillin): antibiotic. Used to treat infections resistant to original forms of penicillin.

Novodigoxin* (digoxin): digitalis preparation. Used to treat CHF and arrhythmias.

Novodipam* (diazepam): benzodiazepine. Used to treat anxiety, muscle spasm, epilepsy, insomnia, and symptoms of alcohol withdrawal.

Novodoparil* (hydrochlorothiazide, methyldopa): diuretic, anti-hypertensive agent. Used to treat HTN.

Novoflupam* (flurazepam): benzodiazepine. Used to treat insomnia.

Novoflurazine* (trifluoperazine): phenothiazine. Used to treat anxiety, paranoia, and schizophrenia.

Novofuran* (nitrofurantoin): anti-infective agent. Used to treat UTIs.

Novohydrazide* (hydrochlorothiazide): thiazide diuretic. Used to treat HTN and fluid retention.

Novolexin* (cephalexin): antibiotic. Used to treat a variety of infections.

Novolin (insulin): anti-diabetic agent. Used to treat insulin-dependent diabetes.

Novometoprol* (metoprolol): beta blocker. Used to treat HTN and angina pectoris.

Novoniacin* (niacin): vitamin B_3. Used to treat high blood levels of cholesterol and vitamin B_3 deficiency.

Novonidazol* (metronidazole): anti-infective agent. Used to treat various infections of the vaginal canal, cervix, male urethra, and intestines.

Novonifedin* (nifedipine): calcium channel blocker. Used to treat angina pectoris and HTN.

NovoPen-VK* (penicillin): antibiotic. Used to treat respiratory tract, middle ear, and skin infections.

Novoperidol* (haloperidol): anti-psychotic agent. Used to treat schizophrenia, manic-depressive disorder, acute psychosis, and Tourette's syndrome.

Novo-Pindol* (pindolol): beta blocker. Used to treat HTN and angina and to prevent migraine headaches.

Novopirocam* (piroxicam): NSAID. Used to treat pain, fever, and inflammation.

Novopranol* (propranolol): beta blocker. Used to treat angina pectoris and HTN and to prevent recurrent heart attack and migraine headaches.

Novo-prazin* (prazosin): anti-hypertensive agent. Used to treat HTN and CHF.

Novoprednisolone* (prednisolone): corticosteroid. Used to treat a variety of allergic and inflammatory problems.

Novoprofen* (ibuprofen): NSAID: Used to treat pain, fever, and inflammation.

Novopropamide* (chlorpropamide): anti-diabetic agent. Used to treat non-insulin-dependent diabetes.

Novopurol* (allopurinol): anti-gout agent. Used to treat gout and prevent gout attacks.

Novoquinidin* (quinidine): anti-arrhythmic agent. Used to treat cardiac arrhythmias.

Novoridazine* (thioridazine): phenothiazine. Used to treat depression, agitation, and anxiety.

Novorythro* (erythromycin): antibiotic. Used to treat general infections.

Novosalmol* (albuterol): bronchodilator. Used to treat asthma.

Novosemide* (furosemide): diuretic. Used to treat HTN and fluid retention.

Novosorbide* (isosorbide dinitrate): nitrate. Used to treat angina and to prevent future attacks.

Novosoxazole* (sulfisoxazole): antibiotic. Used to treat a variety of infections.

Novospiroton* (spironolactone): diuretic. Used to treat HTN and fluid retention.

Novospirozine* (hydrochlorothiazide, spironolactone): diuretic. Used to treat HTN and fluid retention.

Novothalidone* (chlorthalidone): thiazide diuretic. Used to treat HTN and fluid retention.

Novotrimel* (sulfamethoxazole, trimethoprim): antibiotic. Used to treat UTIs.

Novotriphyl* (oxtriphylline): bronchodilator. Used to treat asthma COPD.

Novotriptyn* (amitriptyline): tricyclic antidepressant. Used to treat depression and some pain syndromes.

NPH Iletin I (insulin): anti-diabetic agent. Used to treat insulin-dependent diabetes mellitus.

NPH Iletin II (beef) (insulin): anti-diabetic agent. Used to treat insulin-dependent diabetes mellitus.

NPH Iletin II (pork) (insulin): anti-diabetic agent. Used to treat insulin-dependent diabetes.

NPH Insulin (insulin): anti diabetic agent. Used to treat insulin-dependent diabetes.

NPH Purified Pork (insulin): anti-diabetic agent. Used to treat insulin-dependent diabetes.

Nu-Amoxi* (amoxicillin): antibiotic. Used to treat general infections.

Nubain (nalbuphine): narcotic analgesic. Used to treat moderate to severe pain.

Nucofed (codeine, pseudoephedrine): narcotic, decongestant. Used to treat cold symptoms, especially cough.

Nucofed Expectorant (codeine, guaifenesin, pseudoephedrine): narcotic, expectorant, decongestant. Used to treat cold symptoms, especially cough.

Nu-Loraz* (lorazepam): benzodiazepine. Used to treat anxiety and insomnia.

Nu-Metop* (metoprolol): beta blocker. Used to treat HTN and angina pectoris.

Numorphan* (oxymorphone): narcotic analgesic. Used to treat moderate to severe pain.

Nu-Pinol* (pindolol): beta blocker. Used to treat HTN, to control aggressive behavior, and to prevent migraine headaches.

Nu-Prazo* (prazosin): anti-hypertensive agent. Used to treat HTN and CHF.

Nuprin (ibuprofen): NSAID. Used to treat pain, fever, and inflammation.

Nydrazid (isoniazid): anti-tubercular agent. Used to treat and prevent tuberculosis.

Nytol (diphenhydramine): antihistamine. Used to treat motion sickness and allergic reactions.

Octamide PFS (metoclopramide): anti-emetic agent. Used to treat acid reflux and nausea and vomiting due to migraine headaches or cancer-fighting drugs.

Ocusert Pilo (pilocarpine): anti-glaucoma agent. Used to treat glaucoma.

Ogen (estrogen): female sex hormone. Used to treat gynecological disorders.

Omnicef (cefdinir): antibiotic. Used to treat general infections.

Omnipen (ampicillin): antibiotic. Used to treat general infections and certain types of septicemia and meningitis.

Opticrom (cromolyn): asthma preventive. Used to prevent allergic reactions and asthma attacks.

Optimine (azatadine): antihistamine. Used to treat general allergy symptoms.

Oramide (tolbutamide): anti-diabetic agent. Used to treat type II non-insulin-dependent diabetes mellitus.

Oramorph SR (morphine): narcotic analgesic: Used to treat severe pain.

Orap (pimozide): neuroleptic agent. Used to treat Tourette's syndrome.

Orasone (prednisone): corticosteroid. Used to treat allergic and inflammatory problems, including asthma, colitis, bursitis, tendonitis, and arthritis.

Orbenin* (cloxacillin): antibiotic. Used to treat infections resistant to original forms of penicillin.

Oretic (hydrochlorothiazide): thiazide diuretic. Used to treat HTN and fluid retention

Oreticyl (hydrochlorothiazide): thiazide diuretic. Used to treat HTN and fluid retention.

Orinase (tolbutamide): anti-diabetic agent. Used to treat type II non-insulin-dependent diabetes mellitus.

Orlaam (levomethadyl): narcotic analgesic. Used to treat opioid dependence.

Ornade (chlorpheniramine, phenylpropanolamine): antihistamine. Used to treat symptoms of cold and seasonal allergies.

Ortho-Cept (estrogen and progestin): oral contraceptive. Used to treat menstrual disorders and to prevent pregnancy.

Ortho-Cyclen (estrogen and progestin): oral contraceptive. Used to treat menstrual disorders and to prevent pregnancy.

Ortho-Novum (estrogen and progestin): oral contraceptive. Used to treat menstrual disorders and to prevent pregnancy.

Orudis (ketoprofen): NSAID. Used to treat pain, fever, and inflammation.

Oruvail (ketoprofen): NSAID. Used to treat pain, fever, and inflammation.

Ovcon (estrogen and progestin): oral contraceptive. Used to treat menstrual disorders and to prevent pregnancy.

Ovide (malathion): anti-parasitic agent. Used to treat lice and scabies.

Ovral (estrogen and progestin): oral contraceptive. Used to treat menstrual disorders and to prevent pregnancy.

Ovrette (estrogen and progestin): oral contraceptive. Used to treat menstrual disorders and to prevent pregnancy.

Oxistat (oxiconazole): anti-fungal agent. Used to treat dermal fungal infections.

Oxycocet (acetaminophen, oxycodone): narcotic analgesic. Used to treat moderate to severe pain.

Palaron* (aminophylline): bronchodilator. Used to treat asthma and COPD.

Pamelor (nortriptyline): tricyclic antidepressant. Used to treat depression and chronic pain.

Panmycin (tetracycline): antibiotic. Used to treat severe acne and gum diseaes.

Pantopon (opium alkaloids) narcotic analgesic. Used to treat moderate to severe pain.

Panwarfin (warfarin): anticoagulant. Used to treat blood-clotting disorders.

Paradione (paramethadione): anticonvulsant. Used to treat seizure disorders.

Paraflex (chlorzoxazone): muscle relaxant. Used to treat musculoskeletal pain.

Parafon Forte DSC (acetaminophen, chlorzoxazone): muscle relaxant. Used to treat musculoskeletal pain.

Paregoric (tincture of opium): narcotic analgesic. Used to treat intestinal cramps and diarrhea.

Parepectolin (opium, pectin): narcotic analgesic. Used to treat intestinal cramps and diarrhea.

Parlodel (bromocriptine): ergot alkaloid. Used to treat Parkinson's disease.

Parnate (tranylcypromine): MAO inhibitor. Used to treat depression.

Pavabid (papaverine): vasodilator. Used to treat peripheral vascular diseases.

Paveral* (bromocriptine): ergot alkaloid. Used to treat Parkinson's disease.

Paxil (paroxetine): antidepressant. Used to treat depression, obsessive-compulsive disorder, and panic disorder.

Paxipam (halazepam): benzodiazepine. Used to treat anxiety.

PCE Dispertab (erythromycin): antibiotic. Used to treat general infections.

Pediamycin (erythromycin): antibiotic. Used to treat general infections.

PediaProfen (ibuprofen): NSAID. Used to treat pain, fever, and inflammation.

Pediazole (erythromycin, sulfisoxazole): antibiotic. Used to treat a variety of infections.

Peganone (ethotoin): anticonvulsant. Used to treat epilepsy.

Penapar VK (penicillin): antibiotic. Used to treat respiratory tract, middle ear, and skin infections.

Penbritin* (ampicillin): antibiotic. Used to treat general infections, septicemia, and meningitis.

Penglobe* (bacampicillin): antibiotic. Used to treat general infections.

Pentam 300 (pentamidine): anti-infective agent. Used to treat and prevent *Pneumocystis carinii* pneumonia.

Pentamycetin* (chloramphenicol): antibiotic. Used to treat life-threatening infections.

Pentasa (mesalamine): anti-inflammatory agent. Used to treat intestinal inflammatory disorders.

Pentids (penicillin): antibiotic. Used to treat respiratory tract, middle ear, and skin infections.

Pentritol (pentaerythritol tetranitrate): nitrate. Used to treat angina pectoris.

Pen-Vee K (penicillin V): antibiotic. Used to treat respiratory tract, middle ear, and skin infections.

Pepcid (famotidine): histamine (H$_2$) blocker. Used to treat and prevent ulcers and esophageal reflux.

Peptol* (cimetidine): histamine (H$_2$) blocker. Used to treat and prevent ulcers and esophageal reflux.

Percocet (acetaminophen, oxycodone): narcotic analgesic. Used to treat moderate to severe pain.

Percodan (aspirin, oxycodone): narcotic analgesic. Used to treat moderate to severe pain.

Periactin (cyproheptadine): antihistamine. Used to treat cold and allergy symptoms.

Peridol* (haloperidol): anti-psychotic agent. Used to treat schizophrenia, manic depressive disorder, acute psychosis, and Tourette's syndrome.

Peritrate (pentaerythritol tetranitrate): nitrate. Used to treat angina pectoris.

Permax (pergolide): anti-parkinsonism agent. Used to treat Parkinson's disease.

Permitil (fluphenazine): phenothiazine. Used to treat schizophrenia.

Persantine (dipyridamole): platelet inhibitor. Used to prevent post-cardiac surgery thromboembolism and angina.

Pertofrane (desipramine): tricyclic antidepressant. Used to treat severe depression.

Pethadol (meperidine): narcotic analgesic. Used to treat pain.

Phazyme (simethicone): anti-gas agent. Used to treat abdominal retention of gas.

Phenaphen (acetaminophen): analgesic. Used to treat mild to moderate pain.

Phenaphen with codeine (acetaminophen, codeine): analgesic. Used to treat moderate to severe pain.

Phenazine (perphenazine): phenothiazine. Used to treat psychotic disorders and severe nausea and vomiting, and to calm agitation.

Phenergan (promethazine): antihistamine. Used to treat nausea, vomiting, and motion sickness.

Phenergan with codeine (codeine, promethazine): narcotic, antihistamine. Used to treat nausea, vomiting, and motion sickness.

Phenurone (phenacemide): anticonvulsant. Used to treat seizure disorders.

Phrenilin (acetaminophen, butalbital): analgesic, barbiturate. Used to treat pain and tension headaches.

Phyllocontin (aminophylline): bronchodilator. Used to treat asthma and COPD.

Pilagan (pilocarpine): anti-glaucoma agent. Used to treat glaucoma.

Pilocar (pilocarpine): anti-glaucoma agent. Used to treat glaucoma.

Pilopine HS (pilocarpine): anti-glaucoma agent. Used to treat glaucoma.

Piloptic (pilocarpine): anti-glaucoma agent. Used to treat glaucoma.

Placidyl (ethchlorvynol): hypnotic. Used to treat insomnia.

Plaquenil (hydroxychloroquine): anti-malarial agent.

Used to treat malaria, rheumatoid arthritis, and systemic lupus erythematosus.

Plavix (clopidogrel): platelet inhibitor. Used to reduce risk of complications of atherosclerosis.

Plendil (felodipine): calcium channel blocker. Used to treat angina, CHF, and certain arrhythmias.

PMS Benztropine* (benztropine): anticholinergic. Used to treat parkinsonism.

PMS Carbamazepine* (carbamazepine): anticonvulsant. Used to treat nerve pain, epilepsy, and some psychiatric disorders.

PMS Dopazide* (hydrochlorothiazide, methyldopa): thiazide diuretic, anti-hypertensive agent. Used to treat HTN.

PMS Isoniazid* (isoniazid): anti-tubercular agent. Used to treat and prevent pulmonary tuberculosis.

PMS Levazine* (perphenazine): phenothiazine. Used to treat acute and chronic psychotic disorders and severe nausea and vomiting, and to calm agitation.

PMS Metronidazole* (metronidazole): anti-infective agent. Used to treat various infections of the vaginal canal, cervix, male urethra, and intestines.

PMS Neostigmine* (neostigmine): anti-myasthenic agent. Used to treat myasthenia gravis and to stimulate bowel function after surgery.

PMS Perphenazine* (perphenazine): phenothiazine. Used to treat acute and chronic psychotic disorders and severe nausea and vomiting, and to calm agitation.

PMS Primidone* (primidone): anticonvulsant. Used to treat grand mal and partial seizures.

PMS Prochlorperazine* (prochlorperazine): anti-emetic agent. Used to treat severe nausea and vomiting.

PMS Pyrazinamide* (pyrazinamide): anti-infective agent. Used to treat active tuberculosis.

PMS Sulfasalazine* (sulfasalazine): antibiotic. Used to treat Crohn's disease and ulcerative colitis.

PMS Theophylline* (theophylline): bronchodilator. Used to treat asthma and COPD.

PMS Thioridazine* (thioridazine): phenothiazine. Used to treat depression, agitation, and anxiety.

Pneumopent (pentamidine): anti-infective agent. Used to treat and prevent *Pneumocystis carinii* pneumonia.

Polaramine (dexchlorpheniramine): antihistamine. Used to treat cold and seasonal allergy symptoms.

Polycillin (ampicillin): antibiotic. Used to treat general infections and certain types of septicemia and meningitis.

Ponstan (mefenamic acid): NSAID. Used to treat pain, fever, and inflammation.

Ponstel (mefenamic acid): NSAID. Used to treat pain, fever, and inflammation.

Posicor (mibefradil): calcium channel blocker. Used to treat HTN and angina.

Prandin (repaglinide): anti-diabetic agent. Used to treat non-insulin-dependent diabetes mellitus.

Pravachol (pravastatin): anti-cholesterol agent. Used to treat high blood levels of cholesterol.

Precose (acarbose): anti-diabetic agent. Used to treat non-insulin-dependent diabetes mellitus.

Pred Forte (prednisolone): corticosteroid. Used to treat a variety of allergic and inflammatory problems.

Pred-G (gentamicin, prednisolone): antibiotic, corticosteroid. Used to treat skin infections.

Pred Mild (prednisolone): corticosteroid. Used to treat a variety of allergic and inflammatory problems.

Prelay (troglitazone): anti-diabetic agent. Used to treat non-insulin-dependent diabetes mellitus.

Prelone (prednisolone): corticosteroid. Used to treat a variety of allergic and inflammatory problems.

Premarin (estrogen): female sex hormone. Used to treat gynecological disorders.

Prilosec (omeprazole): anti-ulcer agent. Used to treat GI disorders.

Primatene Mist (epinephrine): sympathomimetic. Used to treat asthma attacks and allergic nasal congestion.

Principen (ampicillin): antibiotic. Used to treat general infections, septicemia, and meningitis.

Prinivil (lisinopril): ACE inhibitor. Used to treat HTN and CHF.

Prinzide (hydrochlorothiazide, lisinopril): diuretic, ACE inhibitor. Used to treat HTN and CHF.

Probalan (probenecid): anti-gout agent. Used to treat gout.

Probampacin (ampicillin, probenecid): anti-gout agent. Used to treat gout.

Pro-Banthine (propantheline): anticholinergic. Used to treat duodenal ulcer and urinary incontinence.

Proben-C (colchicine, probenecid): anti-gout agent. Used to treat gout.

Pro-Biosan (ampicillin): antibiotic. Used to treat general infections and certain types of septicemia and meningitis.

Procamide SR (procainamide): anti-arrhythmic agent. Used to treat and prevent arrhythmias.

Procan SR (procainamide): anti-arrhythmic agent. Used to treat and prevent arrhythmias.

Procardia (nifedipine): calcium channel blocker. Used to treat angina pectoris and HTN.

Procytox* (cyclophosphamide): immunosuppressant. Used to treat cancer and severe rheumatoid arthritis.

Proglycen (diazoxide): vasodilator. Used to treat hypoglycemia.

Prograf (tacrolimus): antibiotic. Used to prevent organ transplant rejection.

Prolixin (fluphenazine): phenothiazine. Used to treat schizophrenia.

Proloid (thyroglobulin): hormone. Used to treat hypothyroidism and goiter.

Proloprim (trimethoprim): anti-infective agent. Used to treat UTIs and eye infections.

Promapar (chlorpromazine): phenothiazine. Used to treat psychotic disorders, tetanus, and vomiting due to toxic chemotherapy.

Promet (promethazine): antihistamine. Used to treat nausea, vomiting, and motion sickness.

Pronestyl (procainamide): anti-arrhythmic agent. Used to treat and prevent premature ventricular contractions, atrial fibrillation, atrial flutter, and tachycardia.

Propacet 100 (acetaminophen, propoxyphene): narcotic analgesic. Used to treat moderate to severe pain.

Propaderm (beclomethasone): corticosteroid. Used to treat asthma.

Propagest (phenylpropanolamine): decongestant. Used to treat symptoms of cold and seasonal allergies.

Propecia (finasteride): Used to treat male pattern baldness.

Propulsid (cisapride): GI stimulant. Used to treat reflux esophagitis and gastroesophageal reflux disease.

Proscar (finasteride): Used to treat benign prostatic hyperplasia (enlarged prostate).

ProSom (estazolam): benzodiazepine. Used to treat insomnia.

ProStep (nicotine): smoking cessation aid. Used to help people quit smoking.

Prostigmin (neostigmine): anti-myasthenic agent. Used to treat myasthenia gravis and to stimulate bowel function after surgery.

Protostat (metronidazole): anti-infective agent. Used to treat various infections of the vaginal canal, cervix, male urethra, and intestines.

Protrin* (sulfamethoxazole, trimethoprim): antibiotic. Used to treat UTIs.

Protropin (somatrem): growth hormone stimulator. Used to treat growth hormone deficiency in children.

Proventil (albuterol): Used to treat asthma and COPD.

Provera (medroxyprogesterone): progestin. Used to treat menstrual disorders and cancer of the breast.

Prozac (fluoxetine): antidepressant. Used to treat depression and bulimia.

Pulmophylline (theophylline): bronchodilator. Used to treat asthma and COPD.

Pulmozyme (dornase alpha): cystic fibrosis agent. Used to treat cystic fibrosis.

Purinethol (mercaptopurine): immunosuppressant. Used to treat cancer.

Purinol (allopurinol): anti-gout agent. Used to treat gout and prevent gout attacks.

PVF (penicillin V): antibiotic. Used to treat respiratory tract, middle ear, and skin infections.

PVF-K* (penicillin V): antibiotic. Used to treat respiratory tract, middle ear, and skin infections.

Pyridamole (dipyridamole): platelet inhibitor. Used to prevent post-cardiac surgery thromboembolism and recurrent heart attacks.

Pyridium (phenazopyridine): analgesic. Used to treat pain and discomfort of UTIs.

Quarzan (clidinium): antispasmodic. Used to treat GI disorders.

Questran (cholestyramine): anti-cholesterol agent. Used to treat high blood levels of LDL cholesterol.

Quibron (guaifenesin, theophylline): bronchodilator. Used to treat asthma and COPD.

Quibron Plus (butabarbital, ephedrine, guaifenesin, theophylline): bronchodilator. Used to treat asthma and COPD.

Quibron-T (theophylline): bronchodilator. Used to treat asthma and COPD.

Quinaglute (quinidine)˙ anti-arrhythmic agent. Used to treat cardiac arrhythmias.

Quinate (quinidine): anti-arrhythmic agent. Used to treat cardiac arrhythmias.

Quinidex (quinidine): anti-arrhythmic agent. Used to treat cardiac arrhythmias.

Quinora (quinidine): anti-arrhythmic agent. Used to treat cardiac arrhythmias.

Rauzide (bendroflumethiazide):˙ thiazide diuretic. Used to treat HTN and fluid retention.

Raxar (grepafloxacin): antibiotic. Used to treat a variety of infections.

Reglan (metoclopramide): anti-emetic agent. Used to treat nausea and vomiting due to migraine headaches or cancer-fighting drugs

Regonol (pyridostigmine): anti-myasthenic agent. Used to treat myasthenia gravis.

Regranex (becaplermin): human-platelet-derived growth factor. Used to treat diabetic ulcers of the lower extremities.

Regroton (chlorthalidone): thiazide diuretic. Used to treat HTN and fluid retention.

Regular Iletin I (insulin): anti-diabetic agent. Used to treat insulin-dependent diabetes.

Regular Iletin II (beef) (insulin): anti-diabetic agent. Used to treat insulin-dependent diabetes.

Regular Iletin II (pork) (insulin): anti-diabetic agent. Used to treat insulin-dependent diabetes.

Regular Iletin II U-500 (insulin): anti-diabetic agent. Used to treat insulin-dependent diabetes.

Relafen (nabumetone): NSAID. Used to treat pain, fever, and inflammation.

Renedil (felodipine): calcium channel blocker. Used to treat angina, CHF, and certain arrhythmias.

Renese (polythiazide): thiazide diuretic. Used to treat HTN and fluid retention.

Renese-R (polythiazide, reserpine): thiazide diuretic, anti-hypertensive agent. Used to treat HTN.

Renormax (spirapril): ACE inhibitor. Used to treat CHF, angina pectoris, and atherosclerosis.

ReQuip (ropinirole): anti-parkinsonism agent. Used to treat Parkinson's disease.

Rescriptor (delavirdine): anti-viral agent. Used to treat HIV-infected patients.

Respbid (theophylline): bronchodilator. Used to treat asthma and COPD.

Restoril (temazepam): benzodiazepine. Used to treat insomnia.

Retet (tetracycline): antibiotic. Used to treat severe acne and gum disease.

Retin-A (tretinoin): vitamin A. Used to treat acne and other skin conditions.

Retrovir (zidovudine): anti-viral agent. Used to treat HIV-infected patients.

Rezulin (troglitazone): anti-diabetic agent. Used to treat non-insulin-dependent diabetes mellitus.

Rheumatrex Dose Pack (methotrexate): antineoplastic agent. Used to treat acute lymphocytic leukemia, cancer, severe psoriasis, and severe rheumatoid arthritis.

RID (pyrethrin): anti-parasitic agent. Used to treat lice.

Ridaura (auranofin): anti-arthritic agent, gold compound. Used to treat severe rheumatoid arthritis in adults.

Rifadin (rifampin): antibiotic. Used to treat and prevent tuberculosis.

Rifamate (isoniazid, rifampin): antibiotic. Used to treat and prevent tuberculosis.

Rifater (isoniazid, pyrazinamide, rifampin): antibiotic. Used to treat and prevent tuberculosis.

Rimactane (rifampin): antibiotic. Used to treat and prevent tuberculosis.

Rimactane/INH (isoniazid, rifampin): antibiotic. Used to treat and prevent tuberculosis.

Riopan (magaldrate): antacid. Used to treat GI disorders.

Riphen-10 (aspirin): analgesic. Used to treat mild pain.

Risperdal (risperidone): anti-psychotic agent. Used to treat schizophrenia, aggression, and Tourette's syndrome.

Ritalin (methylphenidate): amphetamine. Used to treat ADD and narcolepsy.

Rival* (diazepam): benzodiazepine. Used to treat anxiety, muscle spasm, epilepsy, insomnia, and symptoms of alcohol withdrawal.

Rivotril (clonazepam): benzodiazepine. Used to treat epilepsy, panic disorders, and anxiety.

RMS (morphine): narcotic analgesic. Used to treat severe pain.

Robaxin (methocarbamol): muscle relaxant. Used to treat muscle pain and spasm.

Robaxisal (aspirin, methocarbamol): analgesic, muscle relaxant. Used to treat muscle pain and spasm.

Robicillin VK (penicillin V): antibiotic. Used to treat respiratory tract, middle ear, and skin infections.

Robidone* (hydrocodone): narcotic analgesic. Used to treat pain and to control cough.

Robimycin (erythromycin): antibiotic. Used to treat general infections.

Robitet (tetracycline): antibiotic. Used to treat severe acne and gum disease.

Rocephin (ceftriaxone): antibiotic. Used to treat general infections.

Rofact (rifampin): antibiotic. Used to treat active tuberculosis and to prevent tuberculosis in exposed individuals.

Rogaine (minoxidil): anti-hypertensive agent. Used to treat HTN that does not respond to standard therapy and male-pattern baldness.

Ronase (tolazamide): anti-diabetic agent. Used to treat type II non-insulin-dependent diabetes mellitus.

Roubac* (sulfamethoxazole, trimethoprim): antibiotic. Used to treat UTIs.

Rounox with codeine (acetaminophen, codeine): analgesic. Used to treat moderate to severe pain.

Rowasa (mesalamine): anti-inflammatory agent. Used to treat intestinal inflammatory disorders.

Roxanol 100 (morphine): narcotic analgesic. Used to treat severe pain.

Roxicet (acetaminophen, oxycodone): narcotic analgesic. Used to treat moderate to severe pain.

Roxicodone (oxycodone): narcotic analgesic. Used to treat moderate to severe pain.

Roxiprin (aspirin, oxycodone): narcotic analgesic. Used to treat moderate to severe pain.

Rufen (ibuprofen): NSAID. Used to treat pain, fever, and inflammation.

Rynacrom* (cromolyn): asthma preventive. Used to prevent allergic reactions and asthma attacks.

Rynatan (chlorpheniramine, phenylephrine, pyrilamine): antihistamine, sympathomimetic. Used to treat cold and allergy symptoms.

Rythmodan (disopyramide): anti-arrhythmic agent. Used to treat cardiac arrhythmias.

Rythmol (propafenone): anti-arrhythmic agent. Used to treat ventricular arrhythmias.

Sabril (vigabatrin): anticonvulsant. Used to treat seizure disorders.

Sal-Adult (aspirin): analgesic. Used to treat mild pain.

Salazopyrin (sulfasalazine): antibiotic. Used to treat Crohn's disease and ulcerative colitis.

Salflex (salsalate): analgesic. Used to treat pain, fever, and inflammation.

Sal-Infant (aspirin): analgesic. Used to treat mild pain.

Saluron (hydroflumethiazide): thiazide diuretic. Used to treat HTN and fluid retention.

Salutensin (hydroflumethiazide, reserpine): thiazide diuretic, anti-hypertensive agent. Used to treat HTN.

Sandimmune (cyclosporine): immunosuppressant. Used to prevent organ rejection after transplant surgery.

Sansert (methysergide): anti-migraine agent. Used to treat migraine and cluster headaches.

SAS-Enema (sulfasalazine): antibiotic. Used to treat Crohn's disease and ulcerative colitis.

SAS Enteric-500 (sulfasalazine): antibiotic. Used to treat Crohn's disease and ulcerative colitis.

SAS-500 (sulfasalazine): antibiotic. Used to treat Crohn's disease and ulcerative colitis.

Seconal (secobarbital sodium): barbiturate. Used to treat seizure disorders and insomnia.

Sectral (acebutolol): beta blocker. Used to treat HTN and to prevent premature ventricular contractions.

Sedapap-10 (acetaminophen, butalbital): analgesic, barbiturate. Used to treat mild pain and tension headache.

Sedapap #3 (acetaminophen, butalbital, codeine): barbiturate, narcotic analgesic. Used to treat moderate to severe pain and tension headache.

Semilente Insulin (insulin): anti-diabetic agent. Used to treat insulin-dependent diabetes.

Semilente Purified Pork (insulin): anti-diabetic agent. Used to treat insulin-dependent diabetes.

Senokot (senna fruit extract): laxative. Used to treat constipation and irritable bowel syndrome.

Septra (sulfamethoxazole, trimethoprim): antibiotic. Used to treat UTIs.

Ser-Ap-Es (hydralazine, hydrochlorothiazide, reserpine): thiazide diuretic, anti-hypertensive agent. Used to treat HTN.

Serax (oxazepam): benzodiazepine. Used to treat anxiety and alcohol withdrawal.

Serentil (mesoridazine): phenothiazine. Used to treat schizophrenia, behavioral problems, and alcoholism.

Serevent (salmeterol): sympathomimetic agent. Used to treat and prevent asthma attacks and exercise-induced bronchospasm.

Seromycin (cycloserine): anti-infective agent. Used to treat tuberculosis.

Seroquel (quetiapine): anti-psychotic agent. Used to treat schizophrenia.

Serpasil (reserpine): anti-hypertensive agent. Used to treat HTN and psychiatric disorders.

Serpasil-Apresoline (hydralazine, reserpine): diuretic, anti-hypertensive agent. Used to treat HTN.

Sertan (primidone): anticonvulsant. Used to treat grand mal and partial seizures.

Serzone (nafazodone): antidepressant. Used to treat depression.

Silvadene (silver sulfadiazine): topical antibiotic. Used to treat skin infections due to severe burns.

Sincomen (spironolactone): diuretic. Used to treat HTN and fluid retention.

Sinemet (carbidopa, levodopa): anti-parkinsonism agent. Used to treat Parkinson's disease.

Sinequan (doxepin): tricyclic antidepressant. Used to treat depression and sleep disorders.

Sinulin (acetaminophen, chlorpheniramine, phenylpropanolamine): analgesic, antihistamine, decongestant. Used to treat symptoms of cold, seasonal allergies, and respiratory infections.

Skelid (tiludronate): biphosphonate. Used to treat Paget's disease.

SK-penicillin VK (penicillin V): antibiotic. Used to treat respiratory tract, middle ear, and skin infections.

SK-probenecid (probenecid): anti-gout agent. Used to treat gout.

SK-quinidine Sulfate (quinidine): anti-arrhythmic agent. Used to treat cardiac arrhythmias.

SK-soxazole (sulfisoxazole): antibiotic. Used to treat a variety of infections.

SK-tetracycline (tetracycline): antibiotic. Used to treat severe acne and gum disease.

SK-thioridazine (thioridazine): phenothiazine. Used to treat depression, agitation, and anxiety.

SK-triamcinolone (triamcinolone): corticosteroid. Used to treat asthma and other inflammatory problems.

Sleep-Eze 3 (diphenhydramine): antihistamine. Used to treat motion sickness, Parkinson's disease, drug-induced parkinsonism, and allergic reactions.

Slo-bid (theophylline): bronchodilator. Used to treat asthma and COPD.

Slo-Niacin (niacin): vitamin B_3. Used to treat high blood levels of cholesterol and vitamin B_3 deficiency.

Slo-phyllin (theophylline): bronchodilator. Used to treat asthma and COPD.

Slow Fe (ferrous sulfate): iron salt. Used to treat anemia.

Slow-K (potassium chloride): potassium supplement. Used to treat hypokalemia.

Sofarin (warfarin): anticoagulant. Used to treat blood-clotting disorders.

Solalzine (trifluoperazine): phenothiazine. Used to treat psychosis, mania, paranoia, and schizophrenia.

Solfoton (phenobarbital): barbiturate. Used to treat anxiety, nervous tension, insomnia, and epilepsy.

Soma (carisoprodol): muscle relaxant. Used to treat musculoskeletal disorders.

Soma Compound (aspirin, carisoprodol): muscle relaxant. Used to treat musculoskeletal disorders.

Sominex (diphenhydramine): antihistamine. Used to treat motion sickness and allergic reactions.

Somnol (flurazepam): benzodiazepine. Used to treat insomnia.

Somophyllin-12 (aminophylline): bronchodilator. Used to treat asthma and COPD.

Som-Pam* (flurazepam): benzodiazepine. Used to treat insomnia.

Sonazine (chlorpromazine): phenothiazine. Used to treat psychotic disorders, tetanus, and vomiting due to toxic chemotherapy.

Sorbitrate (isosorbide dinitrate): nitrate. Used to treat and prevent angina attacks.

Sotacar (sotalol): beta blocker. Used to treat ventricular arrhythmias.

Span-Niacin (niacin): vitamin B_3. Used to treat high blood levels of cholesterol and vitamin B_3 deficiency.

Sparine (promazine): anti-psychotic agent. Used to treat schizophrenia, psychotic depression, and psychosis.

Spectazole (econazole): anti-fungal agent. Used to treat fungal infections.

Spectrobid (bacampicillin): antibiotic. Used to treat general infections.

Spersacarpine (pilocarpine): anti-glaucoma agent. Used to treat glaucoma.

Sporanox (itraconazole): anti-fungal agent. Used to treat fungal infections.

SSKI (potassium iodide): electrolyte. Used to treat hyperthyroidism.

Stadol (butorphanol): narcotic analgesic. Used to treat postoperative pain.

Stelazine (trifluoperazine): phenothiazine. Used to treat psychosis, mania, paranoia, and schizophrenia.

Stemetil* (prochlorperazine): anti-emetic agent. Used to treat severe nausea and vomiting. Can be used to treat schizophrenia.

Sterapred (prednisone): corticosteroid. Used to treat allergic and inflammatory problems, including asthma, colitis, bursitis, tendonitis, and arthritis.

Sublimaze (fentanyl): narcotic analgesic. Used to treat chronic pain.

Sulcrate* (sucralfate): anti-ulcer agent. Used to treat duodenal ulcer disease.

Sulfatrim DS (sulfamethoxazole, trimethoprim): antibiotic. Used to treat UTIs.

Sumycin (tetracycline): antibiotic. Used to treat severe acne and gum disease.

Supac (acetaminophen, aspirin, caffeine): analgesic. Used to treat mild pain.

Supasa* (aspirin): analgesic. Used to treat mild pain.

Supeudol* (oxycodone): narcotic analgesic. Used to treat moderate to severe pain.

Suprax (cefixime): antibiotic. Used to treat infections of the respiratory tract, ear, or urinary tract and cervical or urethral gonorrhea.

Suprazine (trifluoperazine): phenothiazine. Used to treat psychotic thinking, episodes of mania, paranoia, and schizophrenia.

Surfak (docusate): laxative: Used to treat constipation.

Surmontil (trimipramine): tricyclic antidepressant. Used to treat depression.

Sus-Phrine (epinephrine): sympathomimetic. Used to treat asthma attacks, allergic nasal congestion, glaucoma, and anaphylactic shock.

Sustaire (theophylline): bronchodilator. Used to treat asthma and COPD.

Symadine (amantadine): anti-parkinsonism agent, antiviral agent. Used to treat parkinsonism and respiratory tract infections due to influenza type A virus.

Symmetrel (amantadine): anti-parkinsonism agent, anti-viral agent. Used to treat parkinsonism and respiratory tract infections due to influenza type A virus.

Synalgos-DC (aspirin, caffeine): narcotic analgesic. Used to treat moderate to severe pain.

Synarel (nafarelin): Used to treat endometriosis.

Synthroid (levothyroxine): thyroid hormone. Used to treat thyroid disorders.

Syroxine (levothyroxine): thyroid hormone. Used to treat thyroid disorders.

Tace (estrogens): female sex hormone. Used to treat gynecological disorders.

Tagamet (cimetidine): histamine (H_2) blocker. Used to treat and prevent ulcers and esophageal reflux.

Talacen (acetaminophen, pentazocine): narcotic analgesic. Used to treat moderate to severe pain.

Talwin (pentazocine): narcotic analgesic. Used to treat pain.

Talwin Compound (aspirin, pentazocine): narcotic analgesic. Used to treat moderate to severe pain.

Talwin NX (naloxone, pentazocine): narcotic analgesic. Used to treat pain.

Tambocor (flecainide): anti-arrhythmic agent. Used to treat cardiac arrhythmias.

Tamofen (tamoxifen): antineoplastic agent. Used to treat breast cancer in post-menopausal women and to stimulate ovulation in infertile women.

Tamone (tamoxifen): antineoplastic agent. Used to treat breast cancer in post-menopausal women and to stimulate ovulation in infertile women.

Taractan (chlorprothixene): anti-psychotic agent. Used to treat psychotic disorders.

Tavist (clemastine): antihistamine. Used to treat allergy symptoms.

Tavist-D (clemastine, phenylpropanolamine): antihistamine, decongestant. Used to treat allergy symptoms.

Tazicef (ceftazidime): antibiotic. Used to treat a wide variety of infections.

Tazidime (ceftazidime): antibiotic. Used to treat a wide variety of infections.

Tazorac (tazarotene): retinoid. Used to treat psoriasis.

Tebrazid* (pyrazinamide): anti-infective agent. Used to treat active tuberculosis.

Tedral (ephedrine, phenobarbital, theophylline): barbiturate, bronchodilator. Used to treat asthma and COPD.

Teebaconin (isoniazid): anti-tubercular agent. Used to treat and prevent tuberculosis.

Tegison (etretinate): anti-psoriasis agent. Used to treat psoriasis.

Tegopen (cloxacillin): antibiotic. Used to treat infections resistant to original forms of penicillin.

Tegretol (carbamazepine): anticonvulsant. Used to treat nerve pain, epilepsy, and some psychiatric disorders.

Teldrin (chlorpheniramine): antihistamine. Used to treat symptoms of cold and seasonal allergies.

Tenex (guanfacine): anti-hypertensive agent. potassium supplement. Used to treat HTN.

Ten-K (potassium chloride): potassium supplement. Used to treat hypokalemia.

Tenoretic (atenolol, chlorthalidone): beta blocker, thiazide diuretic. Used to treat HTN.

Tenormin (atenolol): beta blocker. Used to treat exercise-induced angina pectoris and HTN.

Tenuate (diethylpropion): anorexiant agent. Used to treat obesity.

Terazol (terconazole): anti-fungal agent. Used to treat vaginal yeast infections.

Terfluzine* (trifluoperazine): phenothiazine. Used to treat psychotic thinking, episodes of mania, paranoia, and schizophrenia.

Terramycin (oxytetracycline): anti-microbial agent. Used to treat skin disorders and infections.

Teslac (testolactone) hormone: Used to treat breast cancer.

Tessalon (benzonatate): antitussive. Used to treat cough.

Tetra-C (tetracycline): antibiotic. Used to treat severe acne and gum disease.

Tetracyn (tetracycline): antibiotic. Used to treat severe acne and gum disease.

Tetram (tetracycline): antibiotic. Used to treat severe acne and gum disease.

Teveten (eprosartan): anti-hypertensive agent. Used to treat hypertension.

T-Gesic (acetaminophen, hydrocodone): narcotic analgesic. Used to treat moderate and severe pain.

THA (tacrine): cholinesterase inhibitor. Used to treat Alzheimer's disease.

Thalitone (chlorthalidone): thiazide diuretic. Used to treat HTN and fluid retention.

Theobid (theophylline): bronchodilator. Used to treat asthma and COPD.

Theochron (theophylline): bronchodilator. Used to treat asthma and COPD.

Theoclear (theophylline): bronchodilator. Used to treat asthma and COPD.

Theo-Dur (theophylline): bronchodilator. Used to treat asthma and COPD.

Theolair (theophylline): bronchodilator. Used to treat asthma and COPD.

Theo-Organidin (glycerol, theophylline): bronchodilator. Used to treat asthma and COPD.

Theophyl-SR (theophylline): bronchodilator. Used to treat asthma and COPD.

Theo-24 (theophylline): bronchodilator. Used to treat asthma and COPD.

Theovent (theophylline): bronchodilator. Used to treat asthma and COPD.

Theo-X (theophylline): bronchodilator. Used to treat asthma and COPD.

Thiuretic (hydrochlorothiazide): thiazide diuretic. Used to treat HTN and fluid retention.

Thorazine (chlorpromazine): phenothiazine. Used to treat psychotic disorders and vomiting due to toxic chemotherapy.

Thyrolar (levothyroxine, liothyronine): thyroid hormone. Used to treat thyroid disorders.

Ticlid (ticlopidine): platelet aggregation inhibitor. Used to treat and prevent stroke.

Tigan (trimethobenzamide): anti-emetic agent. Used to treat nausea and vomiting.

Timentin (clavulanate, ticarcillin): antibiotic. Used to treat general infections.

Timolide (hydrochlorothiazide, timolol): thiazide diuretic, beta blocker. Used to treat HTN.

Timoptic (timolol): beta blocker. Used to treat angina and HTN.

Tobrex (tobramycin): antibiotic. Used to treat general infections.

Tofranil (imipramine): tricyclic antidepressant. Used to treat depression.

Tolamide (tolazamide): anti-diabetic agent. Used to treat type II non-insulin-dependent diabetes mellitus.

Tolectin (tolmetin): NSAID. Used to treat pain, fever, and inflammation.

Tolinase (tolazamide): anti-diabetic agent. Used to treat type II non-insulin-dependent diabetes mellitus.

Tonocard (tocainide): anti-arrhythmic agent. Used to treat ventricular arrhythmias.

Toprol XL (metoprolol): beta blocker. Used to treat HTN and angina pectoris.

Toradol (ketorolac): NSAID. Used to treat pain, fever, and inflammation.

Torecan (thiethylperazine): phenothiazine. Used to treat nausea and vomiting.

Tornalate (bitolterol): bronchodilator. Used to treat asthma and COPD attacks.

Totacillin (ampicillin): antibiotic. Used to treat general infections, septicemia, and meningitis.

T-Phyl (theophylline): bronchodilator. Used to treat asthma and COPD.

Trancopal (chlormezanone): sedative. Used to treat anxiety.

Trandate (labetalol): beta blocker. Used to treat HTN and angina.

Trandate HCT (labetalol): thiazide diuretic, beta blocker. Used to treat HTN and angina.

Transderm-Nitro (nitroglycerin): nitrate. Used to treat angina pectoris and CHF.

Transderm Scop (scopolamine): anticholinergic. Used to treat motion sickness.

Tranxene (clorazepate): benzodiazepine. Used to treat anxiety, alcohol withdrawal, and epilepsy.

Trasicor (oxprenolol): beta blocker. Used to treat cardiovascular and CNS disorders.

Trecotor-SC (ethionamide): anti-tubercular agent. Used to treat tuberculosis.

Trental (pentoxifylline): bronchodilator. Used to treat peripheral obstructive arterial disease.

Triadapin* (doxepin): tricyclic antidepressant. Used to treat depression and sleep disorders.

Trialodine (trazodone): antidepressant. Used to treat depression and agoraphobia.

Triaminic expectorant with codeine (codeine, guaifenesin, phenylpropanolamine, alcohol): narcotic, expectorant, sympathomimetic. Used to treat cold symptoms, especially cough.

Triaphen-10 (aspirin): analgesic. Used to treat mild pain.

Triavil (amitriptyline, perphenazine): antidepressant, tranquilizer. Used to treat nausea, vomiting, and depression.

Trichlorex (trichlormethiazide): thiazide diuretic. Used to treat HTN and fluid retention.

Tridil (nitroglycerin): nitrate. Used to treat angina pectoris and CHF.

Tridione (trimethadione): anticonvulsant. Used to treat petit mal seizures.

Trikacide* (metronidazole): anti-infective agent. Used to treat various infections of the vaginal canal, cervix, male urethra, and intestines.

Trilafon (perphenazine): phenothiazine. Used to treat acute and chronic psychotic disorders and severe nausea and vomiting and to calm agitation.

Tri-Levlen (estrogen and progestin): oral contraceptive. Used to treat menstrual disorders and to prevent pregnancy.

Trimox (amoxicillin): antibiotic. Used to treat general infections.

Trimpex (trimethoprim): anti-infective agent. Used to treat UTIs and eye infections.

Trinalin (azatadine, pseudoephedrine): antihistamine. Used to treat general allergy symptoms.

Tri-Norinyl (estrogen and progestin): oral contraceptive. Used to treat menstrual disorders and to prevent pregnancy.

Triostat (liothyronine): thyroid hormone. Used to treat thyroid disorders.

Triphasil (estrogen and progestin): oral contraceptive. Used to treat menstrual disorders and to prevent pregnancy.

Triptil (protriptyline): antidepressant. Used to treat depression and bipolar disorders.

Triquilar (estrogen and progestin): oral contraceptive. Used to treat menstrual disorders and to prevent pregnancy.

Trovan (trovafloxacin): antibiotic. Used to treat general infections.

Truphylline (aminophylline): bronchodilator. Used to treat asthma and COPD.

Tuinal (amobarbital, secobarbital): barbiturate. Used to treat seizure disorders and insomnia.

Tussar-2 (pseudoephedrine, codeine, guaifenesin): antihistamine, narcotic, expectorant. Used to treat cold symptoms, especially cough.

Tussar DM (chlorpheniramine, dextromethorphan, pseudoephedrine): antihistamine, expectorant, decongestant. Used to treat symptoms of cold and allergy.

Tussar SF (pseudoephedrine, codeine, guaifenesin): antihistamine, narcotic, expectorant. Used to treat cold symptoms, especially cough.

Tussend (hydrocodone, pseudoephedrine): narcotic analgesic. Used to treat cold symptoms, especially cough.

Tussend Expectorant (hydrocodone, guaifenesin, pseudoephedrine): narcotic analgesic. Used to treat cold symptoms, especially cough.

Tussigon (homatropine, hydrocodone): narcotic analgesic. Used to treat cold symptoms, especially cough.

Tussionex (hydrocodone, phenyltoloxamine): narcotic analgesic. Used to treat cold symptoms, especially cough.

Tussi-Organidin (codeine, glycerol): narcotic analgesic. Used to treat cold symptoms, especially cough.

Tussi-Organidin DMMR (dextromethorphan, iodinated glycerol): antitussive. Used to treat cold symptoms, especially cough.

Twilite (diphenhydramine): antihistamine. Used to treat motion sickness, Parkinson's disease, and allergic reactions and as a sleep aid.

Tycolet (acetaminophen, hydrocodone): narcotic analgesic. Used to treat moderate and severe pain.

Tylenol with codeine (acetaminophen, codeine): narcotic analgesic. Used to treat moderate and severe pain.

Tylox (acetaminophen, oxycodone): narcotic analgesic. Used to treat moderate to severe pain.

Ultracef (cefadroxil): antibiotic. Used to treat infections of the skin, respiratory tract, ear, and urinary tract.

Ultralente Purified Beef (insulin): anti-diabetic agent. Used to treat insulin-dependent diabetes.

Ultram (tramadol): anti-inflammatory. Used to treat pain, fever, and inflammation.

Uniphyl (theophylline): bronchodilator. Used to treat asthma and COPD.

Unipres (hydralazine, hydrochlorothiazide): anti-hypertensive agent, diuretic. Used to treat HTN, CHF, and heart valve insufficiency until surgery.

Unitensen (cryptenamine): anti-hypertensive agent. Used to treat HTN.

Urecholine (bethanechol): cholinergic agent. Used to treat urinary retention.

Uridon (chlorthalidone): thiazide diuretic. Used to treat HTN and fluid retention.

Urispas (flavoxate): anti-spasmodic agent. Used to treat muscle spasms of the bladder.

Uritol* (furosemide): diuretic. Used to treat HTN and fluid retention.

Uroplus DS (sulfamethoxazole, trimethoprim): antibiotic. Used to treat UTIs.

Urozide* (hydrochlorothiazide): thiazide diuretic. Used to treat HTN and fluid retention.

Uticillin VK (penicillin V): antibiotic. Used to treat respiratory tract, middle ear, and skin infections.

Utimox (amoxicillin): antibiotic. Used to treat general infections.

Valdrene (diphenhydramine): antihistamine. Used to

treat motion sickness, Parkinson's disease, and allergic reactions.

Valisone (betamethasone): corticosteroid. Used to treat dermatoses.

Valium (diazepam): benzodiazepine. Used to treat anxiety, muscle spasm, epilepsy, insomnia, and symptoms of alcohol withdrawal.

Valmid (ethinamate): sedative. Used to treat insomnia.

Valtrex (valacyclovir): anti-viral agent. Used to treat shingles (herpes zoster).

Vancenase AQ (beclomethasone): corticosteroid. Used in asthma control for patients who do not respond to bronchodilators.

Vancenase Nasal Inhaler (beclomethasone): corticosteroid. Used in asthma control for patients who do not respond to bronchodilators.

Vanceril (beclomethasone): corticosteroid. Used in asthma control for patients who do not respond to bronchodilators.

Vancocin (vancomycin): anti-infective agent. Used to treat general infections.

Vantin (cefpodoxime): antibiotic. Used to treat general infections.

Vapo-Iso (isoproterenol): sympathomimetic. Used to treat asthma, bronchitis, and emphysema.

Vaponefrin (racepinephrine): sympathomimetic. Used to treat asthma attacks, allergic nasal congestion, glaucoma, and anaphylactic shock.

Vascor (bepridil): calcium channel blocker. Used to treat angina pectoris.

Vaseretic (enalapril, hydrochlorothiazide): ACE inhibitor, thiazide diuretic. Used to treat HTN, renal artery stenosis, and CHF.

Vasocidin (prednisolone, sulfacetamide): corticosteroid. Used to treat a variety of allergic and inflammatory problems.

Vasotec (enalapril). ACE inhibitor. Used to treat HTN, renal artery stenosis, and CHF.

Vazepam (diazepam): benzodiazepine. Used to treat anxiety, muscle spasm, epilepsy, insomnia, and symptoms of alcohol withdrawal.

V-cillin K (penicillin V): antibiotic. Used to treat respiratory tract, middle ear, and skin infections.

VC-K 500 (penicillin V): antibiotic. Used to treat respiratory tract, middle ear, and skin infections.

Veetids (penicillin V): antibiotic. Used to treat respiratory tract, middle ear, and skin infections.

Velosef (cephradine): antibiotic. Used to treat general infections.

Velosulin (insulin): anti-diabetic agent. Used to treat insulin-dependent diabetes.

Ventolin (albuterol): bronchodilator. Used to treat asthma and COPD.

Verelan (verapamil): calcium channel blocker. Used to treat angina pectoris, atrial fibrillation, atrial flutter, atrial tachycardia, and HTN.

Vermox (mebendazole): anthelmintic. Used to treat worm infections—pinworms, roundworms, and hookworms.

Versed (midazolam): benzodiazepine. Used to treat anxiety, insomnia, and psychosis.

Vesprin (triflupromazine): phenothiazine. Used to treat nausea, vomiting, and psychotic disorders.

Viagra (sildenafil): erectile agent. Used to treat impotence.

Vibramycin (doxycycline): tetracycline. Used to treat numerous infections.

Vibra-Tabs (doxycycline): tetracycline. Used to treat numerous infections.

Vicodin (acetaminophen, hydrocodone): narcotic analgesic. Used to treat moderate and severe pain.

Vicoprofen (hydrocodone, ibuprofen): narcotic analgesic. Used to treat pain, fever, and inflammation.

Videx (didanosine): anti-viral agent. Used to treat HIV infection.

Viracept (nelfinavir): anti-viral agent. Used to treat HIV infection.

Virazole (ribavirin): anti-viral agent. Used to treat pneumonia in AIDS patients.

Visken (pindolol): beta blocker. Used to treat HTN and angina and to prevent migraine headaches.

Vistacrom (cromolyn): asthma preventive. Used to prevent allergic reactions and asthma attacks.

Vistaril (hydroxyzine): antihistamine. Used to treat anxiety, nausea, vomiting, and allergy symptoms.

Vivactil (protriptyline): antidepressant. Used to treat depression and bipolar disorders.

Vivol* (diazepam): benzodiazepine. Used to treat anxiety, muscle spasm, epilepsy, insomnia, and symptoms of alcohol withdrawal.

Vivox (doxycycline): tetracycline. Used to treat numerous infections.

Voltaren (diclofenac): NSAID. Used to treat pain, fever, and inflammation.

Vontrol (diphenidol): anti-emetic agent. Used to treat nausea and vomiting.

Warfilone (warfarin): anticoagulant. Used to treat blood-clotting disorders.

Wellbutrin (bupropion): antidepressant. Used to treat depressive disorders and as a smoking cessation aid.

Westcort (hydrocortisone): corticosteroid. Used to treat allergic and inflammatory conditions of the skin.

Wigraine (caffeine, ergotamine): ergot preparation. Used to treat migraine headaches and narcolepsy.

Wigrettes (ergotamine): ergot preparation. Used to treat migraine headaches and narcolepsy.

Winpred* (prednisone): corticosteroid. Used to treat allergic and inflammatory problems, including asthma, colitis, bursitis, tendonitis, and arthritis.

Winstrol (stanozolol): anabolic steroid. Used to treat hereditary angioedema.

Wyamycin (erythromycin): antibiotic. Used to treat general infections.

Wycillin (penicillin V): antibiotic. Used to treat respiratory tract, middle ear, and skin infections.

Wygesic (acetaminophen, propoxyphene): narcotic analgesic. Used to treat moderate to severe pain.

Wymox (amoxicillin): antibiotic. Used to treat general infections.

Wytensin (guanabenz): anti-hypertensive agent. Used to treat HTN.

Xanax (alprazolam): benzodiazepine. Used to treat anxiety, nervous tension, panic attacks, and anxiety associated with depression.

Yocon (yohimbine): erectile agent. Used to treat male impotence.

Yodoxin (iodoquinol): anti-infective agent. Used to treat resistant skin infections and asymptomatic carriers of amebic cysts.

Yohimex (yohimbine): erectile agent. Used to treat male impotence.

Yutopar (ritodrine): preterm labor supplement. Used to treat premature labor and irritable bowel syndrome.

Zantac (ranitidine): histamine (H_2) blocker. Used to treat and prevent ulcers and esophageal reflux.

Zarontin (ethosuximide): anticonvulsant. Used to treat seizure disorders.

Zaroxolyn (metolazone): thiazide diuretic. Used to treat HTN and fluid retention.

Zebeta (bisoprolol): beta blocker. Used to treat HTN.

Zefazone (cefmetazole): antibiotic. Used to treat a wide variety of infections.

Zenapax (dacliximab): immunosuppressant. Used to prevent organ rejection after transplant surgery.

Zerit (stavudine): anti-viral agent. Used to treat HIV infection.

Zestoretic (hydrochlorothiazide, lisinopril): diuretic, ACE inhibitor. Used to treat HTN and CHF.

Zestril (lisinopril): ACE inhibitor. Used to treat HTN and CHF.

Ziac (bisoprolol, hydrochlorothiazide): beta blocker. Used to treat HTN.

Zithromax (azithromycin): antibiotic. Used to treat respiratory tract infections and some skin infections.

Zocor (simvastatin): anti-cholesterol agent. Used to treat high blood levels of cholesterol.

Zofran (ondansetron): anti-emetic agent. Used to treat nausea and vomiting due to cancer treatments.

Zoladex (goserelin): hormone. Used to treat prostate cancer, breast cancer, and endometriosis.

Zoloft (sertraline): antidepressant. Used to treat depression and obsessive-compulsive disorder.

Zomig (zolmitriptan): anti-migraine agent. Used to treat migraine headaches.

ZORprin (aspirin): analgesic. Used to treat mild pain.

Zostrix (capsaicin): plant derivative. Used to treat arthritis pain, neuralgias, and diabetic neuropathy.

Zovirax (acyclovir): anti-viral agent. Used to treat viral infections.

Zurinol (allopurinol): anti-gout agent. Used to treat gout and prevent gout attacks.

Zyban (bupropion): antidepressant. Used as a smoking cessation aid.

Zydone (acetaminophen, hydrocodone): narcotic analgesic. Used to treat moderate and severe pain.

Zyloprim (allopurinol): anti-gout agent. Used to treat gout and prevent gout attacks.

Zyrtec (cetirizine): antihistamine. Used to treat seasonal allergy symptoms.

APPENDIX C

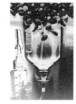

COMMON HERBAL PREPARATIONS

Herbal preparations are now commonly available and used by millions of patients to prevent or treat a wide variety of medical conditions. If a patient is found to be using herbal preparations, it is a good idea to pass the information on to the emergency department staff. Following is a list of some of the more commonly used herbs, along with their uses and side effects.

ALOE	Common uses: Treatment of minor burns Side effects/toxicity: No serious reactions reported
CATNIP	Common uses: Treatment of colds, stomach ailments, hives Side effects/toxicity: No serious reactions reported
CHAMOMILE	Common uses: Treatment of gastrointestinal (GI) disorders, rheumatism Side effects/toxicity: Occasional hypersensitivity
CHAPARRAL	Common uses: Treatment of bronchitis, colds, chickenpox, cancers

Side effects/toxicity: Long-term use may cause liver toxicity

CRANBERRY
Common uses: Urinary tract infections
Side effects/toxicity: Use of large amounts may cause diarrhea

ECHINACEA
Common uses: Treatment of open wounds, to fight infections, as immune system stimulant
Side effects/toxicity: Adverse reactions are very rare

FENNEL
Common uses: Treatment of GI disorders
Side effects/toxicity: Nausea, vomiting, seizures, pulmonary edema (from ingestion of fennel oil)

FEVERFEW
Common uses: Treatment of menstrual pain, asthma, arthritis; also used to prevent migraine headaches
Side effects/toxicity: Mouth ulcerations, loss of taste, dermatitis; withdrawal effects include rebound migraines and anxiety; avoid use by pregnant women

GARLIC
Common uses: Prevention and treatment of hypertension and high cholesterol

Side effects/toxicity: Adverse reactions when used in combination with anticoagulants

GINGER

Common uses: Treatment of dizziness, prevention of motion sickness, as digestive aid
Side effects/toxicity: Large doses may cause arrhythmias or central nervous system (CNS) depression

GINKGO BILOBA

Common uses: Treatment of cerebral insufficiency, cerebral disorders, dementia, asthma
Side effects/toxicity: Headache, dizziness, palpitations, GI disorders

GINSENG

Common uses: Stress reduction, immune stimulant, reduction of cholesterol levels
Side effects/toxicity: Anxiety, sleeplessness

GOLDENSEAL

Common uses: Treatment of infection
Side effects/toxicity: High doses may cause nausea, vomiting, diarrhea, skin rashes, throat irritation

LICORICE

Common uses: Treatment of GI disorders, infection
Side effects/toxicity: Large doses can cause lethargy,

	headache, weakness, facial puffiness
NETTLES	Common uses: As a diuretic Side effects/toxicity: On rare occasions causes gastric irritation and peripheral edema
PAPAYA	Common uses: Treatment of digestive disorders Side effects/toxicity: Occasional hypersensitivity
PENNYROYAL	Common uses: Treatment of digestive disorders, abdominal cramps Side effects/toxicity: May cause uterine contractions; should not be used by pregnant women
PLANTAIN	Common uses: Treatment of high cholesterol levels, as a diuretic Side effects/toxicity: Allergic reactions reported
SAFFRON	Common uses: As a sedative, expectorant Side effects/toxicity: Adverse reactions very rare
SAW PALMETTO	Common uses: Treatment of prostate, urinary disorders Side effects/toxicity: Headache, diarrhea

ST. JOHN'S WORT   Common uses: Treatment of
anxiety, depression
Side effects/toxicity: Rash,
photosensitivity

TURMERIC   Common uses: Treatment of
cancer, prevention of blood
clots
Side effects/toxicity: Adverse
effects rare

APPENDIX D

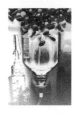

EARLY MANAGEMENT OF PATIENTS WITH CHEST PAIN AND POSSIBLE ACUTE MI

Acute Myocardial Infarction Algorithm
Recommendations for early management of patients with chest pain and possible AMI

COMMUNITY

Community emphasis on
- "Call First, Call Fast, Call 911"
- National Heart Attack Alert Program

EMS SYSTEM

EMS system approach that should address
- Oxygen – IV – cardiac monitor – vital signs
- *Nitroglycerin*
- Pain relief with narcotics
- Notification of emergency department
- Rapid transport to emergency department
- Prehospital screening for *thrombolytic* therapy*
- 12-lead ECG, computer analysis, transmission to emergency department*
- Initiation of *thrombolytic* therapy*

EMERGENCY DEPARTMENT

"Door-to-drug" team protocol approach
- Rapid triage of patients with chest pain
- Clinical decision maker established (emergency physician, cardiologist, or other)

Time interval in emergency department

432

Treatments to consider if there is evidence of coronary thrombosis plus no reasons for exclusion:
(some but not all may be appropriate)

- **Oxygen** at 4 L/min
- **Nitroglycerin** SL, paste or spray
- **Morphine** IV
- **Aspirin** PO
- **Thrombolytic** agents
- **Nitroglycerin** IV
- **β-Blockers** IV
- **Heparin** IV
- **Lidocaine** IV (prophylactic lidocaine not recommended for all patients with AMI)
- **Magnesium sulfate** IV
- **Coronary angiography/angioplasty**

> 30-60 min to **thrombolytic** therapy

Assessment

Immediate:
- Vital signs with automatic or standard BP
- Oxygen saturation
- Start IV
- 12-lead ECG (MD review)
- Brief, targeted history and physical
- Decide on eligibility for **thrombolytic** therapy

Soon:
- Chest x-ray
- Blood studies (electrolytes, enzymes, coagulation studies)
- Consult as needed

*Optional guidelines

433

APPENDIX E

WEIGHT CONVERSION TABLE

1 kilogram = 2.2 pounds
1 pound = 0.45 kilogram
(Conversions are rounded off to the nearest kilogram.)

5 lb = 2.2 kg		85 lb − 38.0 kg
10 lb = 4.5 kg		90 lb = 41.0 kg
15 lb = 7.0 kg		95 lb = 43.0 kg
20 lb − 9.0 kg		100 lb = 45.0 kg
25 lb = 11.0 kg		105 lb = 47.0 kg
30 lb = 14.0 kg		110 lb = 50.0 kg
35 lb = 16.0 kg		115 lb = 52.0 kg
40 lb = 18.0 kg		120 lb = 54.0 kg
45 lb = 20.0 kg		125 lb = 57.0 kg
50 lb = 22.0 kg		130 lb = 59.0 kg
55 lb = 25.0 kg		135 lb = 61.0 kg
60 lb = 27.0 kg		140 lb = 64.0 kg
65 lb = 29.0 kg		145 lb = 66.0 kg
70 lb = 32.0 kg		150 lb = 68.0 kg
75 lb = 34.0 kg		155 lb = 70.0 kg
80 lb = 36.0 kg		160 lb = 73.0 kg

165 lb = 75.0 kg	240 lb = 109.0 kg
170 lb = 77.0 kg	245 lb = 111.0 kg
175 lb = 80.0 kg	250 lb = 114.0 kg
180 lb = 82.0 kg	255 lb = 116.0 kg
185 lb = 84.0 kg	260 lb = 118.0 kg
190 lb = 86.0 kg	265 lb = 120.0 kg
195 lb = 89.0 kg	270 lb = 123.0 kg
200 lb = 91.0 kg	275 lb = 125.0 kg
205 lb = 93.0 kg	280 lb = 127.0 kg
210 lb = 95.0 kg	285 lb = 130.0 kg
215 lb = 98.0 kg	290 lb = 132.0 kg
220 lb = 100.0 kg	295 lb = 134.0 kg
225 lb = 102.0 kg	300 lb = 136.0 kg
230 lb = 105.0 kg	305 lb = 139.0 kg
235 lb = 107.0 kg	310 lb = 141.0 kg

APPENDIX F

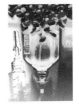

TEMPERATURE CONVERSION TABLE

Fahrenheit	Centigrade (Celsius)
81	27.2
82	27.8
83	28.3
84	28.9
85	29.4
86	30.0
87	30.6
88	31.1
89	31.7
90	32.2
91	32.8
92	33.3
93	33.9
94	34.4
95	35.0
96	35.6
97	36.1

98		36.7
98.6	*Normal*	37.0
99		37.2
100		37.8
101		38.3
102		38.9
103		39.4
104		40.0
105		40.6
106		41.1
107		41.7
108		42.2

Other useful conversions:
1 inch = 2.54 centimeters
1 centimeter = ⅜ inch
1 meter = 39.37 inches

APPENDIX G

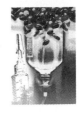

ALGORITHM:
ASYSTOLE
TREATMENT

Asystole Treatment Algorithm

- Continue CPR
- Intubate at once
- Obtain IV access
- Confirm asystole in more than one

↓

Consider possible causes
- Hypoxia
- Hyperkalemia
- Hypokalemia
- Preexisting acidosis
- Drug overdose
- Hypothermia

↓

Consider immediate transcutaneous pacing (TCP)[a]

↓

- **Epinephrine** 1 mg IV push,[b,c] repeat every 3-5 min

↓

- **Atropine** 1 mg IV, repeat every 3-5 min up to a total of 0.03-0.04 mg/kg[d,e]

↓

Consider termination of efforts[f]

Class I:	definitely helpful
Class IIa:	acceptable, probably helpful
Class IIb:	acceptable, possibly helpful
Class III:	not indicated, may be harmful

a. TCP is a Class IIb intervention. Lack of success may be due to delays in pacing. To be effective TCP must be performed early, simultaneously with drugs. Evidence does not support routine use of TCP for asystole.

b. The recommended dose of *epinephrine* is 1 mg IV push every 3-5 min. If this approach fails, several Class IIb dosing regimens can be considered:
   - Intermediate: *epinephrine* 2-5 mg IV push, every 3-5 min
   - Escalating: *epinephrine* 1 mg-3 mg-5 mg IV push, 3 min apart
   - High: *epinephrine* 0.1 mg/kg IV push, every 3-5 min

c. *Sodium bicarbonate* 1 mEq/kg is Class I if patient has known preexisting hyperkalemia.

d. The shorter *atropine* dosing interval (3 min) is Class IIb in asystolic arrest.

e. *Sodium bicarbonate* 1 mEq/kg:
   Class IIa
   - If known preexisting bicarbonate-responsive acidosis
   - If overdose with tricyclic antidepressants
   - To alkalinize the urine in drug overdoses
   Class IIb
   - If intubated and continued long arrest interval
   - Upon return of spontaneous circulation after long arrest interval
   Class III
   - Hypoxic lactic acidosis

f. If patient remains in asystole or other agonal rhythm after successful intubation and initial medications and no reversible causes are identified, consider termination of resuscitative efforts by a physician. Consider interval since arrest.

APPENDIX H

APGAR SCORING SYSTEM

The Apgar scoring system is used to evaluate the status of newborn infants and to determine the need for resuscitation efforts. The infant should be scored 1 minute after birth and then again at 5 minutes.

CRITERIA	0 Points	1 Point	2 Points
Heart rate	Absent	<100	>100
Respirations	Absent	Slow/irregular	Good/crying
Muscle tone	Limp/flaccid	Some flexion	Active motion
Grimace/ irritability	No response	Grimaces	Cry/vigorous motion
Color	Blue/pale	Blue/pink	Fully pink

SCORING SCALE

Total of 7 to 10 is good and requires nothing but supportive care.

Total of 4 to 6 indicates moderate depression and requires some assistance, including oxygenation and stimulation.

Total score below 4 requires aggressive resuscitation efforts, including CPR.

GLASGOW
COMA
SCALE

Adult/Child Scale		Infant Scale
Eye Opening	*Points*	
Spontaneous	4	Spontaneous
To voice	3	To voice/speech
To pain	2	To pain
None	1	None
Verbal Response		
Oriented	5	Coos, babbles
Confused	4	Irritable cries
Inappropriate words	3	Cries to pain
Incomprehensible sounds	2	Moans, grunts
None	1	No response
Motor response		
Obeys commands	6	Spontaneous
Localizes pain	5	Localizes pain

Withdraws from pain	4	Withdraws from pain
Flexion to pain (decorticate)	3	Flexion to pain
Extension to pain (decerebrate)	2	Extension to pain
None	1	None

APPENDIX J

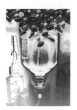

REVISED TRAUMA SCALE

To calculate the revised trauma score, it is necessary to score the patient's respiratory and systolic blood pressure status and then add this score to the converted Glasgow Coma Score, as indicated below.

Respiratory Rate (per minute)	Points	
10–29	4	
>30	3	
6–9	2	
1–5	1	
None	0	_____

Systolic Blood Pressure		
>90	4	
76–89	3	
50–75	2	
1–49	1	
0—no pulse	0	_____

CONVERTED GLASGOW COMA SCORE

Glasgow Score	Points	
13–15	4	
9–12	3	
6–8	2	
4–5	1	
3	0	_____
	TOTAL POINTS	_____

APPENDIX K

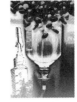

COMMON CAUSES OF COMA

The mnemonic A-E-I-O-U-T-I-P-S is a useful device to help remember the more common causes of coma.

A	Alcohol, acidosis
E	Epilepsy, electrolyte abnormalities
I	Insulin-related problems (diabetic problems)
O	Overdose or poisoning
U	Uremia
T	Trauma
I	Infection
P	Psychosis (hysterical coma)
S	Stroke (cerebrovascular accident [CVA])

APPENDIX II

APPENDIX L

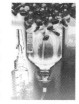

GUIDE TO DIAGNOSTIC SIGNS

Following are some of the more common diagnostic signs that emergency medical services (EMS) providers may be able to observe in the field. Knowledge of these signs can be useful as an aid to assessment and in communicating information to hospital personnel.

Babinski's sign: An upward extension of the big toe and fanning of the remaining toes on stimulation of the sole of the foot; reflects possible brain or central nervous system injury.

Ballance's sign: A resonance detected on the right flank when the patient is lying on the left side; indicates possible splenic rupture.

Battle's sign: Ecchymosis (bluish black bruising) over the mastoid process, which usually indicates a basal skull fracture.

Beck's sign (Beck's triad): Jugular vein distention, muffled heart sounds, and narrowing pulse pressure; indicates cardiac tamponade.

Biot's respiration: A breathing pattern characterized by a number of short breaths followed by long, irregular periods of apnea; indicative of increased intracranial pressure (ICP).

Blumberg's sign: Acute rebound tenderness over the site of a suspected abdominal lesion; indicates possible peritonitis.

Bozzolo's sign: A visual pulsation of the arteries in the nostrils; indicates possible thoracic aortic aneurysm.

Cheyne-Stokes respiration: A pattern of respirations characterized by a period of apnea followed by a series of rapid breaths that start off shallow, become deeper, and then return to shallow; generally indicates brain injury.

Cleeman's sign: A creasing of the skin just above the patella; suggests possible femur fracture.

Cullen's sign: A bluish discoloration around the umbilicus; may indicate peritoneal hemorrhage, which may be caused by ruptured ectopic pregnancy or acute pancreatitis.

Cushing's triad: A combination of increased blood pressure, bradycardia, and decreased respiratory rate; associated with increased ICP.

Kehr's sign: Severe pain in the left shoulder, which can suggest splenic rupture.

Kussmaul's respiration: A pattern of deep, rapid respirations; commonly associated with diabetic ketoacidosis.

Murphy's sign: The inability of the patient to take in a breath when the examiner's fingers are pressed beneath the right costal arch; usually indicates gallbladder inflammation.

Raccoon eyes: Ecchymosis around the eyes after trauma; suggestive of possible skull fracture.

Rovsing's sign: A sensation of acute pain in the lower right quadrant that results from the application of pressure to the lower left quadrant; suggests appendicitis.

APPENDIX M

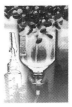

CONSENSUS FORMULA FOR FLUID REPLACEMENT IN BURN MANAGEMENT

In cases of serious burns, fluid replacement is a treatment priority that should be initiated as promptly as possible. In the past, several different formulas were devised to calculate the rate of fluid replacement. Recently, these formulas have been combined into what is commonly known as the *Consensus Formula*. While the purpose of the formula is to establish a fluid replacement rate for a 24-hour period, it is occasionally initiated in the field, depending on local protocol. The formula requires the emergency medical services (EMS) provider to calculate the total body surface area (TBSA) of the burn and to ascertain, as accurately as possible, the patient's body weight in kilograms.

The formula is computed as follows:

(2 to 4 mL of lactated Ringer's) × (Weight in kg) × (TBSA) = Volume to be infused over 24 hours

This formula calculates the amount of fluid to be infused over a 24-hour period. Fifty percent of this total should be infused in the first 8 hours, 25% over the next 8 hours, and 25% over the final 8 hours.

EXAMPLE

A patient weighing 175 pounds has been burned over 40% of his body. Local protocol allows EMS providers to initiate fluid replacement in the field pursuant to the Consensus Formula, using 2 mL of lactated Ringer's (LR) × weight in kilograms × TBSA. The replacement rate is established by proceeding through the following steps:

1. Establish the body weight in kilograms. We know that the patient weights 175 pounds. Since a kilogram equals 2.2 pounds, we divide 175 by 2.2. This gives us a weight of 79.55 kg. To make life easier, this can be rounded out to 80.0 kg.

2. We now have all of the information that we need to apply the Consensus Formula.
(2 mL of LR) × (80 kg) × (40% TBSA) =
Volume to be infused in 24 hours
Multiplying 2 × 80 × 40, we get a total of
6,400 mL.

3. We now know that a total of 6,400 mL of LR is to be infused in 24 hours. Fifty percent of that amount, or 3,200 mL, should be infused in the first 8 hours. To get the hourly rate, we divide by 8. This establishes the rate to be 400 mL per hour.

4. To establish our drip rate per minute, we would use the following formula:
(Volume to be infused) × (Drops [gtt]/mL of infusion set)/Time in minutes = gtt/minute
Our IV administration set delivers fluid at 15 gtt/mL.
Our formula would then be computed as follows:
400 mL × 15 gtt/mL/60 minutes = gtt/minute
400 × 15 = 6,000
We divide 6,000 by 60 and get our rate of 100 gtt/minute.

APPENDIX N

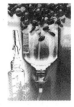

COMMONLY USED MEDICAL AND PHARMACOLOGICAL ABBREVIATIONS

Abbreviation	Meaning
ā	before
ACE	angiotensin-converting enzyme
Ach	acetylcholine
ACLS	advanced cardiac life support
ALS	advanced life support
AMA	against medical advice
amp	ampule
ASA	aspirin
bid	twice daily
BLS	basic life support
BM	bowel movement
BP	blood pressure
BPH	benign prostatic hypertrophy
BSA	body surface area
C	centigrade
c̄	with
cc	cubic centimeter

CABG	coronary artery bypass graft
$CaCl_2$	calcium chloride
CAD	coronary artery disease
caps	capsules
CBC	complete blood count
CC	chief complaint
CHF	congestive heart failure
cm	centimeter
CNS	central nervous system
c/o	complaining of
CO	carbon monoxide
CO_2	carbon dioxide
COPD	chronic obstructive pulmonary disease
CSF	cerebrospinal fluid
CVA	cerebrovascular accident (stroke)
CVP	central venous pressure
D/C	discontinue
DIC	disseminated intravascular coagulation
dig	digitalis
DM	diabetes mellitus
DNR	do not resuscitate
DO	doctor of osteopathic medicine
DVT	deep vein thrombosis
Dx	diagnosis

D₅W	dextrose 5% in water
ECG or EKG	electrocardiogram
EEG	electroencephalogram
EENT	eye, ear, nose, and throat
EGTA	esophageal gastric tube airway
EOA	esophageal obturator airway
et	and
ETOH	alcohol
F	Fahrenheit
FB	foreign body
FUO	fever of unknown origin
Fx	fracture
g or gm	gram
GI	gastrointestinal
gr	grain
gt	drop
gtt	drops
h	hour
Hct	hematocrit
HDL	high density lipoprotein
Hgb	hemoglobin
HIV	human immunodeficiency virus
HR	heart rate
HTN	hypertension

Hx	history
IC	intracardiac
ICP	intracranial pressure
IM	intramuscular
IO	intraosseous
IPPB	intermittent positive pressure breathing
IV	intravenous
JVD	jugular vein distention
kg	kilogram
KO	keep open
KVO	keep vein open
L	liter
L	left
lb	pound
LBBB	left bundle branch block
LDL	low density lipoprotein
LLQ	left lower quadrant
LR	lactated Ringer's
LUQ	left upper quadrant
m	meter
MAO	monoamine oxidase
MD	doctor of medicine
mEq	milliequivalent
mg	milligram

MI	myocardial infarction
mL	milliliter
mm	millimeter
MS	morphine sulfate
MS	multiple sclerosis
μg	microgram
NaHCO$_3$	sodium bicarbonate
NG	nasogastric
NKA	no known allergies
NKDA	no known drug allergies
NPO	nothing by mouth
NS	normal saline
NSAID	nonsteroidal anti-inflammatory drug
NTG	nitroglycerin
N/V	nausea and vomiting
O$_2$	oxygen
OB	obstetric
OD	overdose
OD	right eye
OS	left eye
OTC	over-the-counter
oz	ounce
P	pulse
p̄	after

PAC	premature atrial contraction
PAT	paroxysmal atrial tachycardia
PE	pulmonary emboli
PEARL	pupils equal and reactive to light
PID	pelvic inflammatory disease
PJC	premature junctional contraction
PMH	past medical history
PO	by mouth
prn	as needed, as required
PT	prothrombin time
PTT	partial thromboplastin time
PVC	premature ventricular contraction
q	each, every
qd	every day
qid	four times a day
qt	quart
RBBB	right bundle branch block
RBC	red blood cell
RL	Ringer's lactate
RLQ	right lower quadrant
RUQ	right upper quadrant
Rx	prescription, recipe
s̄	without
SA	sinoatrial

SC (or SQ)	subcutaneous
SL	sublingual
SOB	shortness of breath
s/s	signs and symptoms
STAT	immediately
SVT	supraventricular tachycardia
T	temperature
TB	tuberculosis
TCP	transcutaneous pacing
TIA	transient ischemic attack
tid	three times a day
TKO	to keep open
Tx	treatment
URI	upper respiratory tract infection
UTI	urinary tract infection
vol	volume
WBC	white blood cell
WNL	within normal limits
wt	weight
y.o.	years old

APPENDIX O

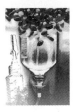

ALGORITHM: VENTRICULAR FIBRILLATION/PULSELESS VENTRICULAR TACHYCARDIA

Ventricular Fibrillation/Pulseless Ventricular Tachycardia (VF/VT) Algorithm

- ABCs
- Perform CPR until defibrillator attached[a]
- VF/VT present on defibrillator

↓

Defibrillate up to 3 times if needed for persistent VF/VT (200 J, 200-300 J, 360 J)

↓

Rhythm after the first 3 shocks?[b]

↓

| Persistent or recurrent VF/VT | Return of spontaneous circulation | PEA Go to Fig 3 | Asystole Go to Fig 4 |

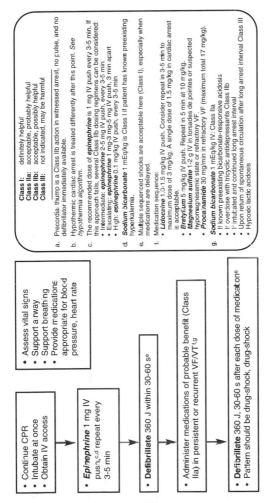

- Continue CPR
- Intubate at once
- Obtain IV access

↓

- **Epinephrine** 1 mg IV push,[c,d] repeat every 3-5 min

↓

- **Defibrillate** 360 J within 30-60 s[e]

↓

- Administer medications of probable benefit (Class IIa) in persistent or recurrent VF/VT[f,g]

↓

- **Defibrillate** 360 J, 30-60 s after each dose of medication[e]
- Pattern should be drug-shock, drug-shock

Side box:

- Assess vital signs
- Support airway
- Support breathing
- Provide medications appropriate for blood pressure, heart rate

Legend and notes:

Class I: definitely helpful
Class IIa: acceptable, probably helpful
Class IIb: acceptable, possibly helpful
Class III: not indicated, may be harmful

a. Precordial thump is a Class IIb action in witnessed arrest, no pulse, and no defibrillator immediately available.

b. Hypothermic cardiac arrest is treated differently after this point. *See hypothermia algorithm.*

c. The recommended dose of *epinephrine* is 1 mg IV push every 3-5 min. If this approach fails, several Class IIb dosing regimens can be considered:
- Intermediate: *epinephrine* 2-5 mg IV push, every 3-5 min
- Escalating: *epinephrine* 1 mg-3 mg-5 mg IV push, 3 min apart
- High: *epinephrine* 0.1 mg/kg IV push, every 3-5 min

d. *Sodium bicarbonate* 1 mEq/kg is Class I if patient has known preexisting hyperkalemia.

e. Multiple sequenced shocks are acceptable here (Class I), especially when medications are delayed.

f. Medication sequence:
- *Lidocaine* 1.0-1.5 mg/kg IV push. Consider repeat in 3-5 min to maximum dose of 3 mg/kg. A single dose of 1.5 mg/kg in cardiac arrest is acceptable.
- *Bretylium* 5 mg/kg IV push. Repeat in 5 min at 10 mg/kg.
- *Magnesium sulfate* 1-2 g IV in torsades de pointes or suspected hypomagnesemic state or refractory VF.
- *Procainamide* 30 mg/min in refractory VF (maximum total 17 mg/kg).

g. *Sodium bicarbonate* 1 mEq/kg IV: Class IIa
- If known preexisting bicarbonate-responsive acidosis
- If overdose with tricyclic antidepressants Class IIb
- If intubated and continued long arrest interval
- Upon return of spontaneous circulation after long arrest interval Class III
- Hypoxic lactic acidosis

465

APPENDIX P

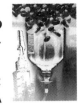

ALGORITHM: TACHYCARDIA

Tachycardia Algorithm

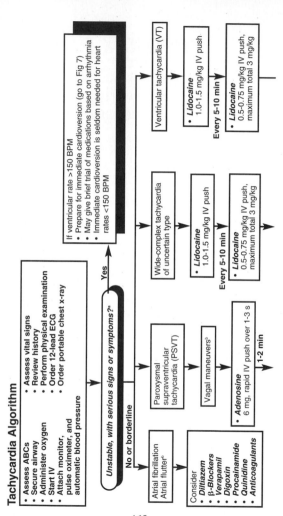

- Assess ABCs
- Secure airway
- Administer oxygen
- Start IV
- Attach monitor, pulse oximeter, and automatic blood pressure
- Assess vital signs
- Review history
- Perform physical examination
- Order 12-lead ECG
- Order portable chest x-ray

Unstable, with serious signs or symptoms?[a]

No or borderline

Yes

If ventricular rate >150 BPM
- Prepare for immediate cardioversion (go to Fig 7)
- May give brief trial of medications based on arrhythmia
- Immediate cardioversion is seldom needed for heart rates <150 BPM

Atrial fibrillation
Atrial flutter[c]

Consider
- *Diltiazem*
- *β-Blockers*
- *Verapamil*
- *Digoxin*
- *Procainamide*
- *Quinidine*
- *Anticoagulants*

Paroxysmal supraventricular tachycardia (PSVT)

Vagal maneuvers[b]

- *Adenosine* 6 mg, rapid IV push over 1-3 s

1-2 min

Wide-complex tachycardia of uncertain type

- *Lidocaine* 1.0-1.5 mg/kg IV push

Every 5-10 min

- *Lidocaine* 0.5-0.75 mg/kg IV push, maximum total 3 mg/kg

Ventricular tachycardia (VT)

- *Lidocaine* 1.0-1.5 mg/kg IV push

Every 5-10 min

- *Lidocaine* 0.5-0.75 mg/kg IV push, maximum total 3 mg/kg

468

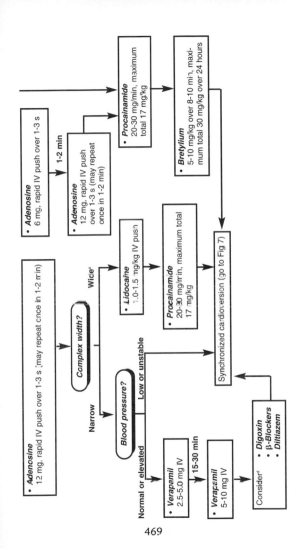

a. Unstable condition must be related to the tachycardia. Signs and symptoms may include chest pain, shortness of breath, decreased level of consciousness, low blood pressure (BP), shock, pulmonary congestion, congestive heart failure, acute myocardial infarction.

b. Carotid sinus pressure is contraindicated in patients with carotid bruits; avoid ice water immersion in patients with ischemic heart disease.

c. If the wide-complex tachycardia is known with certainty to be PSVT and BP is normal/elevated, sequence can include *verapamil.*

d. Use extreme caution with β-blockers after *verapamil.*

GLOSSARY OF PHARMACOLOGICAL TERMS

Absorption: The passage of a substance (medication) through a surface of the body into the fluids and tissues.

Abuse: The improper, inappropriate, or excessive use of a drug in a manner that deviates from medically prescribed or indicated use.

Acetylcholine: A substance produced by the body that facilitates the transmission of nerve impulses at the synapse.

Acidosis: The excessive buildup of acid or loss of bicarbonate.

Adrenergic: A classification of drugs that produce epinephrine-like effects; a term applied to nerve fibers that, when stimulated, produce epinephrine.

Adsorption: Adhesion by a liquid gas to the surface of a solid. *Example:* Activated charcoal works by adsorption.

Agonist: A drug that binds with a receptor to produce a physiological response.

Analgesic: A medication or substance that relieves pain.

Antagonist: A drug that blocks or interferes with the action of another drug. *Example:* Naloxone (Narcan) is a narcotic antagonist.

Anti-arrhythmic agent: A drug used to control or prevent cardiac arrhythmias.

Anticholinergic: A drug that blocks parasympathetic nerve impulses. *Example:* Atropine sulfate.

Anticoagulant: A drug that prevents or delays blood clotting.

Antidote: A substance that neutralizes poisons or their effects.

Anti-emetic: A substance used to relieve or prevent nausea and vomiting. *Example:* Prochlorperazine (Compazine).

Antihistamine: A drug that counters the effect of histamines, amines released by mast cells that promote inflammation. *Example:* Diphenhydramine (Benadryl).

Antipyretic: A drug that reduces fever.

Benzodiazepine: A class of drugs primarily used to treat anxiety and to induce sedation and/or sleep. *Example:* Diazepam (Valium).

Bronchodilator: A drug that has the effect of dilating the bronchi and bronchioles. *Example:* Albuterol (Proventil).

Calcium channel blocker: A class of drugs that slow the absorption of calcium ions into muscle tissues. The result is decreased arterial resistance and decreased myocardial oxygen demand. These drugs are used to treat hypertension, tachyarrhythmias, and angina. *Example:* Verapamil (Calan).

Catalyst: A substance that speeds up a chemical reaction.

Chronotropic: Having an effect on heart rate. A positive chronotropic drug increases heart rate.

Colloid: A substance of high molecular weight. Molecules contained in colloids are too large to pass through the capillary membrane. *Example:* Plasma.

Cumulative effect: The effect produced when a subsequent dose of a drug is administered before the original dose is eliminated or metabolized.

Depressant: A drug that depresses a body function or activity.

Diffusion: The movement of solutes from an area of high concentration to an area of lower concentration.

Dromotropic: Having an effect on conduction velocity. A drug that increases conduction velocity is said to have a positive dromotropic effect.

Emetic: A drug or agent that causes vomiting.

Enteral: By way of the gastrointestinal tract.

Excitability: The sensitivity of a cell to stimulation.

Habituation: The physical or psychological dependence on a drug that develops after repeated use. Also known as *dependence*.

Half-life: The time required to reduce a drug's concentration in the blood by 50%.

Hypercalcemia: An excessive amount of calcium in the blood.

Hyperglycemia: An excessive amount of glucose in the blood. Usually associated with diabetes.

Hypersensitivity: An exaggerated, unanticipated response to a drug.

Hypertonic: Having a higher solute concentration or osmolar pressure than a compared solution.

Hypoglycemia: Lower than normal blood glucose level.

Idiosyncratic response: An unusual, unanticipated response to a drug.

Inotropic: Having an influence on the force of the heart's contraction. A drug that increases the force of contraction is said to have a positive inotropic effect.

Intramuscular: Into or within the muscle.

Intraosseous: Into the bone; refers to a route of medication administration whereby a drug is injected into the medullary canal of a long bone.

Isotonic: Having the same solute concentration or osmotic pressure as another solution.

Medullary canal: The canal within a long bone that contains marrow.

Miosis: Abnormal constriction of the pupils of the eyes.

Opioid: A class of synthetic narcotics that are not derived from opium.

Parasympatholytic: An agent that blocks the effects of the parasympathetic nervous system. *Example:* Atropine sulfate.

Parenteral: Any route of medication administration that is outside of the alimentary canal.

Phlebitis: Inflammation of a vein.

Polydipsia: Excessive thirst.

Polyuria: Excessive urination.

Potentiation: The enhanced effect that occurs when one drug increases the effect of another drug.

Receptor: The component of a cell that combines with a drug to produce a physiological response.

Side effect: The action or effect of a drug other than that which is desired.

Slurry: A thin, watery mixture.

Sublingual: Beneath or under the tongue.

Sympathomimetic: A substance that imitates the action of the sympathetic nervous system. *Example:* Epinephrine.

Synergism: The combined effect of two drugs that is greater than the sum of the two drugs acting independently.

Tolerance: The decreased sensitivity or response to a drug that occurs after repeated doses.

Vasoconstrictor: A drug that causes constriction or narrowing of blood vessels.

Vasodilator: A drug that causes relaxation or widening of blood vessels.

INDEX

Note: Page numbers in *italics* refer to illustrations; page numbers followed by a t refer to tables.

Abbreviations, 455–461

Absorption, drug, 1–3, 471
    circulation and, 2–3
    rate of, 2–3
    surface area and, 2
    tissue thickness and, 2

Acarbose (Precose), 21, 22, 301

Accolate (zafirlukast), 337

Accupril (quinapril), 19–20, 337

Accurbron. See *Theophylline.*

Accutane (isotretinoin), 337

ACE (angiotensin converting enzyme) inhibitors, 19–20
    toxicity of, 20

Acebutolol (Monitan, Sectral), 26–27, 301

Acetaminophen, 301
    oxycodone with, 34–35, 324

Acetazolam (acetazolamide), 337

Acetazolamide (Diamox), 301

Acetohexamide (Dymelor), 21, 22, 301

Acetylcholine, 471

Achromycin (tetracycline), 337

Actidil (triprolidine), 337

Actidose-Aqua. See *Activated charcoal.*

Actifed (pseudoephedrine and triprolidine), 337

Actigall (ursodiol), 337

Actisite (tetracycline), 337

Activated charcoal, 53–55
    angiotensin converting enzyme inhibitors and, 20
    antihistamines and, 23
    beta blockers and, 27
    contraindications to, 54
    dosage for, 54
    for barbiturate abuse, 272–273
    for ingested narcotics, 34–35
    for sedative abuse, 272–273
    for stimulant abuse, 271
    ipecac and, 138, 139
    mechanism of, 471
    nonsteroidal anti-inflammatory drugs and, 36
    poisoning and, 294
    serotonin re-uptake inhibitors and, 21
    toxicity of, 54
    tricyclic antidepressants and, 38

Acular (ketorolac), 338

Acute myocardial infarction algorithm, 432–433

Acyclovir (Zovirax), 301

Adalat. See *Nifedipine (Adalat, Procardia).*

Adapin (doxepin), 338

Adenosine (Adenocard), 55–58
    administration of, 254
    contraindications to, 55

Adenosine (Adenocard) (*Continued*)
  dosage of, 56–57
  for paroxysmal
      supraventricular
      tachycardia, 285, 468,
      469
  interactions with, 56
  toxicity of, 57
Adrenalin Chloride
    (epinephrine), 111–116,
    338. See also *Epinephrine*.
  1:1000, 113–116
    dosage of, 114
    for anaphylaxis, 279
    for respiratory distress,
        296
    toxicity of, 115
  1:10,000, 111–113
    dosage of, 112
    for anaphylaxis, 279
    for bradycardia, 284
    for cardiac arrest, 282
    interactions with, 111
    toxicity of, 112–113
Adrenergic agents, 471
β-Adrenergic blockers. See *Beta
    blockers*.
Adverse effects, of drugs, 16–17,
    48, 49
Advil (ibuprofen), 338
AeroBid (flunisolide), 296, 338
Aerolate. See *Theophylline*.
Aerolone. See *Isoproterenol
    (Isuprel)*.
Aerosporin (polymyxin), 327,
    338
Agonists, 5, 471
Agrylin (anagrelide), 338
Akarpine (pilocarpine), 338
AK-Chlor (chloramphenicol), 338

AK-Cide (prednisolone and
    sulfacetamide), 338
AK-Dex. See *Dexamethasone
    (Decadron, Dexasone,
    Maxidex)*.
Akineton (biperiden), 338
AK-Pred (prednisolone), 338
Ak-Tate (prednisolone), 338
AK-Zol (acetazolamide), 338–339
Alatone (spironolactone), 339
Alazine. See *Hydralazine (Alazine,
    Apresoline)*.
Albuterol (Proventil, Ventolin),
    17, 28–29, 58–60, 301
  contraindications to, 58
  dosage of, 59
  for anaphylaxis, 279
  for bronchospasm, 28, 58, 71,
      161, 296
  interactions with, 59
  toxicity of, 59–60
Albuterol and ipratropium
    (Combivent), 28, 29, 353
Alcaine (proparacaine), 205–206
Alclometasone, 301
Alcohol, abuse of, 274–275
  butorphanol and, 80
  chlorpromazine and, 84–85
  diazepam and, 90
  dimenhydrinate and, 99
  diphenhydramine and,
      100–101
  fosphenytoin and, 121
  haloperidol and, 127
  hydromorphone and, 133
  lorazepam and, 149
  magnesium sulfate and,
      151–152
  meperidine and, 156
  midazolam and, 162

476

Alcohol (*Continued*)
  pentazocine and, 190
  phenobarbital and, 192
  phenytoin and, 194
  promethazine and, 204
Aldactazide (hydrochlorothiazide
    and spironolactone), 339
Aldactone (spironolactone), 32,
    33, 339
Aldoclor-150 (chlorothiazide,
    methyldopa), 339
Aldomet (methyldopa), 339
Aldoril (chlorothiazide,
    methyldopa), 339
Aleve (naproxen), 339
Allegra (fexofenadine), 339
Allerdryl. See *Diphenhydramine*
    (*Benadryl*).
Allergic reactions, and drugs,
    17–18
  treatment of. See specific
    drugs.
Alloprin (allopurinol), 339
Allopurinol (Purinol, Zurinol),
    302
Almocarpine (pilocarpine), 339
Aloe, 425
Alpha methyl fentanyl ("China
    white"), 269–270
Alprazolam (Xanax), 24–25, 302
  abuse of, 272–273
Altace (ramipril), 19–20, 339
Alteplase (tissue plasminogen
    activator, tPA), 60–63
  dosage of, 62
  exclusion criteria for, 61
  for thrombolytic therapy, 288
  interactions with, 62
  toxicity of, 62
Aluminum hydroxide, 302

Alupent. See *Metaproterenol*
    (*Alupent, Metaprel*).
Alurate (aprobarbital), 272–273,
    339
Alvosulfon (dapsone), 339
Amantadine (Symadine,
    Symmetrel), 302
Amaryl (glimepiride), 39, 339
Ambenyl Cough syrup (codeine,
    bromodiphenhydramine),
    340
Ambien (zolpidem), 340
Amcill (ampicillin), 340
Amen (medroxyprogesterone),
    340
Amersol (ibuprofen), 340
Amesec (ephedrine,
    aminophylline), 340
Amikacin (Amikin), 302
Amikin (amikacin), 340
Amiloride (Midamor, Moduretic),
    32, 33, 302
Aminophylline, 20, 29, 63–65,
    302
  contraindications to, 63
  dosage of, 64
  erythromycin and, 64
  for congestive heart failure,
    290
  for respiratory distress,
    296
  interactions with, 64
  pralidoxime and, 199
  toxicity of, 64–65
Amiodarone (Cordarone), 42,
    302
Amitriptyline (Amitril, Elavil),
    37–38, 302
Amlodipine (Norvasc), 29–30,
    302

477

Amobarbital (Amytal, Tuinal), 272–273, 302
Amoline. See *Aminophylline.*
Amoxapine (Asendin), 37–38, 302
Amoxicillin (Amoxil, Trimox), 302
Amoxil (amoxicillin), 340
Amphetamine (Benzedrine), 271–272, 302
Amphotericin B (Amphotec-F), 302
Ampicillin (Omnipen, Polycillin), 302
Ampicin (ampicillin), 340
Ampicin PRB (ampicillin, probenecid), 340
Ampules, 237, 239–240, 239
Amrinone (Inocor), 65–67
  contraindications to, 66
  dosage of, 66
  for congestive heart failure, 288, 290
  interactions with, 66
  toxicity of, 66–67
Amyl nitrite (Vaporole), 67–69
  dosage of, 68–69
  for cyanide poisoning, 294
  interactions with, 68
  toxicity of, 69
  Viagra and, 68
Amytal sodium (amobarbital), 272–273, 340
Anacin (aspirin and caffeine), 340
Anacin w/codeine (aspirin, caffeine, codeine), 340
Anadrol-50 (oxymetholone), 340
Anafranil (clomipramine), 37–38, 340
Anagrelide (Agrylin), 303

Analgesics, 471
Anaphylactic reactions, 278–279
Anaprox (naproxen), 341
Ancasal. See *Aspirin (A.S.A.).*
Ancobon (flucytosine), 314, 341
Ancotil (flucytosine), 341
Android-10 (methyltestosterone), 341
Anexsia (hydrocodone, acetaminophen), 341
Angiotensin converting enzyme (ACE) inhibitors, 19–20
  toxicity of, 20
Ansaid (flurbiprofen), 35–36, 341
Antabuse (disulfiram), 341
Antagonists, 5–6, 471
Antiarrhythmic agents, 42–43, 471
  bretylium tosylate and, 76
Anticholinergics, 471
Anticoagulants, 472
  aspirin and, 70
  dextran and, 261
  glucagon and, 125
  hetastarch and, 263
  streptokinase and, 211
  tissue plasminogen activator and, 62
Anticonvulsants, for isoproterenol–induced tremors, 142–143
Antidepressants, diazepam and, 90
  midazolam and, 162
  morphine and, 164
  serotonin re-uptake inhibitor, 20–21
  toxicity of, 21
  tricyclic, 37–38
    activated charcoal and, 38

478

Antidepressants (*Continued*)
 antagonists for, 38, 196,
  209
 butorphanol and, 80
 fosphenytoin and, 121
 meperidine and, 156
 racemic epinephrine and,
  116–117
 toxicity of, 37–38
Antidiabetic agents, 21–22
 toxicity of, 22
Antidote, 472
Anti-emetic agents, 472
Antihistamines, 23–24, 472
 activated charcoal and, 23
 hydromorphone and, 133
 ipecac and, 23
 meperidine and, 156
 pentazocine and, 190
 racemic epinephrine and,
  116–117
 seizure treatment for, 23
 toxicity of, 23
Antihypertensives, amyl nitrite
  and, 68
 haloperidol and, 127
 labetalol and, 144
 nitroprusside and, 177
 procainamide and, 201–202
 verapamil and, 221
Antilipid agents, 30–31
Antilirium. See *Physostigmine*
  (Antilirium).
Antipsychotic agents, and
  magnesium sulfate, 151–152
Antipyretics, 472
Antispasmodic (atropine,
  hyoscyamine,
  phenobarbital,
  scopolamine), 341

Antivert (meclizine), 341
Anturane (sulfinpyrazone), 341
Anxiety attacks, 280
Anzemet (dolasetron), 341
Apgar scoring system, 443
Apo-Allopurinol (allopurinol),
  341
Apo-Amitriptyline (amitriptyline),
  341
Apo-Amoxi (amoxicillin), 341
Apo-Ampi (ampicillin), 342
Apo-Benztropine (benztropine),
  342
Apo-Carbamazepine. See
  Carbamazepine (Tegretol).
Apo-Chlorpropamide
  (chlorpropamide), 342
Apo-Chlorthalidone
  (chlorthalidone), 342
Apo-Cimetidine. See *Cimetidine*
  (Tagamet).
Apo-Cloxi (cloxacillin), 342
Apo-Diazepam. See *Diazepam*
  (Meval, Valium, Vivol).
Apo-Dipyridamole. See
  Dipyridamole (Persantine).
Apo-Erythro Base. See
  Erythromycin.
Apo-Erythro-ES. See
  Erythromycin.
Apo-Fluphenazine
  (fluphenazine), 342
Apo-Flurazepam. See *Flurazepam*
  (Dalmane).
Apo-Furosemide. See *Furosemide*
  (Lasix, Uritol).
Apo-Haloperidol. See *Haloperidol*
  (Haldol, Peridol).
Apo-Hydro
  (hydrochlorothiazide), 343

Apo-Ibuprofen (ibuprofen), 343

Apo-Indomethacin
(indomethacin), 343

Apo-ISDN (isosorbide dinitrate),
343

Apo-Lorazepam. See *Lorazepam
(Ativan)*.

Apo-Methazide
(hydrochlorothiazide,
methyldopa), 343

Apo-Metoclop (metoclopramide),
343

Apo-Metoprolol. See *Metoprolol
(Lopressor)*.

Apo-Nadol (nadolol), 343

Apo-Naproxen (naproxen), 343

Apo-Nifed. See *Nifedipine (Adalat,
Procardia)*.

Apo-Nitrofurantoin
(nitrofurantoin), 343

Apo-Oxtriphylline
(oxtriphylline), 343

Apo-Penicillin VK (penicillin V),
343

Apo-Perphenazine
(perphenazine), 343

Apo-Piroxicam (piroxicam), 344

Apo-Prazo (prazosin), 344

Apo-Prednisone (prednisone),
344

Apo-Primidone (primidone),
344

Apo-Procainamide. See
Procainamide (Pronestyl).

Apo-Propranolol. See *Propranolol
(Detensol, Inderal)*.

Apo-Quinidine (quinidine), 344

Apo-Ranitidine. See *Ranitidine*.

Apo-Sulfamethoxazole
(sulfamethoxazole), 344

Apo-Sulfatrim (sulfamethoxazole,
trimethoprim), 344

Apo-Tetra (tetracycline), 344

Apo-Thioridazine (thioridazine),
344

Apo-Timolol (timolol), 344

Apo-Tolbutamide (tolbutamide),
344

Apo-Triazide
(hydrochlorothiazide,
trimethoprim), 344

Apo-Trifluoperazine
(trifluoperazine), 344

Apresazide (hydralazine,
hydrochlorothiazide), 345

Apresoline. See *Hydralazine
(Alazine, Apresoline)*.

Apresoline-Esidrix (hydralazine,
hydrochlorothiazide), 345

Aprobarbital (Alurate), 272–273,
303

Aquatensen (methyclothiazide),
345

Aralen (chloroquine), 307, 345

Ardeparin (Normiflo), 303

Aricept (donepezil), 311, 345

Aristocort (triamcinolone), 345

Arm-a-Med. See *Metaproterenol
(Alupent, Metaprel)*.

Artane (trihexyphenidyl), 333,
345

Arthrotec (diclofenac,
misoprostol), 345

Asacol (mesalamine), 345

Asantine (aspirin, dipyridamole),
345

Asendin (amoxapine), 37–38, 345

Aspergum. See *Aspirin (A.S.A.)*.

Aspirin (A.S.A.), 69–71

    contraindications to, 70

Aspirin (*Continued*)
dosage of, 70–71
for chest pain, 287
interactions with, 70
magnesium sulfate and,
151–152
oxycodone with, 34–35
toxicity of, 71
Astemizole (Hismanal), 23–24,
303
Asthma, 295, 296
Astramorph PF. See *Morphine*
(*Duramorph, MS Contin,*
Roxanol).
Astrin. See *Aspirin (A.S.A.)*.
Asystole treatment algorithm,
440–441
Atabrine hydrochloride
(quinacrine), 346
Atarax (hydroxyzine), 346
Atenolol (Tenormin), 26–27,
303
Ativan. See *Lorazepam (Ativan)*.
Atorvastatin calcium (Lipitor),
303
Atovaquone (Mepron), 303
Atromid-S (clofibrate), 308,
346
Atropine, 71–74, 303
dosage of, 73–74, 284
for asystole, 223, 283, 440,
441
for bradycardia, 25, 27, 30,
72, 145, 284
for organophosphate
poisoning, 294
for physostigmine toxicity,
196, 197
for propranolol toxicity, 208
interactions with, 73

Atropine (*Continued*)
pralidoxime and, 199–200
toxicity of, 74
Atrovent (ipratropium), 28, 29,
296, 346
Augmentin (amoxicillin,
clavulanate), 346
Auranofin (Ridaura), 303
Avapro (irbesartan), 346
Aventyl (nortriptyline), 346
Axid (nizatidine), 346
Axotal (aspirin, butalbital), 346
Azaline (sulfasalazine), 346
Azatadine (Optimine, Trinalin),
23, 24, 303
Azathioprine, 303
Azdone (aspirin, hydrocodone),
346
Azithromycin (Zithromax), 303
Azmacort (triamcinolone), 296,
346
Azo Gantanol (phenazopyridine,
sulfamethoxazole), 346
Azo Gantrisin (phenazopyridine,
sulfisoxazole), 346
AZT (zidovudine), 303, 346
Azulfidine (sulfasalazine), 346

Babinski's sign, 451
Bacampicillin (Perglobe), 303
Bacitracin (Neosporin), 303
Bactocill (oxacillin), 346
Bactrim (sulfamethoxazole,
trimethoprim), 347
Ballance's sign, 451
Bancap HC (hydrocodone,
acetaminophen), 347
Barbita. See *Phenobarbital*
(*Barbita, Luminal, Solfoton*).

Barbiturates, abuse of, 272–273
butorphanol and, 80
chlorpromazine and, 84–85
dexamethasone and, 86
diazepam and, 90
dimenhydrinate and, 99
for isoproterenol–induced tremors, 142–143
haloperidol and, 127
hydrocortisone and, 131
lorazepam and, 149
magnesium sulfate and, 151
meperidine and, 156
midazolam and, 162
nalbuphine and, 167
pentazocine and, 190
phenytoin and, 194
promethazine and, 204
Battle's sign, 451
Baycol (cerivastatin), 30–31, 347
Bayer Aspirin. See *Aspirin (A.S.A.)*.
Becaplermin (Regranex), 304
Beck's sign, 451
Beclomethasone (Vancenase AQ), 304
Beclovent (beclomethasone), 296, 347
Beconase AQ (beclomethasone), 347
Beepen-VK (penicillin V), 347
Behavioral emergencies, 279–282
treatment for, 280–281
Belladenal (belladonna, phenobarbital), 347
Belladonna (Bellafoline), 304
Bellergal (ergotamine, phenobarbital), 347
Benadryl. See *Diphenhydramine (Benadryl)*.

Benazepril (Lotensin), 19–20, 304
Bendroflumethiazide (Naturetin, Rauzide), 32, 33, 304
Benemid (probenecid), 347
Bensylate (benztropine), 347
Bentyl (dicyclomine), 310, 347
Benuryl (probenecid), 347
Benylin. See *Diphenhydramine (Benadryl)*.
Benzamycin (erythromycin, benzoyl peroxide), 347
Benzodiazepines, 24–25, 118, 472
antagonist for, 25, 118
for seizure, 65
meperidine and, 156
pancuronium and, 189
succinylcholine with, 214–215
toxicity of, 25
vecuronium with, 220
Benzonatate (Tessalon), 304
Benzphetamine, 304
Benzthiazide (Exna), 32, 33, 304
Benztropine, 304
Bepadin (bepridil), 347
Bepridil (Vascor), 29–30, 304
Beta blockers, 26–27
activated charcoal and, 27
albuterol and, 59
aminophylline and, 64
amyl nitrite and, 68
chlorpromazine and, 85
digoxin and, 95
diltiazem and, 97
for arrhythmia, 43
heart rate and, 26
insulin and, 135
lidocaine and, 146
nifedipine and, 172

Beta blockers (*Continued*)
  norepinephrine and, 181
  terbutaline and, 216
  toxicity of, 27
  verapamil and, 221, 469, 470
Betaloc. See *Metoprolol*
  (*Lopressor*).
Betamethasone (Celestone,
  Lotrisone), 304, 351
Betapace (sotalol), 26–27, 348
Betapen-VK (penicillin), 348
Betaxolol (Betoptic, Kerlone),
  26–27, 304
Bethanechol, 304
Bethaprim (sulfamethoxazole,
  trimethoprim), 348
Betoptic (betaxolol), 348
Biaxin (clarithromycin), 348
Bicillin C-R (penicillin), 348
Biohisdex DHC
  (diphenylpyraline,
  hydrocodone,
  phenylephrine), 348
Biohisdine DHC
  (diphenylpyraline,
  hydrocodone,
  phenylephrine), 348
Biotransformation, of drugs, 4
Biot's respiration, 451
Biperiden (Akineton), 304
Biphetamine
  (dextroamphetamine,
  amphetamine), 348
Biquin Durules (quinidine), 348
Bisacodyl (Dulcolax), 304
Bisoprolol (Zebeta), 26–27, 304
Bitolterol (Tornalate), 28, 29, 304
Blephamide (prednisolone), 348
Blocadren (timolol), 26–27, 348
Blood-brain barrier, 4

Blumberg's sign, 451
Bozzolo's sign, 452
Bradycardia treatments, 284–285
Brethaire. See *Terbutaline*
  (*Brethine*).
Brethine. See *Terbutaline*
  (*Brethine*).
Bretylate. See *Bretylium tosylate*
  (*Bretylate, Bretylol*).
Bretylium tosylate (Bretylate,
  Bretylol), 75–77
  dosage of, 76–77
  for ventricular arrhythmia,
    283, 285, 465, 469
  interactions with, 76
  toxicity of, 77
Brevicon (norethindrone), 348
Bricanyl. See *Terbutaline*
  (*Brethine*).
Bromfenac (Duract), 305
Bromocriptine (Parlodel), 305
Bromodiphenhydramine
  (Ambenyl), 305
Brompheniramine (Bromfed,
  Diamine), 23, 24, 305
Bronalide (flunisolide), 349
Bronchodilators, 28–29, 472
  toxicity of, 28
Brondecon (guaifenesin,
  oxtriphylline), 349
Bronitin Mist. See *Epinephrine*.
Bronkaid Mist. See *Epinephrine*.
Bronkephrine
  (ethylnorepinephrine), 349
Bronkodyl. See *Theophylline*.
Bronkometer. See *Isoetharine*
  (*Bronkosol*).
Bronkosol. See *Isoetharine*
  (*Bronkosol*).
Bucladin-S (buclizine), 349

483

Buclizine (Bucladin-S), 305
Bumetanide (Bumex), 32, 33,
    77–79, 305
  contraindications to, 78
  dosage of, 78
  for congestive heart failure,
    210, 287–288, 289
  interactions with, 78
  toxicity of, 79
Bumex. See *Bumetanide (Bumex)*.
Buprenex (buprenorphine), 349
Buprenorphine, 305
Bupropion (Wellbutrin, Zyban),
    305
Burn management, fluid therapy
    for, 453–454
BuSpar (buspirone), 349
Buspirone (BuSpar), 305, 349
Butabarbital (Buticaps, Butisol),
    272–273, 305
Butalbital, 305
Butazolidin (phenylbutazone),
    349
Buticaps (butabarbital), 349
Butisol sodium (butabarbital),
    272–273, 349
Butorphanol (Stadol), 79–81,
    305
  contraindications to, 80
  dosage of, 80
  for pain management, 79, 299
  interactions with, 80
  toxicity of, 81

Cafergot (caffeine, ergotamine),
    349
Cafergot PB (atropine, caffeine,
    ergotamine, phenobarbital),
    349–350

Caladryl (calamine,
    diphenhydramine), 350
Calan. See *Verapamil (Calan,
    Isoptin, Verelan)*.
Calcimar (calcitonin), 350
Calcipotriene (Dovonex), 305
Calcitonin (Calcimar), 305
Calcium, 81–84, 305
  contraindications to, 82
  digoxin and, 82, 94–95
  diltiazem and, 98
  dosages of, 82–83
  for black widow spider
    reaction, 294
  for calcium channel
    blocker–induced reaction,
    222, 294
  for magnesium
    sulfate–induced reaction,
    152–153, 294
  interactions with, 82
  toxicity of, 83
Calcium channel blockers,
    29–30, 472
  for arrhythmia, 43
  propranolol and, 207
  toxicity of, 29–30
Canesten (clotrimazole), 350
Capital with/Codeine
    (acetaminophen, codeine),
    350
Capoten (captopril), 19–20,
    350
Capozide (captopril,
    hydrochlorothiazide),
    350
Capsaicin (Zostrix), 305
Captopril (Capoten, Capozide),
    19–20, 305
Carafate (sucralfate), 350

Carbamazepine (Tegretol), 39, 305
  adenosine and, 56
Carbenicillin (Geocillin), 306
Carbidopa, 306
Carbolith. See Lithium.
Cardene (nicardipine), 29–30, 350
Cardiac arrest, 282–283
  epinephrine metabolization and, 4
  treatment algorithm for, 440–441
Cardiac dysrhythmias, 283–286
  tachycardia algorithm for, 468–470
  treatment for, 284–286
  ventricular VF/VT algorithm for, 464–465
Cardioquin (quinidine), 350
Cardiovascular disease, medications for, 40–43
Cardiovascular function, drug absorption and, 2–3
  drug distribution and, 3
Cardizem. See Diltiazem (Cardizem).
Cardura (doxazosin), 312, 350
Carfin. See Warfarin (Coumadin, Sofarin).
Carisoprodol (Soma), 306
Carteolol (Cartrol), 26–27, 306
Cartrol (carteolol), 26–27, 350
Cataflam (diclofenac), 350
Catalyst, 472
Catapres (clonidine), 350
Catheters, 250
Catnip, 425
Ceclor (cefaclor), 351
Cefaclor (Ceclor), 306

Cefadroxil (Duricef), 306
Cefdinir (Omnicef), 306
Cefixime (Suprax), 306
Cefmetazole (Zefazone), 306
Cefotaxime (Claforan), 306
Cefoxitin (Mefoxin), 306
Cefpodoxime (Vantin), 306
Cefprozil (Cefzil), 306
Ceftazidime (Fortaz), 306
Ceftin (cefuroxime), 351
Ceftriaxone (Rocephin), 306
Cefuroxime (Ceftin), 306
Cefzil (cefprozil), 351
Celestone (betamethasone), 304, 351
Celontin (methsuximide), 351
Centrax (prazepam), 24–25, 327, 351
Cephalexin (Ceporex, Keflex), 306
Cephanex (cephalexin), 351
Cephradine (Velosef), 307
Ceporex (cephalexin), 351
Cerebyx. See Fosphenytoin (Cerebyx).
Cerivastatin (Baycol), 30–31, 307
Cetirizine (Zyrtec), 307
Chamomile, 425
Chaparral, 425–426
Chardonna-2 (belladonna, phenobarbital), 351
Cheyne-Stokes respiration, 452
Child birth, and Apgar scoring system, 443
Chloral hydrate, 307
Chlorambucil (Leukeran), 307
Chloramphenicol (Chloroptic, Fenicol), 307
Chlordiazepoxide (Libritabs, Librium), 272–273, 307

485

Chlormezanone (Trancopal),
307
Chloromycetin
(chloramphenicol), 351
Chloronase (chlorpropamide),
351
Chloroptic (chloramphenicol),
351
Chloroquine (Aralen), 307, 345
Chlorothiazide (Diachlor,
Diupres, Diuril), 32, 33,
307
Chlorpheniramine (Atrohist
Pediatric, Chlorspan,
Chlor-Trimeton), 23, 24,
307
Chlor-Promanyl. See
Chlorpromazine.
Chlorpromazine, 84–86, 307
contraindications to, 84
dosage of, 85
for agitation, 281
for hallucinogen abuse, 274
interactions with, 84–85
toxicity of, 85
Chlorpropamide (Chloronase,
Diabinese), 21, 22, 307
Chlorprothixene, 307
Chlorthalidone (Hygroton,
Hylidone, Regroton), 32, 33,
307
Chlor-Trimeton
(chlorpheniramine), 23, 24,
351
Chlorzoxazone (Paraflex), 307
Choledyl (oxtriphylline), 28, 29,
351
Cholesterol lowering agents,
30–31
toxicity of, 31

Cholestyramine (Questran),
30–31, 307
Choloxin (dextrothyroxine), 351
Cholybar (cholestyramine), 352
Chronic obstructive pulmonary
disease (COPD), 295, 296
Chronotropic, 472
Cibalith-S. See Lithium.
Cimetidine (Tagamet), 308
lidocaine and, 146
Cin-Quin (quinidine), 352
Cipro. See Ciprofloxacin (Cipro).
Ciprofloxacin (Cipro), 308
Circulation, and drug absorption,
2–3
drug distribution and, 3
Cisapride (Propulsid), 308
Claforan (cefotaxime), 352
Clarithromycin (Biaxin), 308
Claritin (loratadine), 23, 24, 352
Claritin-D, 352
Clavulin (amoxicillin,
clavulanate), 352
Cleeman's sign, 452
Clemastine (Tavist), 23, 24, 308
Cleocin. See Clindamycin
(Cleocin).
Clidinium (Quarzan), 308
Clindamycin (Cleocin), 308
magnesium sulfate and,
151–152
Clinoril (sulindac), 35–36, 37,
352
Clofibrate (Atromid-S), 308, 346
Clomipramine (Anafranil),
37–38, 308
Clonazepam (Klonopin), 24–25,
39, 308
abuse of, 272–273
Clonidine (Catapres), 308

486

Clopidogrel (Plavix), 308
Clorazepate (Tranxene), 24–25, 308
    abuse of, 272–273
Clotrimazole (Gyne-Lotrimin), 308
Cloxacillin (Cloxapen), 308
Cloxapen (cloxacillin), 352
Clozapine (Clozaril), 308
Clozaril (clozapine), 352
Co-Advil (ibuprofen, pseudoephedrine), 352
Co-Betaloc (hydrochlorothiazide, metoprolol), 352
Cocaine, 271–272
Codeine (Empirin with codeine, Tylenol with codeine), 34–35, 308
    abuse of, 269–270
Codiclear DH (guaifenesin, hydrocodone), 352
Codimal DH (hydrocodone, phenylephrine, pyrilamine), 352
Codimal DM (dextromethorphan, phenylephrine, pyrilamine), 352–353
Codimal PH (codeine, phenylephrine, pyrilamine), 353
Codimal-L.A. (chlorpheniramine, pseudoephedrine), 353
Cogentin (benztropine), 353
Co-Gesic (acetaminophen, codeine), 353
Cognex (tacrine), 353
Colace (docusate), 353
ColBenemid (colchicine, probenecid), 353
Colchicine, 308

Colestid (colestipol), 30–31, 353
Colestipol (Colestid), 30–31, 309
Colloid fluids, 253, 472
Coma, causes of, 449
Coma scale, 445–446
Combipres (chlorthalidone, clonidine), 353
Combivent (albuterol and ipratropium), 28, 29, 353
Comoxol (sulfamethoxazole), 353
Compazine (prochlorperazine), 353
Compoz. See Diphenhydramine (Benadryl).
Congess JR/SR (guaifenesin, pseudoephedrine), 353
Congestive heart failure (CHF), 288–290
    treatment for, 289–290
Conjugated estrogens, 309
Consensus Formula, for burn management, 453, 454
Constant-T. See Theophylline.
Coptin (sulfadiazine, trimethoprim), 353
Cordarone (amiodarone), 42, 354
Corgard (nadolol), 26–27, 354
Coronex (isosorbide dinitrate), 354
Corzide (nadolol, bendroflumethiazide), 354
Cotrim (sulfamethoxazole, trimethoprim), 354
Coumadin. See Warfarin (Coumadin, Sofarin).
Cozaar (losartan), 354
Cranberry, 426
Cromolyn (Gastrocrom), 309
Crystalloid fluids, 253–254
Crystodigin (digitoxin), 354

Cullen's sign, 452

Cumulative effect, of medication, 6, 472

Cuprimine (penicillamine), 354

Curretab (medroxyprogesterone), 354

Cushing's triad, 452

Cutivate (fluticasone), 354

Cyanocobalamin (vitamin B_{12}), 309

Cyclacillin, 309

Cyclandelate (Cyclospasmol), 309

Cyclobenzaprine (Flexeril), 309

Cyclopar (tetracycline), 354

Cyclophosphamide (Cytoxan), 309

Cycloserine (Seromycin), 309

Cyclospasmol (cylandelate), 354

Cyclosporine (Sandimmune), 309

Cycrin (medroxyprogesterone), 354

Cylert (pemoline), 354

Cyproheptadine (Periactin), 23, 24, 309

Cystospaz (hyoscyamine), 354

Cytomel (liothyronine), 354

Cytotec (misoprostol), 355

Cytovene (ganciclovir), 355

Cytoxan (cyclophosphamide), 355

D_5W (Dextrose 5% in water), 258–259

$D_{10}W$ (Dextrose 10% in water), 253–254, 259–260

Dacliximab (Zenapax), 309

Dalacin C. See Clindamycin (Cleocin).

Dalgan (dezocine), 355

Dallergy (chlorpheniramine, methscopolamine, phenylephrine), 355

Dalmane. See Flurazepam (Dalmane).

Damason-P (aspirin, hydrocodone), 355

Dantrium (dantrolene), 355

Dantrolene (Dantrium), 309

Dapsone (Alvosulfon), 309

Daranide (dichlorphenamide), 355

Daraprim (pyrimethamine), 355

Darvocet-N (acetaminophen, propoxyphene), 355

Darvon. See Propoxyphene (Darvon, Dolene).

Darvon w/ aspirin (aspirin, propoxyphene), 355

Daypro (oxaprozin), 35–36, 37, 355

Dazamide (acetazolamide), 355

DDAVP (desmopressin), 356

Decaderm. See Dexamethasone (Decadron, Dexasone, Maxidex).

Decadron. See Dexamethasone (Decadron, Dexasone, Maxidex).

Decadron with Xylocaine (dexamethasone, lidocaine), 356

Decaspray. See Dexamethasone (Decadron, Dexasone, Maxidex).

Declomycin (demeclocycline), 356

Deconamine (chlorpheniramine, pseudoephedrine), 356

Defibrillation, for ventricular
    fibrillation, 464, 465
Delavirdine (Rescriptor), 309
Delestrogen (estradiol), 356
Delsym (dextromethorphan),
    356
Delta-Cortef (prednisolone), 356
Deltasone (prednisone), 356
Demadex (torsemide), 32, 33,
    356
Demecarium (Humorsol), 309
Demeclocycline (Declomycin),
    309
Demerol. See Meperidine
    (Demerol, Pethadol).
Demi-Regroton (chlorthalidone,
    reserpine), 356
Demser (metyrosine), 356
Demulen (ethynodiol), 356
Depa (valproic acid), 356
Depakene (valproic acid), 39,
    357
Depakote (divalproex sodium),
    39, 311, 357
Depen (penicillamine), 357
Depo Provera
    (medroxyprogesterone),
    357
Deponit. See Nitroglycerin.
Depressants, 472
Deproic (valproic acid), 357
Deronil. See Dexamethasone
    (Decadron, Dexasone,
    Maxidex).
Deserpidine (Harmonyl), 309
Desipramine (Norpramin),
    37–38, 310
Desmopressin (DDAVP), 310
Desoxyn (methamphetamine),
    271–272, 357

Desyrel (trazodone), 357
Detensol. See Propranolol
    (Detensol, Inderal).
Dexamethasone (Decadron,
    Dexasone, Maxidex), 86–87,
    310
    dosage of, 86–87
    for head injury, 299
    interactions with, 86
    lidocaine with, 356
    toxicity of, 87
Dexasone. See Dexamethasone
    (Decadron, Dexasone,
    Maxidex).
Dexbrompheniramine, 310
Dexchlorpheniramine, 310
Dexedrine (dextroamphetamine),
    271–272, 357
Dexone. See Dexamethasone
    (Decadron, Dexasone,
    Maxidex).
Dextran, 260–261
    contraindications to, 260
    dosage of, 261
    interactions with, 261
Dextroamphetamine (Dexedrine),
    271–272, 310
Dextromethorphan, 310
Dextrose 5% in water (D_5W),
    258–259
    contraindication to, 258
    interactions with, 259
Dextrose 10% in water ($D_{10}W$),
    253–254, 259–260
    contraindications to, 259
    interactions with, 260
Dextrose 50% ($D50$), 87–89
    adverse reactions and, 89
    dosage of, 88
    for alcohol abuse, 274

489

Dextrose (Continued)
for antidiabetic agent
overdose, 22
for diabetic hypoglycemia,
291–292, 298
for insulin overdose, 136
for narcotic abuse, 270
for seizure, 298
phenytoin and, 194
poisoning and, 294
precautions with, 88
thiamine with, 88, 217, 218
Dextrothyroxine (Choloxin),
310
Dezocine (Dalgan), 310
DiaBeta (glyburide), 21, 22,
357
Diabetes, insulin and, 13–14
medications for, 21–22, 39–40
Diabetic emergency, 290–292
treatment for, 291–292
Diabinese (chlorpropamide), 21,
22, 357
Diachlor (chlorothiazide), 357
Diagnostic signs, 451–452
Dialose (docusate), 357
Diamox (acetazolamide), 358
Diazemuls. See Diazepam (Meval,
Valium, Vivol).
Diazepam (Meval, Valium, Vivol),
89–92, 310
abuse of, 272–273
antagonist for, 91
contraindications to, 90
dosage of, 90
for alcohol abuse, 275
for anxiety, 281
for hallucinogen abuse, 274
for isoproterenol–induced
tremors, 142–143

Diazepam (Continued)
for seizure, 23, 28, 38, 85, 89,
148, 298
for stimulant abuse, 272
interactions with, 90
intubation with, 300
poisoning and, 294
succinylcholine and, 213
toxicity of, 91
Diazepam Intensol, 358
Diazoxide (Hyperstat), 92–94,
310
contraindications to, 92
dosage of, 93
for hypertensive crisis, 298
interactions with, 93
toxicity of, 93
Dibenzyline
(phenoxybenzamine), 358
Dichlorphenamide, 310
Diclofenac (Arthrotec, Voltaren),
35–36, 310
Dicloxacillin (Dycill, Dynapen),
310
Dicumarol
(bishydroxycoumarin), 358
Dicyclomine (Bentyl), 310
Didanosine (Videx), 310
Didrex (benzphetamine), 358
Didronel (etidronate), 358
Diethylpropion (Tenuate), 310
Difenoxine (Motofen), 34–35
Diffusion, 473
Diflucan (fluconazole), 358
Diflunisal (Dolobid), 311
Digitalis, and furosemide, 123
Digitoxin (Crystodigin), 311
Digoxin (Lanoxin), 94–96, 311
calcium and, 82, 94–95
contraindications to, 94

Digoxin (*Continued*)
  dosage of, 95
  for atrial dysrhythmia, 285,
    311
  for congestive heart failure,
    290, 311
  interactions with, 94–95
  succinylcholine and, 213
  toxicity of, 95
Dihydrocodeine, 311
Dilacor XR. See *Diltiazem*
    (Cardizem).
Dilantin. See *Phenytoin (Dilantin,*
    Diphenylan).
Dilatrate-SR (isosorbide
    dinitrate), 358
Dilaudid. See *Hydromorphone*
    (Dilaudid).
Dilor (dyphylline), 358
Dilor-G (dyphylline, guaifenesin),
    358
Diltiazem (Cardizem), 29–30,
    96–98, 311
  calcium and, 98
  contraindications to, 96
  dosage of, 97
  for atrial dysrhythmia, 285
  interactions with, 97
  toxicity of, 97–98
Dimenhydrinate (Dramamine,
    Travamine), 98–100, 311
  contraindications to, 98
  dosage of, 99
  for nausea, 300
  interactions with, 99
  toxicity of, 99
Dimetane Expectorant-DC
    (brompheniramine,
    hydrocodone,
    phenylpropanolamine), 358

Dimetane-DC, 34–35
Dimetane-DC Cough
    (brompheniramine, codeine,
    phenylpropanolamine),
    358
Dimetapp-C (brompheniramine,
    codeine), 359
Diovan (valsartan), 359
Dipentum (olsalazine), 359
Diphenhist. See *Diphenhydramine*
    (Benadryl).
Diphenhydramine (Benadryl),
    100–101, 311, 347
  contraindications to, 100
  dosage of, 101
  for anaphylaxis, 279
  for diazepam allergy, 91
  for furosemide allergy, 124
  for lidocaine allergy, 148
  for magnesium sulfate allergy,
    153
  for meperidine allergy, 157
  for morphine allergy, 165–166
  for promethazine allergy, 204
  interactions with, 100–101
  toxicity of, 101
Diphenidol (Vontrol), 311
Diphenoxylate, 34–35, 311
Diphenylan sodium. See
    Phenytoin (Dilantin,
    Diphenylan).
Dipyridamole (Persantine), 311
  adenosine and, 56
Disalcid (salsalate), 359
Disopyramide (Norpace), 42, 311
Distribution, drug, 3–4
    blood-brain barrier and, 4
    circulation and, 3
    plasma in, 3
    protein binding in, 3

Disulfiram (Antabuse), 311
Ditropan (oxybutynin), 359
Diucardin (hydroflumethiazide), 32, 33, 359
Diuchlor-H (hydrochlorothiazide), 359
Diulo (metolazone), 359
Diupres (chlorothiazide), 359
Diurese (trichlormethiazide), 32, 33, 359
Diuretics, 32–33
   digoxin and, 94–95
   for congestive heart failure, 32, 131, 208, 210
   hydralazine and, 129
   toxicity of, 32–33
Diurigen (chlorothiazide), 359
Diuril (chlorothiazide), 32, 33, 359
Diutensen (cryptenamine, methyclothiazide), 359
Diutensen-R (methyclothiazide, reserpine), 359
Divalproex sodium (Depakote), 39, 311
Dixarit (clonidine), 359
Dizac. See Diazepam (Meval, Valium, Vivol).
Dobutamine (Dobutrex), 101–106
   contraindications to, 102
   dosage of, 102–103, 104t–105t
   for congestive heart failure, 288, 290
   interactions with, 102
   magnesium sulfate and, 151–152
   toxicity of, 103
Docusate (Surfak), 311

Dolasetron (Anzemet), 311
Dolene. See Propoxyphene (Darvon, Dolene).
Dolobid (diflunisal), 360
Dolophine hydrochloride. See Methadone (Dolophine).
Donepezil (Aricept), 311, 345
Dopamine (Intropin, Revimine), 106–109
   contraindications to, 106–107
   dosage of, 107–108, 109
   for bradycardia, 284
   for bretylium–induced reaction, 77
   for hypotension, 91, 101, 148, 150, 153, 222
   interactions with, 107
   oxytocin and, 187
   toxicity of, 108
Dopar (levodopa), 360
Doral (quazepam), 24–25, 360
Dornase alfa (Pulmozyme), 311
Doryx (doxycycline), 360
Dovonex (calcipotriene), 360
Doxazosin (Cardura), 312
Doxepin (Adapin, Sinequan), 37–38, 312
Doxidan (docusate), 360
Doxychel (doxycycline hyclate), 360
Doxycycline (Doryx), 312
Dramamine. See Dimenhydrinate (Dramamine, Travamine).
Drixoral (dexbrompheniramine), 360
Dromotropic, 473
Dronabinol, 312
Droperidol (Inapsine), 109–110, 312
   contraindication to, 109

Droperidol (Inapsine) (*Continued*)
  dosage of, 110
  interactions with, 110
  toxicity of, 110
Drug(s). See also *Fluid therapy*.
  absorption of, 1–3, 471
    circulation and, 2–3
    surface area and, 2
    tissue thickness and, 2
  action of, 47
  administration of, 227–236
    ampules in, 237, 239–240,
      239
    buccal, 229
    endotracheal tube, 230–231,
      245
    inhalation, 232
    intracardiac, 232–233
    intramuscular, 230,
      241–243, 242
      needles for, 241
      syringes for, 241
    intraosseous, 233–234,
      246–247, 473
    intravenous line, 244–245,
      247–248
    oral, 228
    parenteral, 474
    pre-filled syringes in, 237,
      240
    rectal, 231–232
    subcutaneous, 229–230,
      243, 244
      needles for, 243
      syringes for, 243
    sublingual, 228–229, 474
    transdermal, 234
    Tubex cartridges in, 237,
      240–241
    vials in, 237–239, 237–238

Drug(s) (*Continued*)
  allergic reactions with, 17–18
  antagonism of, 5–6, 471
  binding capacity of, 3
  biotransformation of, 4
  class of, 47
  concentration of, 2
  container labels and, 11,
    12–14
  contraindications to, 47–48
  cumulative action of, 6, 472
  distribution of, 3–4
    blood-brain barrier and, 4
    plasma in, 3
    protein binding in, 3
  excretion of, 4–5
  habituation and, 7, 473
  history taking and, 9, 10–11
  idiosyncrasy and, 7, 473
  indications for, 47
  interaction of, 6–7, 18–19, 48
  metabolism of, 4
  names of, 46
    generic, 301–335
    trade, 337–424
  overdose of, 14–15, 49
  pH of, 2
  potentiation of, 6, 474
  precautions for, 48
  receptors of, 5, 474
  reservoirs of, 3
  routes for, 49. See also *Drug(s)*,
    administration of.
  side effects of, 16–17, 48,
    474
  solubility of, 2
  synergism of, 6, 474
  tolerance to, 6, 7, 474
  toxicity and, 6, 49
  underdosing of, 15–16

Drug abuse, 265–266
  assessment of, 266–268
  treatment of, 268
Drug box, 235, 237
Dulcolax (bisacodyl), 360
Duocet (acetaminophen, hydrocodone), 360
Duo-Medihaler (isoproterenol, phenylephrine), 360
Duotrate (pentaerythritol tetranitrate), 360
Duract (bromfenac), 360
Duradyne (acetaminophen, hydrocodone), 360
Duragesic. See *Fentanyl (Sublimaze, Duragesic)*.
Duralith. See *Lithium*.
Duramorph. See *Morphine (Duramorph, MS Contin, Roxanol)*.
Durapam. See *Flurazepam (Dalmane)*.
Duraquin (quinidine), 361
Duratuss (guaifenesin, hydrocodone, pseudoephedrine), 361
Duretic (methyclothiazide), 361
Duricef (cefadroxil), 361
DV (dienestrol), 361
Dyazide (hydrochlorothiazide, triamterene), 361
Dycill (dicloxacillin), 361
Dymelor (acetohexamide), 21, 22, 361
DynaCirc (isradipine), 29–30, 361
Dynapen (dicloxacillin), 361
Dyphylline (Dilor), 312

Dyrenium (triamterene), 32, 33, 361
Dysne-Inhal. See *Epinephrine*.

Easprin. See *Aspirin (A.S.A.)*.
Echinacea, 426
Econazole (Spectazole), 312
Econopred (prednisolone), 361–362
Ecotrin. See *Aspirin (A.S.A.)*.
Edecrin (ethacrynic acid), 32, 33, 362
E.E.S. See *Erythromycin*.
Effexor (venlafaxine), 20–21, 362
Elavil (amitriptyline), 37–38, 362
Eldepryl (selegiline), 362
Elimite (permethrin), 362
Elixomin. See *Theophylline*.
Elixophyllin. See *Theophylline*.
Elocon (mometasone), 362
Eltroxin (levothyroxine), 362
Emadine (emedastine), 362
Emedastine (Emadine), 312
Emetics, 473
Emex (metoclopramide), 362
Emitrip (amitriptyline), 362
Emla (lidocaine, prilocaine), 362
Emphysema, 295
Empirin. See *Aspirin (A.S.A.)*.
Empirin with Codeine (aspirin, codeine), 362
Empracet (acetaminophen, codeine), 363
Emtec (acetaminophen, codeine), 363
E-Mycin. See *Erythromycin*.
Enalapril (Vasotec), 19–20, 312
Encainide (Enkaid), 312
Endep (amitriptyline), 36

494

Endocet (acetaminophen, oxycodone), 363

Endodan (aspirin, oxycodone), 363

Endotracheal intubation, 300
in drug administration, 230–231, 245

Enduron (methyclothiazide), 32, 33, 363

Enduronyl (methyclothiazide, deserpidine), 363

Enovid (mestranol, norethynodrel), 363

Enteral route, 473

Entex LA (phenylpropanolamine, guaifenesin), 363

Entrophen. See Aspirin (A.S.A.).

E-Pam. See Diazepam (Meval, Valium, Vivol).

Ephed II (ephedrine), 363

Ephedrine (Vicks Vatronol), 28, 29, 312

Epifrin. See Epinephrine.

Epimorph. See Morphine (Duramorph, MS Contin, Roxanol).

Epinephrine, 29, 111–118, 312
1:1000, 113–116
dosage of, 114
for anaphylaxis, 279
for diazepam allergy, 91
for furosemide allergy, 124
for lidocaine allergy, 148
for magnesium sulfate allergy, 153
for morphine allergy, 165–166
for respiratory distress, 296
toxicity of, 115

Epinephrine (Continued)
1:10,000, 111–113
dosage of, 112
for anaphylaxis, 279
for bradycardia, 284
for cardiac arrest, 282
interactions with, 111
toxicity of, 112–113
albuterol and, 59
chlorpromazine and, 85
for asystole, 222, 440, 441
for meperidine allergy, 157
for ventricular fibrillation, 465
glucagon and, 125
isoetharine and, 140
isoproterenol and, 142
metabolization of, 4
oxytocin and, 186
promethazine and, 204
racemic, 116–118, 329
contraindications to, 116
dosage of, 117
for anaphylaxis, 279
for respiratory distress, 296
interactions with, 116–117
toxicity of, 117–118

Epipen. See Epinephrine.

Epitol. See Carbamazepine (Tegretol).

Epitrate. See Epinephrine.

Epival (valproic acid), 364

Eprosartan (Teveten), 312

Equagesic (aspirin, meprobamate), 364

Equanil (meprobamate), 364

Ercaf (caffeine, ergotamine), 364

Ergoloid mesylate (Hydergine), 312

Ergomar (ergotamine), 364

Ergostat (ergotamine), 364

Ergotamine, 312
ERYC. See *Erythromycin.*
EryDerm. See *Erythromycin.*
Erygel. See *Erythromycin.*
Erypar. See *Erythromycin.*
EryPed. See *Erythromycin.*
Ery-Tab. See *Erythromycin.*
Erythrityl tetranitrate (Cardilate), 312
Erythrocin stearate. See *Erythromycin.*
Erythromid. See *Erythromycin.*
Erythromycin, 313
  aminophylline and, 64
Eryzole (erythromycin, sulfisoxazole), 364
Esgic (acetaminophen, butalbital, caffeine), 364
Esgic with codeine (acetaminophen, butalbital, caffeine, codeine), 364–365
Esidrix (hydrochlorothiazide), 365
Esimil (guanethidine, hydrochlorothiazide), 365
Eskalith. See *Lithium.*
Estazolam (ProSom), 24–25, 313
Estinyl (estrogen), 365
Estrace (estrogen), 365
Estraderm (estrogen), 365
Estradiol, 313
Estraguard (estrogen), 365
Estratab (estrogen), 365
Estrogen(s), 313
  conjugated, 309
Estropipate, 313
Estrovis (estrogen), 365
Ethacrynic acid (Edecrin), 32, 33, 313
Ethambutol, 313

Ethatab (ethaverine), 365
Ethaverine (Ethatab), 313
Ethchlorvynol (Placidyl), 313
Ethionamide (Trecator-SC), 313
Ethmozine (moricizine), 42, 365
Ethosuximide (Zarontin), 313
Ethotoin, 313
Ethylnorepinephrine (Bronkephrine), 313
Etidronate (Didronel), 313
Etodolac (Lodine), 35–36, 313
Etrafon (amitriptyline, perphenazine), 365
Etretinate (Tegison), 313
Euflex, 365
Euglucon (glyburide), 365
Eulexin (flutamide), 365
Euthroid (levothyroxine, liothyronine), 365
E-Vista (hydroxyzine), 365
Excedrin (acetaminophen, aspirin, caffeine), 366
Excedrin P.M. (acetaminophen, diphenhydramine), 366
Excitability, 473
Excretion, of drugs, 4–5
Exdol (acetaminophen, caffeine, codeine), 366
Exna (benzthiazide), 32, 33, 366

Factor VIII (Monoclate-P), 313
Fahrenheit to Centigrade, 437t–438t
Famciclovir (Famvir), 313
Famotidine (Pepcid), 313
Famvir (famciclovir), 366
Fansidar (pyrimethamine, sulfadoxine), 366
Felbamate (Felbatol), 39, 314

Felbatol (felbamate), 39, 366
Feldene (piroxicam), 35–36, 37, 366
Felodipine (Plendil), 29–30, 314
Femara (letrozole), 366
Femazole (metronidazole), 366
Femcet (acetaminophen, butalbital, caffeine), 366
Feminone (estrogen), 366
Femogen (estrogen), 366
Femogex (estrogen), 366
Fenicol (chloramphenicol), 366
Fennel, 426
Fenoprofen (Nalfon), 35–36, 314
Fentanyl (Sublimaze, Duragesic), 314
    abuse of, 269–270
    naloxone and, 170
Fentanyl (Duragesic transdermal) patch, 34–35
Feosol (ferrous sulfate), 366
Fergon (ferrous sulfate), 366
Ferrous gluconate, 314
Ferrous sulfate, 314
Feverfew, 426
Fevernol (acetaminophen), 366
Fexofenadine (Allegra), 314
Finasteride (Propecia, Proscar), 314
Fioricet (acetaminophen, butalbital, caffeine), 367
Fiorinal (aspirin, butalbital, caffeine), 367
Fiorinal with Codeine (acetaminophen, butalbital, caffeine, codeine), 367
Flagyl (metronidazole), 367
Flavoxate (Urispas), 314
Flecainide (Tambocor), 42, 314
Flexeril (cyclobenzaprine), 367

Flomax (tamsulosin), 367
Floropryl (isoflurophate), 367
Floxin (ofloxacin), 367
Fluconazole (Diflucan), 314
Flucytosine (Ancobon), 314, 341
Fluid therapy, 249–263
    administration sets in, 250–251
    catheters in, 250
    colloid solutions in, 253, 472
    crystalloid solutions in, 253–254
    diffusion and, 473
    for burn management, 453–454
    infusion rate for, 251–252, 263t
    sites for, 254
Flumadine (rimantadine), 367
Flumazenil (Romazicon), 91, 118–120
    contraindications to, 119
    dosage of, 119–120
    for benzodiazepine antagonism, 25, 118, 150, 273, 294
    for midazolam–induced reaction, 162
    toxicity of, 120
Flunisolide (AeroBid), 314
Fluocinolone (Lidex), 314
Fluoxetine (Prozac), 20–21, 314
Fluphenazine (Permitil), 314
Flurazepam (Dalmane), 24–25, 314
    abuse of, 272–273
Flurbiprofen (Ansaid), 35–36, 315
Flutamide (Eulexin), 315
Fluticasone (Cutivate), 315
Fluvastatin (Lescol), 30–31, 315

497

Fluvoxamine (Luvox), 315
Folex (methotrexate), 367
Fortaz (ceftazidime), 367
Fosinopril (Monopril), 19–20, 315
Fosphenytoin (Cerebyx), 120–122
  contraindications to, 121
  dosage of, 121
  for seizure, 120–121, 210
  interactions with, 121
  toxicity of, 122
Fructose, 315
Fulvicin (griseofulvin), 367
Furadantin (nitrofurantoin), 367
Furalan (nitrofurantoin), 367
Furanite (nitrofurantoin), 367
Furosemide (Lasix, Uritol), 32, 33, 122–125, 315
  amrinone and, 66
  contraindications to, 123
  digoxin and, 94–95
  dosage of, 123
  for chest pain, 287–288
  for congestive heart failure, 27, 32, 131, 139, 173, 289
  for pulmonary edema, 145, 160–161
  interactions with, 123
  toxicity of, 124
Furoside. See Furosemide (Lasix, Uritol).

Gabapentin (Neurontin), 39, 315
Gabitril (tiagabine), 368
Ganciclovir (Cytovene), 315
Gantanol (sulfamethoxazole), 368
Gantrisin (sulfisoxazole), 368

Gardenal. See Phenobarbital (Barbita, Luminal, Solfoton).
Garlic, 426–427
Gastrocrom (cromolyn), 368
Gemfibrozil (Lopid), 30–31, 315
Gemnisyn (acetaminophen, aspirin), 368
Genahist. See Diphenhydramine (Benadryl).
Generic drug names, 301–335
Genora (norethindrone, mestranol), 368
Gentamicin, 315
Geocillin (carbenicillin), 368
Ginger, 427
Ginkgo biloba, 427
Ginseng, 427
Glasgow coma scale, 445–446
  in revised trauma scale, 448
Glaucon. See Epinephrine.
Glimepiride (Amaryl), 39, 315
Glipizide (Glucotrol), 21, 22, 315
Glossary of terms, 471–474
Glucagon, 125–126, 315
  contraindication to, 125
  dosage of, 125–126
  for diabetic hypoglycemia, 292
  interactions with, 125
  toxicity of, 126
Glucopaste (glucose), 291
Glucophage (metformin), 21–22, 368
Glucose, 315
Glucotrol (glipizide), 21, 22, 368
Glyburide (DiaBeta, Micronase), 21, 22, 315
Glynase (glyburide), 368
Goldenseal, 427
Goserelin (Zoladex), 315
Grepafloxacin (Raxar), 315

Grifulvin (griseofulvin), 368

Grisactin (griseofulvin), 368

Griseofulvin (Fulvicin), 316

Grisovin FP (griseofulvin), 368

Grisp-PEG (griseofulvin), 368

Guaifed (guaifenesin, pseudoephedrine), 369

Guaifenesin, 316

Guanabenz (Wytensin), 316

Guanadrel (Hylorel), 316

Guanethidine (Esimil), 316

Guanfacine (Tenex), 316

Gyne-Lotrimin (clotrimazole), 369

Gynergen (ergotamine), 369

Habitrol (nicotine), 369

Habituation, drug, 7, 473

Halazepam (Paxipam), 24–25, 316

Halcion. See Triazolam (Halcion).

Haldol. See Haloperidol (Haldol, Peridol).

Half-life, 473

Halfprin. See Aspirin (A.S.A.).

Hallucinogens, 273–274

Haloperidol (Haldol, Peridol), 126–128, 316
  contraindications to, 127
  dosage of, 127
  for psychoses, 281
  interactions with, 127
  toxicity of, 128

Halperon. See Haloperidol (Haldol, Peridol).

Haltran (ibuprofen), 369

Head injury, 299

Heparin. See also Ardeparin (Normiflo).
  dextran and, 261

Herbal preparations, 425–429

Heroin, 269–270

Hetastarch (Hespan), 262–263
  contraindications to, 262
  dosage of, 263
  interactions with, 263

Hexadrol. See Dexamethasone (Decadron, Dexasone, Maxidex).

Hismanal (astemizole), 23–24, 369

Histanil. See Promethazine (Histanil, Phenergan).

History taking, medications and, 9, 10–11

Hivid (zalcitabine), 369

Homatropine, 316

Humorsol (demecarium), 369

Humulin. See Insulin.

Hycodan (homatropine, hydrocodone), 369

Hycomine Compound (acetaminophen, caffeine, chlorpheniramine, hydrocodone, phenylephrine), 369

Hycomine syrup (hydrocodone, phenylpropanolamine), 370

Hycomine-S (ammonium chloride, hydrocodone, phenylephrine, pyrilamine), 369–370

Hycotuss Expectorant (guaifenesin, hydrocodone), 370

Hydergine (ergoloid mesylate), 370

Hydralazine (Alazine, Apresoline), 128–130, 316, 339
  contraindications to, 129

Hydralazine (Alazine, Apresoline) (*Continued*)
dosage of, 129
for congestive heart failure, 209
for hypertensive crisis, 299
interactions with, 129
toxicity of, 129–130
Hydrex (benzthiazide), 370
Hydro Z (hydrochlorothiazide), 370
Hydrocet (acetaminophen, hydrocodone), 370
Hydro-Chlor (hydrochlorothiazide), 370
Hydrochlorothiazide (Aprozide, HydroDIURIL), 32, 33, 316
Hydrocodone (Hycodan, Lortab, Vicodin), 34–35, 316
Hydrocortisone (Solu-Cortef, Westcort), 130–132, 316
dosage of, 131
for anaphylaxis, 279
interactions with, 131
magnesium sulfate and, 151–152
toxicity of, 131
HydroDIURIL (hydrochlorothiazide), 32, 33, 370
Hydroflumethiazide (Diucardin, Saluron), 32, 33, 316
Hydromorphone (Dilaudid), 34–35, 132–134, 316
abuse of, 269–270
contraindications to, 132
dosage of, 133
for pain management, 299
interactions with, 133
toxicity of, 133–134

Hydromox (quinethazone), 32, 33, 370
Hydromox R (quinethazone, reserpine), 370
Hydropres (hydrochlorothiazide, reserpine), 370
Hydroxychloroquine, 316
Hydroxyzine (Vistaril), 317
Hygroton (chlorthalidone), 32, 33, 370
Hylidone (chlorthalidone), 370
Hylorel (guanadrel), 370
Hyoscyamine (Cystospaz), 317
Hypercalcemia, 473
Hyperglycemia, 473
Hypersensitivity, 473
Hyperstat. See *Diazoxide (Hyperstat)*.
Hypertensive crisis, 298–299
Hypertonic solutions, 253–254, 473
Hypoglycemia, 473
Hypotonic solutions, 254
Hytrin (terazosin), 370
Hyzaar (hydrochlorothiazide, losartan), 371

Ibuprofen (Advil, Motrin, Nuprin), 35–36, 317
Ibuprohm (ibuprofen), 371
Ibu-Tab (ibuprofen), 371
Idiosyncrasy, drug, 7, 473
Iletin II NPH. See *Insulin*.
Ilosone. See *Erythromycin*.
Ilotycin. See *Erythromycin*.
Imdur (isosorbide mononitrate), 371
Imipramine (Tofranil), 37–38, 317

Imitrex (sumatriptan), 371
Imodium (loperamide), 371
Imodium A-D (loperamide), 371
Imuran (azathioprine), 371
Inapsine. See Droperidol
    (Inapsine).
Indameth (indomethacin), 371
Indapamide (Lozol), 32, 33, 317
Inderal. See Propranolol (Detensol,
    Inderal).
Inderide (hydrochlorothiazide,
    propranolol), 371
Indochron E-R (indomethacin),
    371
Indocid (indomethacin), 372
Indocin (indomethacin), 35–36,
    372
Indomethacin (Indameth,
    Indocin), 35–36, 317
Infergen (interferon alfacon-1),
    372
Inflamase (prednisolone), 372
Infusion rate, for intravenous
    fluid therapy, 251–252,
    263t
Initard. See Insulin.
Inocor. See Amrinone (Inocor).
Inotropics, 473
Insomnal. See Diphenhydramine
    (Benadryl).
Insta-Char. See Activated charcoal.
Insulatard NPH. See Insulin.
Insulin, 40, 134–136, 317
    contraindications to, 134
    dosage of, 135
    for diabetic ketoacidosis, 292
    interactions with, 135
    toxicity of, 135–136
Intal (cromolyn), 372
Intestines, drug excretion and, 4

Intramuscular injections, 230,
    241–243, 242
    needles for, 241
    syringes for, 241
Intraosseous access, for drug
    administration, 233–234,
    246–247, 473
Intravenous fluid therapy. See
    Fluid therapy.
Intravenous line, in drug
    administration, 244–245
    piggyback procedure with,
    247–248
Intropin. See Dopamine (Intropin,
    Revimine).
Intubation, 300
Inversine (mecamylamine), 372
Iodoquinol (Diquinol), 317
Ipecac, 136–139
    antihistamines and, 23
    contraindications to, 137
    dosage of, 138
    for ingested narcotics, 34–35
    interactions with, 138
    nonsteroidal anti-inflammatory
    drugs and, 36
    poisoning and, 294
    toxicity of, 138–139
Ipran. See Propranolol (Detensol,
    Inderal).
Ipratropium (Atrovent), 28, 29,
    296, 317
Ipratropium and albuterol
    (Combivent), 28, 29, 353
Irbesartan (Avapro), 317
Iron salt(s), 314
Ismelin (guanethidine), 372
Ismelin-Esidrix (guanethidine,
    hydrochlorothiazide),
    372

501

Ismo (isosorbide mononitrate), 372

Iso-Bid (isosorbide dinitrate), 372

Isocarboxazid (Marplan), 317

Isoclor Expectorant (codeine, guaifenesin, pseudoephedrine, alcohol), 372

Isodil (isosorbide dinitrate), 372

Isoetharine (Bronkosol), 28, 29, 139–141, 317
  contraindication to, 139–140
  dosage of, 140
  for respiratory distress, 296
  interactions with, 140
  toxicity of, 140–141

Isoflurophate (Floropryl), 317

Isomethteptene, 317

Isonate (isosorbide dinitrate), 372

Isoniazid, 317

Isoproterenol (Isuprel), 141–143, 317
  contraindications to, 141
  dosage of, 142
  for bradycardia, 284–285
  interactions with, 142
  toxicity of, 142–143

Isoptin. See Verapamil (Calan, Isoptin, Verelan).

Isopto Carpine (pilocarpine), 373

Isopto Fenicol (chloramphenicol), 373

Isordil (isosorbide dinitrate), 373

Isordil Tembids (isosorbide dinitrate), 373

Isordil Titradose (isosorbide dinitrate), 373

Isosorbide dinitrate (Iso-Bid), 317

Isosorbide mononitrate (Imdur, Monoket), 318

Isotamine (isoniazid), 373

Isotonic solutions, 254

Isotonics, 473

Isotretinoin, 318

Isoxsuprine (Vasodilan), 318

Isradipine (DynaCirc), 29–30, 318

Isuprel. See Isoproterenol (Isuprel).

Itraconazole (Sporanox), 318

Kaolin, 318

Kaon-Cl (potassium chloride), 373

Kaopectate (kaolin, pectin), 373

Kay-Ciel (potassium chloride), 373

K-Dur (potassium chloride), 373

Keflet (cephalexin), 373

Keflex (cephalexin), 373

Keftab (cephalexin), 374

Kefurox (cefuroxime), 374

Kehr's sign, 452

Kemadrin (procyclidine), 374

Kenacort (triamcinolone), 374

Kenalog (triamcinolone), 374

Kerlone (betaxolol), 26–27, 374

Ketoconazole (Nizoral), 318

Ketoprofen (Orudis), 35–36, 318

Ketorolac (Toradol), 35–36, 318

Kidney(s), and drug excretion, 4

Kinesed (atropine, phenobarbital), 374

Klonopin. See Clonazepam (Klonopin).

K-Lor (potassium chloride), 373

Klor-Con (potassium chloride), 374

Klotrix (potassium chloride), 374
K-Lyte (potassium chloride), 373
K-Norm (potassium), 373
Kolyum (potassium chloride),
    374
Korvess (potassium chloride),
    374
K-Tab (potassium chloride), 373
Kussmaul's respiration, 452
Kwell (lindane), 374

Labetalol (Normodyne,
    Trandate), 143–145, 318
    contraindications to, 143
    dosage of, 144
    for hypertensive crisis, 299
    interactions with, 144
    toxicity of, 145
Lactated Ringer's solution,
    256–257
    contraindications to, 256
    dosage of, 257
Lamictal (lamotrigine), 39, 374
Lamotrigine (Lamictal), 39, 318
Laniazide (isoniazid), 374
Lanoxicaps. See Digoxin
    (Lanoxin).
Lanoxin. See Digoxin (Lanoxin)
Largactil. See Chlorpromazine.
Larodopa (levodopa), 374
Larotid (amoxicillin), 375
Lasix. See Furosemide (Lasix,
    Uritol).
Ledercillin VK (penicillin V), 375
Lenoltec with codeine
    (acetaminophen, caffeine,
    codeine), 375
Lente Iletin I. See Insulin.
Lente Iletin II (beef). See Insulin.

Lente Iletin III (pork). See Insulin.
Lente Insulin. See Insulin.
Lescol (fluvastatin), 30–31, 375
Letrozole (Femara), 318
Leukeran (chlorambucil), 375
Levate (amitriptyline), 375
Levatol (penbutolol), 26–27, 375
Levlen (estrogen), 375
Levodopa (Larodopa, Sinemet),
    318
Levo-Dromoran (levorphanol),
    34–35, 375
Levomethadyl (Orlaam), 318
Levophed. See Norepinephrine
    (Levophed).
Levorphan (levorphanol), 375
Levorphanol (Levo-Dromoran),
    34–35, 318
Levothroid (levothyroxine), 375
Levothyroxine (Eltroxin,
    Levothroid, Synthroid), 318
Levoxine (levothyroxine), 375
Levsin (hyoscyamine), 376
Librax (chlordiazepoxide,
    clidinium), 376
Libritabs (chlordiazepoxide), 376
Librium (chlordiazepoxide),
    272–273, 376
Licorice, 427–428
Lidex (fluocinolone), 376
Lidocaine (Xylocaine), 145–148
    contraindications to, 146
    dexamethasone with, 356
    dosage of, 147
    for paroxysmal
        supraventricular
        tachycardia, 285, 469
    for ventricular arrhythmia,
        145–146, 283, 285, 286,
        468

503

Lidocaine (*Continued*)
for ventricular fibrillation, 283, 465
interactions with, 146–147
intubation with, 300
toxicity of, 148
Limbitrol (amitriptyline, chlordiazepoxide), 376
Lindane (Kwell), 318
Liothyronine (Cytomel), 318
Lipitor (atorvastatin calcium), 376
Lisinopril (Prinivil, Zestril), 19–20, 319
Lithane. See *Lithium*.
Lithium, 319
furosemide and, 123
Lithizine. See *Lithium*.
Lithobid. See *Lithium*.
Lithonate. See *Lithium*.
Lithotabs. See *Lithium*.
Liver, drug elimination and, 4–5
drug metabolization and, 4
Lodine (etodolac), 35–36, 376
Lodrane. See *Theophylline*.
Loestrin, 376
Loestrin Fe, 376
Lomotil (atropine, diphenoxylate), 376
Loniten (minoxidil), 377
Loop diuretics, 32, 33
digoxin and, 94–95
Lo/Ovral (estrogen), 377
Loperamide (Imodium), 319
Lopid (gemfibrozil), 30–31, 377
Lopressor. See *Metoprolol (Lopressor)*.
Lopressor HCT (hydrochlorothiazide, metoprolol), 377

Lopurin (allopurinol), 377
Loratadine (Claritin), 23, 24, 319
Lorazepam (Ativan), 24–25, 149–150, 319
abuse of, 272–273
contraindications to, 149
dosage of, 149, 150
for anxiety, 281
for seizure, 298
for stimulant abuse, 272
interactions with, 149
toxicity of, 150
Lorazepam Intensol. See *Lorazepam (Ativan)*.
Lorcet (acetaminophen, hydrocodone), 377
Lorelco (probucol), 377
Lortab (acetaminophen, hydrocodone), 377
Lortab ASA (aspirin, hydrocodone), 377
Losartan (Cozaar), 319
Losec (omeprazole), 377
Lotensin (benazepril), 19–20, 377
Lotrel (benazepril, amlodipine), 377
Lotrimin (clotrimazole), 377
Lotrisone (betamethasone, clotrimazole), 377
Lovastatin (Mevacor), 30–31, 319
Loxapine (Loxitane), 319
Loxitane (loxapine), 377
Lozol (indapamide), 32, 33, 378
Ludiomil (maprotiline), 37–38, 378
Lufyllin (dyphylline), 378
Luminal. See *Phenobarbital (Barbita, Luminal, Solfoton)*.
Lung(s), and drug elimination, 5

Luvox (fluvoxamine), 378
Lysergic acid diethylamide (LSD), 273–274

Macrobid (nitrofurantoin), 378
Macrodantin (nitrofurantoin), 378
Macrodrip intravenous sets, 250
Magaldrate (Riopan), 319
Magan (magnesium salicylate), 378
Magnesium gluconate, 319
Magnesium hydroxide, 319
Magnesium salicylate (Magan), 319
Magnesium sulfate, 150–153
  contraindications to, 151
  dosage of, 152
  for eclampsia, 151, 152, 298
  for seizure, 298
  for ventricular arrhythmia, 283, 286, 465
  interactions with, 151–152
  pancuronium and, 188
  toxicity of, 152–153
Magonate (magnesium gluconate), 378
Malathion (Ovide), 319
Mammary(ies), and drug excretion, 5
Mandelamine (methenamine), 378
Mannitol (Osmitrol), 153–155
  contraindications to, 154
  dosage of, 154
  for closed head injury, 299
  interactions with, 154
  toxicity of, 154–155

MAO (monoamine oxidase) inhibitors, morphine and, 164
Maprotiline (Ludiomil), 37–38, 319
Marax (ephedrine, hydroxyzine, theophylline), 378
Marijuana, 273–274
Marinol (dronabinol), 378
Marplan (isocarboxazid), 378
Maxair (pirbuterol), 28, 29, 378
Maxidex. See Dexamethasone (Decadron, Dexasone, Maxidex).
Maxolon (metoclopramide), 378
Maxzide (hydrochlorothiazide, triamterene), 378
Mazepine. See Carbamazepine (Tegretol).
Measurin. See Aspirin (A.S.A.).
Mebaral (mephobarbital), 272–273, 379
Mebendazole (Vermox), 319
Mecamylamine (Inversine), 319
Meclizine (Antivert), 319
Meclodium (meclofenamate), 379
Meclofenamate (Meclomen), 35–36, 37, 320
Meclomen (meclofenamate), 35–36, 37, 379
Medication. See also Drug(s); Fluid therapy.
  administration of. See Drug(s), administration of.
  generic names for, 301–335
  interaction of, 6–7, 18–19, 48
  overdose of, 14–15, 49
  trade names for, 337–424
Medication labels, 11, 12–14
Medicycline (tetracycline), 379

Medihaler-Epi. See *Epinephrine*.
Medipren (ibuprofen), 379
Medrol. See *Methylprednisolone
  (Medrol, Solu-Medrol)*.
Medroxyprogesterone (Curretab,
  Provera), 320
Medullary canal, 473
Mefenamic acid (Ponstel), 35–36,
  37, 320
Mefoxin (cefoxitin), 379
Megace (megestrol), 379
Megestrol, 320
Mellaril (thioridazine), 379
Menest (estrogen), 379
Menrium (chlordiazepoxide,
  estrogen), 379
Mepergan (meperidine,
  promethazine), 379
Meperidine (Demerol, Pethadol),
  34–35, 155–157, 320
  abuse of, 269–270
  contraindications to, 155
  dosage of, 156
  for pain management, 299
  interactions with, 156
  promethazine with, 205
  toxicity of, 156–157
  versus morphine, 157
Mephenytoin (Mesantoin), 320
Mephobarbital (Mebaral),
  272–273, 320
Meprobamate (Equanil,
  Miltown), 320
Mepron (atovaquone), 379
Meprospan (meprobamate), 379
Meridia (sibutramine), 379
Mesalamine (Asacol), 320
Mesantoin (mephenytoin), 380
Mescaline, 273–274
Mesoridazine (Serentil), 320

Mestinon (pyridostigmine), 380
Mestranol, 320
Metabolism, of drugs, 4
Metabolite, 4
Metahydrin (trichlormethiazide),
  380
Metaprel. See *Metaproterenol
  (Alupent, Metaprel)*.
Metaproterenol (Alupent,
  Metaprel), 28, 29, 320
  for respiratory distress, 296
Metastron (strontium), 380
Metatensin (reserpine,
  trichlormethiazide), 380
Metformin (Glucophage), 21–22,
  320
Methadone (Dolophine), 34–35,
  320
  abuse of, 269–270
Methamphetamine (Desoxyn,
  Methedrine), 271–272, 320
Methazolamide (Neptazane), 320
Methdilazine (Tacaryl), 23, 24
Methenamine (Mandelamine), 321
Methergine (methylergonovine),
  380
Methocarbamol (Robaxin), 321
Methotrexate (Folex), 321
Methscopolamine (Dallergy), 321
Methsuximide (Celontin), 321
Methyclothiazide (Diutensen-R,
  Enduron), 32, 33, 320,
  321
Methyldopa (Aldomet), 321
Methylergonovine (Methergine),
  321
Methylphenidate (Ritalin), 321
Methylprednisolone (Medrol,
  Solu-Medrol), 157–159, 321
  contraindications to, 158

Methylprednisolone (Medrol,
    Solu-Medrol) (Continued)
  dosage of, 158
  for anaphylaxis, 279
  for respiratory distress, 296
  toxicity of, 158
Methyltestosterone (Android),
    321
Methysergide (Sansert), 321
Meticorten (prednisone), 380
Metizol (metronidazole), 380
Metoclopramide (Emex, Reglan),
    321
Metolazone (Zaroxolyn), 32, 33,
    321
Metoprolol (Lopressor), 26–27,
    159–161, 321
  contraindications to, 159
  dosage of, 160
  for chest pain, 287
  for hypertensive crisis, 299
  interactions with, 160
  toxicity of, 160–161
MetroGel (metronidazole), 380
Metronidazole (Femazole, Flagyl),
    321
Metryl (metronidazole), 380
Metyrosine (Demser), 322
Mevacor (lovastatin), 30–31,
    380
Meval. See Diazepam (Meval,
    Valium, Vivol).
Mexate (methotrexate), 380
Mexiletine (Mexitil), 42, 322
Mexitil (mexiletine), 42, 380
Mibefradil (Posicor), 322
Miconazole, 322
Microdrip intravenous sets, 250
Micro-K (potassium chloride),
    381

Micronase (glyburide), 21, 22,
    381
Micronor, 381
Microsulfon (sulfadiazine), 381
Midamor (amiloride), 32, 33, 381
Midazolam (Versed), 24–25,
    161–163, 322
  contraindications to, 161
  dosage of, 162
  interactions with, 162
  intubation with, 300
  toxicity of, 162–163
Midol (aspirin, caffeine), 381
Midol 200 (ibuprofen), 381
Midol PMS (acetaminophen,
    pamabrom, pyrilamine), 381
Millazine (thioridazine), 381
Milontin (phensuximide), 381
Miltown (meprobamate), 381
Minestrin, 381
Minims (pilocarpine), 381
Minipress (prazosin), 381
Minitran. See Nitroglycerin.
Minizide (polythiazide, prazosin),
    381
Minocin (minocycline), 381
Minocycline (Minocin), 322
Minodyl (minoxidil), 381
Minoxidil (Loniten, Minodyl,
    Rogaine), 322
Miocarpine (pilocarpine), 382
Miosis, 474
Mirapex (pramipexole), 382
Misoprostol (Cytotec), 322
Mixtard. See Insulin.
Moban. See Molindone (Moban).
Mobenol (tolbutamide), 382
Modecate (fluphenazine), 382
Modicon (estrogen, progestin),
    382

507

Moditen (fluphenazine), 382

Moduret (amiloride, hydrochlorothiazide), 382

Moduretic (amiloride, hydrochlorothiazide), 382

Molindone (Moban), 322
  morphine and, 164

Mometasone (Elocon), 322

Monistat 7 (miconazole), 382

Monitan (acebutolol), 382

Monoamine oxidase (MAO) inhibitors, morphine and, 164

Monoclate-P (factor VIII), 382

Mono-Gesic (salsalate), 382

Monoket (isosorbide mononitrate), 382

Monopril (fosinopril), 19–20, 382

Moricizine (Ethmozine), 42, 322

Morphine (Duramorph, MS Contin, Roxanol), 34–35, 163–166, 322
  abuse of, 269–270
  antagonism of, 5–6
  contraindications to, 164
  dosage of, 164–165
  for chest pain, 287
  for congestive heart failure, 139, 173, 289
  for pain management, 299
  for pulmonary edema, 145
  interactions with, 164
  pralidoxime and, 199
  promethazine and, 6
  toxicity of, 165–166
  versus meperidine, 157

Morphine HP. See Morphine (Duramorph, MS Contin, Roxanol).

Morphitec. See Morphine (Duramorph, MS Contin, Roxanol).

M.O.S. See Morphine (Duramorph, MS Contin, Roxanol).

Motofen (atropine, difenoxin), 383

Motrin (ibuprofen), 383

MS Contin. See Morphine (Duramorph, MS Contin, Roxanol).

MSIR. See Morphine (Duramorph, MS Contin, Roxanol).

Mudrane GG Elixir (ephedrine, phenobarbital, theophylline, guaifenesin), 383

Mudrane GG Tablets (aminophylline, ephedrine, phenobarbital, guaifenesin), 383

Murphy's sign, 452

Muscle relaxants, bronchodilator, 28–29
  meperidine and, 156

Myambutol (ethambutol), 383

Mycelex (clotrimazole), 383

Myclo (clotrimazole), 383

Mycobutin (rifabutin), 383

Mycolog II (nystatin, triamcinolone), 383

Mycostatin (nystatin), 383

Myidone (primidone), 383

Mykrox (metolazone), 383

Myocardial infarction, 286–288
  management of, 432–433

Mysoline (primidone), 39, 383

Nabumetone (Relafen), 35–36, 37, 322

Nadolol (Corgard), 26–27, 322
Nadopen-V (penicillin), 384
Nafarelin (Synarel), 322
Naftifine (Naftin), 322
Naftin (naftifine), 384
Nalbuphine (Nubain), 166–168, 323
  contraindications to, 166
  dosage of, 167
  for pain management, 299
  interactions with, 167
  toxicity of, 167–168
Nalcrom (cromolyn), 384
Naldecon CX (codeine, guaifenesin, phenylpropanolamine), 384
Nalfon (fenoprofen), 35–36, 384
Nalmefene (Revex), 166
Naloxone (Narcan), 5–6, 168–171
  alcohol abuse and, 274–275
  contraindication to, 169
  diabetic emergency and, 292
  dosage of, 170
  fentanyl and, 170, 269
  for hydromorphone overdose, 133
  for meperidine overdose, 156
  for morphine, 165
  for nalbuphine reversal, 168
  for narcotic depression, 35, 269
  for respiratory depression, 80, 168, 191
  poisoning and, 294
  seizures and, 298
  toxicity of, 170–171
Naltrexone (Trexan), 323
Napamide (disopyramide), 384
Naprosyn (naproxen), 35–36, 37, 384

Naproxen (Aleve, Naprosyn), 35–36, 37, 323
Naqua (trichlormethiazide), 384
Naquival (reserpine, trichlormethiazide), 384
Narcan. See Naloxone (Narcan).
Narcotics, 34–35, 474. See also Opium.
  abuse of, 268–269
    treatment for, 269–270
  antagonism of, 5–6, 166, 168
  butorphanol and, 80
  diazepam and, 90
  dimenhydrinate and, 99
  droperidol and, 110
  fosphenytoin and, 121
  haloperidol and, 127
  ingested, activated charcoal for, 34–35
    ipecac for, 34–35
  lorazepam and, 149
  magnesium sulfate and, 151–152
  midazolam and, 162
  morphine and, 164
  nalbuphine and, 167
  pancuronium and, 188, 189
  phenobarbital and, 192
  phenytoin and, 194
  succinylcholine with, 214–215
  toxicity of, 34–35
  vecuronium and, 219, 220
Nardil (phenelzine), 384
Nasacort (triamcinolone), 384
Nasalcrom (cromolyn), 384
Nasalide (flunisolide), 384
Natrimax (hydrochlorothiazide), 384
Naturetin (bendroflumethiazide), 32, 33, 384

Nausea, 300
Navane (thiothixene), 384
Naxen (naproxen), 384
NebuPent (pentamidine), 385
Nefazodone (Serzone), 20–21, 323
Nelfinavir (Viracept), 323
Nelova, 385
Nembutal (pentobarbital), 272–273, 385
Neo-Codema (hydrochlorothiazide), 385
Neomycin, 323
Neonates, and Apgar scoring system, 443
Neosar (cyclophosphamide), 385
Neosporin ointment (bacitracin, neomycin, polymyxin), 385
Neostigmine (Prostigmin), 323
Neo-Tetrine (tetracycline), 385
Neothylline-GG (dyphylline, guaifenesin), 385
Nephronex (nitrofurantoin), 385
Neptazane (methazolamide), 385
Nettles, 428
Neumega (oprelvekin), 385
Neurontin (gabapentin), 39, 385
Neuro-Spasex (homatropine, phenobarbital), 385
NeuTrexin (trimetrexate), 385
Nia-Bid (niacin), 385
Niac (niacin), 385
Niacels (niacin), 386
Niacin (Niac, Nicobid), 30–31, 323
Nicardipine (Cardene), 29–30, 323
Nico-400 (niacin), 386
Nicobid (niacin), 386

Nicoderm (nicotine), 386
Nicolar (niacin), 386
Nicorette (nicotine), 386
Nicotine (Habitrol, Nicoderm), 323
Nicotinex (niacin), 386
Nicotrol (nicotine), 386
Nifedipine (Adalat, Procardia), 29–30, 171–173, 323
  contraindications to, 171
  dosage of, 172
  for hypertensive crisis, 299
  interactions with, 172
  toxicity of, 172–173
Nilstat (nystatin), 386
Nimodipine, 323
Nimotop (nimodipine), 386
Nipride. See Nitroprusside (Nipride).
Nisentil (alphaprodine), 386
Nitro-Bid. See Nitroglycerin.
Nitrocap. See Nitroglycerin.
Nitrocine. See Nitroglycerin.
Nitrodisc. See Nitroglycerin.
Nitro-Dur. See Nitroglycerin.
Nitrofurantoin (Macrodantin), 323
Nitrogard. See Nitroglycerin.
Nitroglycerin, 173–176, 323
  contraindications to, 173–174
  dosage of, 174
  for chest pain, 287, 299
  for congestive heart failure, 139, 173, 289
  for hypertensive crisis, 298
  for pulmonary edema, 145
  headache with, 16–17, 175
  interactions with, 174
  toxicity of, 175
  Viagra and, 174

Nitroglyn. See Nitroglycerin.

Nitrol. See Nitroglycerin.

Nitrolingual Spray. See Nitroglycerin.

Nitrong. See Nitroglycerin.

Nitronox. See Nitrous oxide (Nitronox).

Nitroprusside (Nipride), 176–178
contraindications to, 176
dosage of, 177
for congestive heart failure, 290
for hypertensive crisis, 299
interactions with, 177
toxicity of, 177–178
Viagra and, 176

Nitrospan. See Nitroglycerin.

Nitrostabilin. See Nitroglycerin.

Nitrostat. See Nitroglycerin.

Nitrous oxide (Nitronox), 178–180
contraindications to, 179
dosage of, 179–180
for pain management, 300
interactions with, 179
toxicity of, 180

Nix (permethrin), 387

Nizatidine (Axid), 323

Nizoral (ketoconazole), 387

Nolamine (chlorpheniramine, phenindamine, phenylpropanolamine), 387

Nolvadex (tamoxifen), 387

Nonsteroidal anti-inflammatory drugs (NSAIDs), 35–37
activated charcoal and, 36
bumetanide and, 78
ipecac and, 36
toxicity of, 36

Norcept-E 1/35, 387

Norcet (acetaminophen, hydrocodone), 387

Norcuron. See Vecuronium (Norcuron).

Nordette (estrogen and progestin), 387

Norepinephrine (Levophed), 180–183
contraindications to, 181
dosage of, 181–182
interactions with, 181
toxicity of, 182

Norflex (orphenadrine), 387

Norfloxacin (Noroxin), 323

Norgesic (aspirin, caffeine), 387

Norinyl (estrogen and progestin), 388

Norisodrine Aerotrol. See Isoproterenol (Isuprel).

Norlestrin (estrogen and progestin), 388

Normal saline, 255–256
half, 257–258
contraindications to, 257

Normiflo (ardeparin), 388

Normodyne. See Labetalol (Normodyne, Trandate).

Normozide (hydrochlorothiazide, labetalol), 388

Noroxin (norfloxacin), 388

Norpace (disopyramide), 42, 388

Norpramin (desipramine), 37–38, 388

Nor-Q.D. (progestogen), 388

Nor-Tet (tetracycline), 388

Nortriptyline (Pamelor), 37–38, 323

Norvasc (amlodipine), 29–30, 388

511

Novahistex C (codeine, phenylephrine), 388

Novahistex DH (diphenylpyraline, hydrocodone, phenylephrine), 388

Novahistine DH (chlorpheniramine, codeine, pseudoephedrine), 388

Novahistine Expectorant (codeine, guaifenesin, pseudoephedrine), 389

Novamoxin (amoxicillin), 389

Novasen. See *Aspirin (A.S.A.)*.

Novo-Ampicillin (ampicillin), 389

Novoanaprox (naproxen), 389

Novobutamide (tolbutamide), 389

Novochlorpromazine. See *Chlorpromazine*.

Novocimetine. See *Cimetidine (Tagamet)*.

Novocloxin (cloxacillin), 389

Novodigoxin. See *Digoxin (Lanoxin)*.

Novodipam. See *Diazepam (Meval, Valium, Vivol)*.

Novodoparil (hydrochlorothiazide, methyldopa), 389

Novoflupam. See *Flurazepam (Dalmane)*.

Novoflurazine (trifluoperazine), 389

Novofuran (nitrofurantoin), 389

Novohydrazide (hydrochlorothiazide), 389

Novolexin (cephalexin), 390

Novolin. See *Insulin*.

Novometoprol. See *Metoprolol (Lopressor)*.

Novoniacin (niacin), 390

Novonidazol (metronidazole), 390

Novonifedin. See *Nifedipine (Adalat, Procardia)*.

NovoPen-VK (penicillin), 390

Novoperidol. See *Haloperidol (Haldol, Peridol)*.

Novo-Pindol (pindolol), 390

Novopirocam (piroxicam), 390

Novopranol. See *Propranolol (Detensol, Inderal)*.

Novo-prazin (prazosin), 390

Novoprednisolone (prednisolone), 390

Novoprofen (ibuprofen), 390

Novopropamide (chlorpropamide), 390

Novopurol (allopurinol), 390

Novoquinidin (quinidine), 391

Novoridazine (thioridazine), 391

Novorythro. See *Erythromycin*.

Novosalmol. See *Albuterol (Proventil, Ventolin)*.

Novosemide. See *Furosemide (Lasix, Uritol)*.

Novosorbide (isosorbide dinitrate), 391

Novosoxazole (sulfisoxazole), 391

Novospiroton (spironolactone), 391

Novospirozine (hydrochlorothiazide, spironolactone), 391

Novothalidone (chlorthalidone), 391

Novotrimel (sulfamethoxazole, trimethoprim), 391

Novotriphyl (oxtriphylline), 391
Novotriptyn (amitriptyline), 391
NPH Iletin I. See *Insulin*.
NPH Iletin II (beef). See *Insulin*.
NPH Iletin II (pork). See *Insulin*.
NPH Insulin. See *Insulin*.
NPH Purified Pork. See *Insulin*.
Nu-Amoxi (amoxicillin), 392
Nubain. See *Nalbuphine (Nubain)*.
Nucofed (codeine,
    pseudoephedrine), 392
Nucofed Expectorant (codeine,
    guaifenesin,
    pseudoephedrine), 392
Nu-Loraz. See *Lorazepam
    (Ativan)*.
Nu-Metop. See *Metoprolol
    (Lopressor)*.
Numorphan (oxymorphone),
    34–35, 392
Nu-Pinol (pindolol), 392
Nu-Prazo (prazosin), 392
Nuprin (ibuprofen), 392
Nydrazid (isoniazid), 392
Nylidrin, 324
Nystatin (Nilstat), 324
Nytol. See *Diphenhydramine
    (Benadryl)*.

Octamide PFS (metoclopramide),
    392
Ocusert Pilo (pilocarpine), 392
Ofloxacin (Floxin), 324
Ogen (estrogen), 392
Olsalazine (Dipentum), 324
Omeprazole (Losec, Prilosec),
    324
Omnicef (cefdinir), 392
Omnipen (ampicillin), 393

Ondansetron (Zofran), 324
Opioids. See *Narcotics*.
Opium, 324. See also *Pantopon
    (opium alkaloids); Paregoric
    (opium)*.
    tincture of, 332
Opticrom (cromolyn), 393
Optimine (azatadine), 23, 24, 393
Oramide (tolbutamide), 393
Oramorph SR. See *Morphine
    (Duramorph, MS Contin,
    Roxanol)*.
Orap (pimozide), 393
Orasone (prednisone), 393
Orbenin (cloxacillin), 393
Oretic (hydrochlorothiazide), 393
Oreticyl (hydrochlorothiazide),
    393
Orinase (tolbutamide), 21, 22,
    393
Orlaam (levomethadyl), 393
Ornade (chlorpheniramine,
    phenylpropanolamine), 393
Orphenadrine (Norflex), 324
Ortho-Cept (estrogen and
    progestin), 393
Ortho-Cyclen (estrogen and
    progestin), 393
Ortho-Novum (estrogen and
    progestin), 394
Orudis (ketoprofen), 35–36, 394
Oruvail (ketoprofen), 394
Osmitrol. See *Mannitol (Osmitrol)*.
Osmotic diuretics, 32. See also
    Mannitol (Osmitrol).
Ovcon (estrogen and progestin),
    394
Overdose, drug, 14–15, 49
    poisoning in, 292–294
    treatment for, 293–294

513

Over-the-counter drugs, and
generic names, 301–335
trade names of, 337–424
Ovide (malathion), 394
Ovral (estrogen and progestin),
394
Ovrette (estrogen and progestin),
394
Oxacillin (Bactocill), 324
Oxaprozin (Daypro), 35–36, 37,
324
Oxazepam (Serax), 24–25, 324
abuse of, 272–273
Oxiconazole (Oxistat), 324
Oxistat (oxiconazole), 394
Oxprenolol (Trasicor), 324
Oxtriphylline (Choledyl), 28, 29,
324
Oxybutynin (Ditropan), 324
Oxycocet (acetaminophen,
oxycodone), 394
Oxycodone (Roxicodone), 34–35,
324
Oxycodone with acetaminophen
(Percocet), 34–35, 324
Oxycodone with aspirin
(Percodan), 34–35, 324
abuse of, 269–270
Oxygen, 183–185
chronic obstructive pulmonary
disease and, 184, 185
dosage for, 184–185
toxicity of, 185
Oxymetholone (Anadrol-50), 324
Oxymorphone (Numorphan),
34–35, 325
Oxytetracycline (Terramycin),
325
Oxytocin (Pitocin), 185–187
contraindication to, 186

Oxytocin (Pitocin) (Continued)
dosage of, 186
interactions with, 186
toxicity of, 187

Pain, chest, algorithm for,
432–433
Pain management, 299–300
Palaron. See Aminophylline.
Pamelor (nortriptyline), 37–38,
394
Pancuronium (Pavulon),
188–189
benzodiazepine before, 189
contraindications to, 188
dosage of, 188–189
interactions with, 188
narcotics and, 188, 189
toxicity of, 189
Panmycin (tetracycline), 394
Pantopon (opium alkaloids), 394
Panwarfin. See Warfarin
(Coumadin, Sofarin).
Papaverine (Pavabid), 325
Papaya, 428
Paradione (paramethadione), 394
Paraflex (chlorzoxazone), 394
Parafon Forte DSC
(acetaminophen,
chlorzoxazone), 394–395
Paramedic drug box, 235, 237
Paramethadione (Paradione), 325
Parasympatholytics, 474
Paregoric (opium), 395
Parenteral route, 474
Parepectolin (opium, pectin), 395
Parlodel (bromocriptine), 395
Parnate (tranylcypromine), 395
Paroxetine (Paxil), 20–21, 325

Patient assessment, medication labels in, 11, 12–14
Pavabid (papaverine), 395
Paveral (bromocriptine), 395
Pavulon. See *Pancuronium (Pavulon)*.
Paxil (paroxetine), 20–21, 395
Paxipam (halazepam), 24–25, 395
PCE Dispertab. See *Erythromycin*.
Pediamycin. See *Erythromycin*.
PediaProfen (ibuprofen), 395
Pediazole (erythromycin, sulfisoxazole), 395
Peganone (ethotoin), 395
Pemoline, 325
Penapar VK (penicillin), 395
Penbritin (ampicillin), 395
Penbutolol (Levatol), 26–27, 325
Penglobe (bacampicillin), 395
Penicillamine (Cuprimine), 325
Penicillin V (V-Cillin K, Veetids), 325
Pennyroyal, 428
Pentaerythritol tetranitrate (Duotrate), 325
Pentam 300 (pentamidine), 396
Pentamidine (Pentam 300, Pneumopent), 325
Pentamycetin (chloramphenicol), 396
Pentasa (mesalamine), 396
Pentazocine (Talwin), 34–35, 190–191, 325
  contraindications to, 190
  dosage of, 190
  for pain management, 300
  interactions with, 190
  morphine and, 164
  toxicity of, 191

Pentids (penicillin), 396
Pentobarbital (Nembutal), 272–273, 325
Pentoxifylline (Trental), 325
Pentritol (pentaerythritol tetranitrate), 396
Pen-Vee K (penicillin V), 396
Pepcid (famotidine), 396
Peptol. See *Cimetidine (Tagamet)*.
Percocet (acetaminophen, oxycodone), 34–35, 396
Percodan (aspirin, oxycodone), 34–35, 396
Pergolide (Permax), 325
Periactin (cyproheptadine), 23, 24, 396
Peridol. See *Haloperidol (Haldol, Peridol)*.
Peritrate (pentaerythritol tetranitrate), 396
Permax (pergolide), 396
Permethrin (Elimite, Nix), 325
Permitil (fluphenazine), 396
Perphenazine (Phenazine, Trilafon), 326
Persantine. See *Dipyridamole (Persantine)*.
Pertofrane (desipramine), 397
Pethadol. See *Meperidine (Demerol, Pethadol)*.
pH, 2
Pharmacodynamics, 1, 5–6
Pharmacokinetics, 1–5
Phazyme (simethicone), 397
Phenacemide (Phenurone), 326
Phenaphen (acetaminophen), 397
Phenaphen with Codeine (acetaminophen, codeine), 397
Phenazine (perphenazine), 397

Phenazopyridine (Pyridium), 326
Phencyclidine (PCP), 273–274
Phenelzine (Nardil), 326
Phenergan. See *Promethazine (Histanil, Phenergan).*
Phenergan with Codeine (codeine, promethazine), 397
Phenindamine, 326
Phenobarbital (Barbita, Luminal, Solfoton), 16, 39, 191–193, 326
  abuse of, 272–273
  contraindications to, 192
  dosage of, 192
  for isoproterenol–induced tremors, 142–143
  for seizure, 39, 85, 191, 210, 298
  interactions with, 192
  toxicity of, 193
Phenothiazines, and morphine, 164
  pralidoxime and, 199
Phenoxybenzamine (Dibenzyline), 326
Phensuximide (Milontin), 326
Phenurone (phenacemide), 397
Phenylbutazone (Butazolidin), 326
Phenylephrine, 326
Phenylpropanolamine, 326
Phenyltoloxamine, 326
Phenytoin (Dilantin, Diphenylan), 39, 42, 193–196, 326
  contraindications to, 194
  dexamethasone and, 86
  dextrose and, 194, 259, 260
  digitalis and, 194

Phenytoin (Dilantin, Diphenylan) (*Continued*)
  dopamine and, 107
  dosage of, 194–195
  for seizure, 16, 39, 99, 193, 194, 298
  hydrocortisone and, 131
  interactions with, 194
  morphine and, 164
  toxicity of, 195
Phlebitis, 474
Phrenilin (acetaminophen, butalbital), 397
Phyllocontin. See *Aminophylline.*
Physostigmine (Antilirium), 196–198
  contraindications to, 196
  dosage of, 197
  for atropine antagonism, 74
  for tricyclic antagonism, 38, 196, 294
  interactions with, 197
  toxicity of, 197
Pilagan (pilocarpine), 397
Pilocar (pilocarpine), 397
Pilocarpine (Pilagan, Pilocar), 326
Pilopine HS (pilocarpine), 397
Piloptic (pilocarpine), 397
Pimozide (Orap), 326
Pindolol (Visken), 326
Pirbuterol (Maxair), 28, 29, 327
Piroxicam (Feldene), 35–36, 37, 327
Pitocin. See *Oxytocin (Pitocin).*
Placenta barrier, 4
Placidyl (ethchlorvynol), 397
Plantain, 428
Plaquenil (hydroxychloroquine), 397–398

Plasma, and drug distribution, 3
Plasma protein fraction
    (Plasmanate), 261–262
    dosage of, 262
Plavix (clopidogrel), 398
Plendil (felodipine), 29–30, 398
PMS Benztropine (benztropine),
    398
PMS Carbamazepine. See
    Carbamazepine (Tegretol).
PMS Dopazide
    (hydrochlorothiazide,
    methyldopa), 398
PMS Isoniazid (isoniazid), 398
PMS Levazine (perphenazine),
    398
PMS Metronidazole
    (metronidazole), 398
PMS Neostigmine (neostigmine),
    398
PMS Perphenazine
    (perphenazine), 398
PMS Primidone (primidone), 398
PMS Prochlorperazine
    (prochlorperazine), 398
PMS Pyrazinamide
    (pyrazinamide), 398
PMS Sulfasalazine (sulfasalazine),
    398
PMS Theophylline. See
    Theophylline.
PMS Thioridazine (thioridazine),
    399
Pneumopent (pentamidine), 399
Poisoning/overdose, 14–15, 49,
    292–294
    treatments for, 293–294
Polaramine
    (dexchlorpheniramine), 399
Polycillin (ampicillin), 399

Polydipsia, 474
Polymyxin (Aerosporin), 327,
    338
Polythiazide (Renese), 32, 33,
    327
Polyuria, 474
Ponstan (mefenamic acid), 399
Ponstel (mefenamic acid), 35–36,
    37, 399
Posicor (mibefradil), 399
Potassium chloride (K-Dur,
    Slow-K), 327
Potassium iodide (SSKI), 327
Potassium-sparing diuretics,
    32, 33
Potentiation, drug, 6, 474
Pounds to kilograms, 435t–436t
Pralidoxime (Protopam
    Chloride), 198–200
    atropine and, 199–200
    contraindication to, 198
    dosage of, 199
    for organophosphate
        poisoning, 299
    interactions with, 199
    toxicity of, 199–200
Pramipexole (Mirapex), 327
Prandin (repaglinide), 399
Pravachol (pravastatin), 30–31,
    399
Pravastatin (Pravachol), 30–31,
    327
Prazepam (Centrax), 24–25, 327,
    351
Prazosin (Minipress), 327
Precose (acarbose), 21, 22, 399
Pred Forte (prednisolone), 399
Pred Mild (prednisolone), 399
Pred-G (gentamicin,
    prednisolone), 399

Prednisolone (Prelone, Vasocidin), 327

Prednisone (Winpred, Orasone), 327

Pregnancy, and Apgar scoring system, 443

Prelay (troglitazone), 399

Prelone (prednisolone), 399

Premarin (estrogen), 399

Prescription drugs, and generic names, 301–335
    trade names of, 337–424

Prilosec (omeprazole), 399

Primatene. See Epinephrine.

Primatene Mist. See Epinephrine.

Primidone (Mysoline, Sertan), 39, 327

Principen (ampicillin), 400

Prinivil (lisinopril), 19–20, 400

Prinzide (hydrochlorothiazide, lisinopril), 400

Probalan (probenecid), 400

Probampacin (ampicillin, probenecid), 400

Pro-Banthine (propantheline), 400

Proben-C (colchicine, probenecid), 400

Pro-Biosan (ampicillin), 400

Probucol (Lorelco), 327

Procainamide (Pronestyl), 200–202, 327
    bretylium tosylate and, 76
    contraindications to, 201
    dosage of, 201–202
    for ventricular arrhythmia, 283, 285, 469
    interactions with, 201
    toxicity of, 202

Procaine, and magnesium sulfate, 151–152

Procamide SR. See Procainamide (Pronestyl).

Procan SR. See Procainamide (Pronestyl).

Procardia. See Nifedipine (Adalat, Procardia).

Prochlorperazine (Stemetil, Compazine), 327

Procyclidine (Kemadrin), 328

Procytox (cyclophosphamide), 400

Proglycem. See Diazoxide (Hyperstat).

Prograf (tacrolimus), 400

Prolixin (fluphenazine), 400

Proloid (thyroglobulin), 400

Proloprim (trimethoprim), 401

Promapar, 401. See also Chlorpromazine.

Promazine (Sparine), 328

Prometh. See Promethazine (Histanil, Phenergan).

Promethazine (Histanil, Phenergan), 23, 24, 203–205, 328
    codeine with, 35
    contraindications to, 203
    dosage of, 204
    epinephrine and, 204
    for vomiting, 65, 79, 203, 217, 300
    interactions with, 204
    morphine and, 6
    toxicity of, 204

Pronestyl. See Procainamide (Pronestyl).

Propacet 100 (acetaminophen, propoxyphene), 401

Propaderm (beclomethasone), 401

Propafenone (Rythmol), 42, 328

Propagest (phenylpropanolamine), 401

Propantheline, 328

Proparacaine (Alcaine), 205–206
    contraindication to, 205
    dosage of, 205

Propecia (finasteride), 401

Propoxyphene (Darvon, Dolene), 34–35, 328
    abuse of, 269–270

Propranolol (Detensol, Inderal), 14, 26–27, 206–208, 328
    contraindications to, 206
    dosage of, 207
    for atrial dysrhythmia, 285
    for chest pain, 287
    for hypertensive crisis, 299
    interactions with, 207
    toxicity of, 207–208

Propulsid (cisapride), 401

Propylthiouracil, 328

Proscar (finasteride), 401

ProSom (estazolam), 24–25, 401

ProStep (nicotine), 401

Prostigmin (neostigmine), 401

Protopam Chloride. See Pralidoxime (Protopam Chloride).

Protostat (metronidazole), 401

Protrin (sulfamethoxazole, trimethoprim), 401

Protriptyline (Triptil), 37–38, 328

Protropin (somatrem), 402

Proventil. See Albuterol (Proventil, Ventolin).

Provera (medroxyprogesterone), 402

Prozac (fluoxetine), 20–21, 402

Pseudoephedrine, 328

Psilocybin, 273–274

Pulmophylline. See Theophylline.

Pulmozyme (dornase alfa), 402

Purinethol (mercaptopurine), 402

Purinol (allopurinol), 402

PVF (penicillin V), 402

PVF-K (penicillin V), 402

Pyrazinamide, 328

Pyrethrin (RID), 328

Pyridamole. See Dipyridamole (Persantine).

Pyridium (phenazopyridine), 402

Pyridostigmine (Regonol, Mestinon), 328

Pyrilamine, 328

Pyrimethamine (Daraprim), 328

Quarzan (clidinium), 402

Quazepam (Doral), 24–25, 328

Questran (cholestyramine), 30–31, 402

Quetiapine (Seroquel), 328

Quibron (guaifenesin, theophylline), 402

Quibron Plus (butabarbital, ephedrine, guaifenesin, theophylline), 402

Quibron-T. See Theophylline.

Quinaglute (quinidine), 403

Quinapril (Accupril), 19–20, 329

Quinate (quinidine), 403

Quinethazone (Hydromox), 32, 33, 328

Quinidex (quinidine), 42, 403

Quinidine (Quinaglute, Quinate, Quinidex), 42, 329

Quinora (quinidine), 403

Raccoon eyes, 452

Racepinephrine. See *Vaponefrin (racemic epinephrine, racepinephrine).*

Raloxifene (E-Vista), 329

Ramipril (Altace), 19–20, 329

Ranitidine, 329
  lidocaine and, 146

Rauzide (bendroflumethiazide), 403

Raxar (grepafloxacin), 403

Receptors, drug, 5, 474

Reglan (metoclopramide), 403

Regonol (pyridostigmine), 403

Regranex (becaplermin), 403

Regroton (chlorthalidone), 403

Regular Iletin I. See *Insulin.*

Regular Iletin II (beef). See *Insulin.*

Regular Iletin II (pork). See *Insulin.*

Regular Iletin II U-500. See *Insulin.*

Relafen (nabumetone), 35–36, 37, 403

Renedil (felodipine), 403

Renese (polythiazide), 32, 33, 403

Renese-R (polythiazide, reserpine), 404

Renormax (spirapril), 19–20, 404

Repaglinide (Prandin), 329

ReQuip (ropinirole), 404

Rescriptor (delavirdine), 404

Reserpine, 329

Respbid. See *Theophylline.*

Respiratory disease, medications for, 40

Respiratory distress, 295–296

Restoril (temazepam), 24–25, 404

Retet (tetracycline), 404

Retin-A (tretinoin), 404

Retrovir (zidovudine), 404

Revex (nalmefene), 166

Revimine. See *Dopamine (Intropin, Revimine).*

Rezulin (troglitazone), 21, 22, 404

Rheumatrex Dose Pack (methotrexate), 404

Ribavirin (Virazole), 329

RID (pyrethrin), 404

Ridaura (auranofin), 404

Rifabutin (Mycobutin), 329

Rifadin (rifampin), 404

Rifamate (isoniazid, rifampin), 404

Rifampin (Rifadin, Rofact), 329

Rifarer (isoniazid, pyrazinamide, rifampin), 404

Rimactane (rifampin), 404

Rimactane/INH (isoniazid, rifampin), 405

Rimantadine (Flumadine), 329

Riopan (magaldrate), 405

Riphen-10. See *Aspirin (A.S.A.).*

Risperdal (risperidone), 405

Risperidone (Risperdal), 329

Ritalin (methylphenidate), 405

Ritodrine (Yutopar), 329

Rituximab (Rituxan), 329

Rival. See *Diazepam (Meval, Valium, Vivol).*

Rivotril. See *Clonazepam*
  (*Klonopin*).
RMS. See *Morphine* (*Duramorph,*
  MS Contin, Roxanol).
Robaxin (methocarbamol), 405
Robicillin VK (penicillin V), 405
Robidone (hydrocodone), 405
Robimycin. See *Erythromycin.*
Robitet (tetracycline), 405
Rocephin (ceftriaxone), 405
Rofact (rifampin), 405
Rogaine (minoxidil), 405
Romazicon. See *Flumazenil*
  (*Romazicon*).
Ronase (tolazamide), 406
Ropinirole (ReQuip), 329
Roubac (sulfamethoxazole,
  trimethoprim), 406
Rounox with codeine
  (acetaminophen, codeine),
  406
Rovsing's sign, 452
Rowasa (mesalamine), 406
Roxanol. See *Morphine*
  (*Duramorph, MS Contin,*
  Roxanol)
Roxanol 100. See *Morphine*
  (*Duramorph, MS Contin,*
  Roxanol).
Roxicet (acetaminophen,
  oxycodone), 406
Roxicodone (oxycodone), 34–35,
  406
Roxiprin (aspirin, oxycodone),
  406
Rufen (ibuprofen), 406
Rynacrom (cromolyn), 406
Rynatan (chlorpheniramine,
  phenylephrine, pyrilamine),
  406

Rythmodan (disopyramide), 406
Rythmol (propafenone), 42, 406

Sabril (vigabatrin), 406
Saffron, 428
St. John's wort, 429
Sal-Adult. See *Aspirin (A.S.A.).*
Salazopyrin (sulfasalazine), 406
Salbutamol (Volmax), 28–29,
  58–60. See also *Albuterol*
  (*Proventil, Ventolin*).
  contraindications to, 58
  dosage of, 59
  for anaphylaxis, 279
  for bronchospasm, 28, 58, 71,
    161, 296
  interactions with, 59
  toxicity of, 59–60
Salflex (salsalate), 406
Salicylamide, 329
Sal-Infant. See *Aspirin (A.S.A.).*
Salivary glands, drug excretion
  and, 5
Salmeterol (Serevent), 28, 29,
  330
Salsalate (Disalcid, Salflex), 330
Saluron (hydroflumethiazide),
  407
Salutensin (hydroflumethiazide,
  reserpine), 407
Sandimmune (cyclosporine), 407
Sansert (methysergide), 407
SAS Enteric-500 (sulfasalazine),
  407
SAS-Enema (sulfasalazine), 407
SAS-500 (sulfasalazine), 407
Saw palmetto, 428
Schizophrenia, 280
Scopolamine, 330

521

Secobarbital (Seconal), 272–273, 330

Seconal (secobarbital), 272–273, 407

Sectral (acebutolol), 26–27, 407

Sedapap #3 (acetaminophen, butalbital, codeine), 407

Sedapap-10 (acetaminophen, butalbital), 407

Sedatives, abuse of, 272–273
  chlorpromazine and, 84–85
  diphenhydramine and, 100–101
  hydromorphone and, 133
  lorazepam and, 149
  morphine and, 164
  nalbuphine and, 167
  phenobarbital and, 192

Seizure disorders, 297–298
  medications for, 39, 298

Selegiline (Eldepryl), 330

Selenium, 330

Semilente Insulin. See Insulin.

Semilente Purified Pork. See Insulin.

Senna fruit extract (Senokot), 330

Senokot (senna fruit extract), 407

Septra (sulfamethoxazole, trimethoprim), 407

Ser-Ap-Es (hydralazine, hydrochlorothiazide, reserpine), 407

Serax (oxazepam), 24–25, 272–273, 408

Serentil (mesoridazine), 408

Serevent (salmeterol), 28, 29, 408

Seromycin (cycloserine), 408

Seroquel (quetiapine), 408

Serotonin re-uptake inhibitors, 20–21
  toxicity of, 21

Serpasil (reserpine), 408

Serpasil-Apresoline (hydralazine, reserpine), 408

Sertan (primidone), 408

Sertraline (Zoloft), 20–21, 330

Serzone (nefazodone), 20–21, 408

Sibutramine (Meridia), 330

Side effects, drug, 16–17, 48, 474

Signs in diagnosis, 451–452

Sildenafil (Viagra), 330
  amyl nitrite and, 68
  nitroglycerin and, 174
  nitroprusside and, 176

Silvadene (silver sulfadiazine), 408

Silver sulfadiazine (Silvadene), 330

Simethicone, 330

Simvastatin (Zocor), 30–31, 330

Sincomen (spironolactone), 408

Sinemet (carbidopa, levodopa), 408

Sinequan (doxepin), 37–38, 408

Sinulin (acetaminophen, chlorpheniramine, phenylpropanolamine), 408

Skelid (tiludronate), 408

Skin, and drug excretion, 5

SK-penicillin VK (penicillin V), 408

SK-probenecid (probenecid), 409

SK-quinidine sulfate (quinidine), 409

SK-soxazole (sulfisoxazole), 409

SK-tetracycline (tetracycline), 409

SK-thioridazine (thioridazine), 409

SK-triamcinolone (triamcinolone), 409

Sleep-Eze 3. See Diphenhydramine (Benadryl).

Slo-bid. See Theophylline.

Slo-Niacin (niacin), 409

Slo-phyllin. See Theophylline.

Slow Fe (ferrous sulfate), 409

Slow-K (potassium chloride), 409

Slurry, 474

Sodium bicarbonate, 208–210
  calcium and, 82, 209
  contraindications to, 209
  diabetic emergency with, 292
  dopamine and, 107
  dosage of, 209
  for cardiac arrest, 283, 441
  for sedative abuse, 273
  for tricyclic overdose, 209, 283, 294, 465
  interactions with, 209
  toxicity of, 209–210

Sofarin. See Warfarin (Coumadin, Sofarin).

Solalzine (trifluoperazine), 409

Solfoton. See Phenobarbital (Barbita, Luminal, Solfoton).

Solubility, of drugs, 2

Solu-Cortef. See Hydrocortisone (Solu-Cortef).

Solu-Medrol. See Methylprednisolone (Medrol, Solu-Medrol).

Soma (carisoprodol), 409

Soma Compound (aspirin, carisoprodol), 409

Somatrem (Protropin), 330

Sominex. See Diphenhydramine (Benadryl).

Somnol. See Flurazepam (Dalmane).

Somophyllin-12. See Aminophylline.

Somophylline. See Aminophylline

Som-Pam. See Flurazepam (Dalmane).

Sonazine. See Chlorpromazine.

Sorbitrate (isosorbide dinitrate), 410

Sotacor (sotalol), 410

Sotalol (Betapace, Sotacor), 26–27, 330

Span-Niacin (niacin), 410

Sparine (promazine), 410

Spectazole (econazole), 410

Spectrobid (bacampicillin), 410

Spersacarpine (pilocarpine), 410

Spirapril (Renormax), 19–20, 330

Spironolactone (Alatone, Aldactone), 32, 33, 330

Sporanox (itraconazole), 410

SSKI (potassium iodide), 410

Stadol. See Butorphanol (Stadol).

Stanozolol (Winstrol), 330

Status epilepticus, 297

Stavudine (Zerit), 331

Stelazine (trifluoperazine), 410

Stemetil (prochlorperazine), 410–411

Sterapred (prednisone), 411

Stimulants, 271–272

Streptokinase (Streptase), 210–212
  contraindications to, 210
  dosage of, 211
  for thrombolytic therapy, 288

Streptokinase (Streptase)
(*Continued*)
interactions with, 211
toxicity of, 211–212
Strontium chloride-89
(Metastron), 331
Sublimaze. See *Fentanyl*
(*Sublimaze, Duragesic*).
Succinylcholine (Anectine),
212–215
benzodiazepine with, 214–215
contraindications to, 213
dosage of, 213
interactions with, 213
intubation with, 300
lidocaine and, 146–147
narcotics with, 214–215
physostigmine and, 197
pralidoxime and, 199
toxicity of, 213–214
Sucralfate (Carafate, Sulcrate),
331
Suicidal behavior, 280
Sulcrate (sucralfate), 411
Sulfacetamide, 331
Sulfadiazine (Microsulfon), 331
Sulfadoxine (Fansidar), 331
Sulfamethoxazole (Gantanol), 331
Sulfasalazine (Azaline,
Salazopyrin), 331
Sulfatrim DS (sulfamethoxazole,
trimethoprim), 411
Sulfinpyrazone, 331
Sulfisoxazole (Gantrisin), 331
Sulindac (Clinoril), 35–36, 37,
331
Sumatriptan (Imitrex), 331
Sumycin (tetracycline), 411
Supac (acetaminophen, aspirin,
caffeine), 411

Supasa. See *Aspirin (A.S.A.)*.
Supeudol (oxycodone), 411
Suprax (cefixime), 411
Suprazine (trifluoperazine),
411
Surfak (docusate), 411
Surmontil (trimipramine), 37–38,
411
Sus-Phrine. See *Epinephrine*.
Sustaire. See *Theophylline*.
Sweat glands, and drug
excretion, 5
Symadine (amantadine), 411
Symmetrel (amantadine),
411–412
Sympathomimetic agents, 474
abuse of, 271–272
aminophylline and, 64
isoetharine and, 140
isoproterenol and, 142
Synalgos-DC (aspirin, caffeine,
dihydrocodeine), 412
Synarel (nafarelin), 412
Synergism, of drugs, 6, 474
Synthroid (levothyroxine), 412
Syringes, intramuscular injection,
241
pre-filled, 237, 240
subcutaneous injection, 243
Syroxine (levothyroxine), 412

Tace (estrogens), 412
Tachycardia algorithm, *468–470*.
See also *Ventricular
dysrhythmias*.
Tacrine (THA, Cognex), 331
Tacrolimus (Prograf), 331
Tagamet. See *Cimetidine
(Tagamet)*.

Talacen (acetaminophen,
    pentazocine), 412
Talwin. See Pentazocine (Talwin).
Talwin Compound (aspirin,
    pentazocine), 412
Talwin NX (naloxone,
    pentazocine), 412
Tambocor (flecainide), 42, 412
Tamofen (tamoxifen), 412
Tamone (tamoxifen), 412
Tamoxifen (Tamofen, Nolvadex),
    331
Tamsulosin (Flomax), 331
Taractan (chlorprothixene), 412
Tavist (clemastine), 23, 24, 412
Tavist-D (clemastine,
    phenylpropanolamine), 412
Tazarotene (Tazorac), 331
Tazicef (ceftazidime), 413
Tazidime (ceftazidime), 413
Tazorac (tazarotene), 413
Tebrazid (pyrazinamide), 413
Tedral (ephedrine, phenobarbital,
    theophylline), 413
Teebaconin (isoniazid), 413
Tegison (etretinate), 413
Tegopen (cloxacillin), 413
Tegretol. See Carbamazepine
    (Tegretol)
Teldrin (chlorpheniramine), 413
Temazepam (Restoril), 24–25,
    331
Temperature conversion table,
    437t–438t
Tenex (guanfacine), 413
Ten-K (potassium chloride), 413
Tenoretic (atenolol,
    chlorthalidone), 413
Tenormin (atenolol), 26–27, 413
Tenuate (diethylpropion), 413

Terazol (terconazole), 413
Terazosin (Hytrin), 331
Terbutaline (Brethine), 28, 29,
    215–217, 332
    contraindications to, 215
    dosage of, 216
    for respiratory distress, 296
    interactions with, 216
    toxicity of, 216–217
Terconazole (Terazol), 332
Terfenadine (Seldane), 23, 24,
    332
Terfluzine (trifluoperazine), 413
Terramycin (oxytetracycline), 414
Teslac (testolactone), 414
Tessalon (benzonatate), 414
Testolactone (Teslac), 332
Tetra-C (tetracycline), 414
Tetracycline (Retet, Sumycin),
    332
Tetracyn (tetracycline), 414
Tetram (tetracycline), 414
Teveten (eprosartan), 414
T-Gesic (acetaminophen,
    hydrocodone), 414
THA (tacrine), 414
Thalitone (chlorthalidone), 414
Theobid. See Theophylline.
Theochron. See Theophylline.
Theoclear. See Theophylline.
Theo-Dur. See Theophylline.
Theolair. See Theophylline.
Theo-Organidin (glycerol,
    theophylline), 414
Theophylline, 28, 29, 332
    adenosine and, 56
Theophyl-SR. See Theophylline.
Theo-24. See Theophylline.
Theovent. See Theophylline.
Theo-X. See Theophylline.

Thiamine (vitamin B$_1$), 217–218
  dosage of, 218
  for alcohol abuse, 274
  for diabetic emergency, 291
  for narcotic abuse, 270
  for seizure, 298
  poisoning and, 294
  toxicity of, 218
Thiazide diuretics, 32, 33
Thiethylperazine (Torecan), 332
Thiothixene (Navane), 332
Thiuretic (hydrochlorothiazide), 415
Thorazine. See Chlorpromazine.
Thyroglobulin (Proloid), 332
Thyrolar (levothyroxine, liothyronine), 415
Tiagabine (Gabitril), 332
Ticarcillin, 332
Ticlid (ticlopidine), 415
Ticlopidine (Ticlid), 332
Tigan (trimethobenzamide), 415
Tiludronate (Skelid), 332
Timentin (clavulanate, ticarcillin), 415
Timolide (hydrochlorothiazide, timolol), 415
Timolol (Blocadren, Timoptic), 26–27, 332
Timoptic (timolol), 415
Tincture of opium (Paregoric), 332
Tissue plasminogen activator (Alteplase, tPA), 60–63
  dosage of, 62
  exclusion criteria for, 61
  for thrombolytic therapy, 288
  interactions with, 62
  toxicity of, 62
Tobramycin (Tobrex), 332

Tobrex (tobramycin), 415
Tocainide (Tonocard), 42, 332
Tofranil (imipramine), 37–38, 415
Tolamide (tolazamide), 415
Tolazamide (Ronase, Tolinase), 21, 22, 333
Tolbutamide (Orinase), 21, 22, 333
Tolectin (tolmetin), 35–36, 37, 415
Tolerance, drug, 6–7, 474
Tolinase (tolazamide), 21, 22, 415
Tolmetin (Tolectin), 35–36, 37, 333
Tonocard (tocainide), 42, 415
Toprol XL. See Metoprolol (Lopressor).
Toradol (ketorolac), 35–36, 416
Torecan (thiethylperazine), 416
Tornalate (bitolterol), 28, 29, 416
Torsemide (Demadex), 32, 33, 333
Totacillin (ampicillin), 416
Toxicity, drug, 49
  cumulative action and, 6
tPA. See Tissue plasminogen activator (Alteplase, tPA).
T-Phyl. See Theophylline.
Trade drug names, 337–424
Tramadol (Ultram), 333
Trancopal (chlormezanone), 416
Trandate. See Labetalol (Normodyne, Trandate).
Trandate HCT. See Labetalol (Normodyne, Trandate).
Tranquilizers, butorphanol and, 80
  chlorpromazine and, 84–85

Tranquilizers (*Continued*)
  dimenhydrinate and, 99
  diphenhydramine and,
      100–101
  haloperidol and, 127
  hydromorphone and, 133
  midazolam and, 162
  morphine and, 164
  phenobarbital and, 192
  phenytoin and, 194
  promethazine and, 204
Transderm-Nitro. See
    Nitroglycerin.
Transderm-Scop (scopolamine),
    416
Tranxene (clorazepate), 24–25,
    272–273, 416
Tranylcypromine (Parnate),
    333
Trasicor (oxprenolol), 416
Trauma scale, 447–448
Travamine. See *Dimenhydrinate
    (Dramamine, Travamine).*
Trazodone (Desyrel, Trialodine),
    333
Trecator-SC (ethionamide), 416
Trental (pentoxifylline), 416
Tretinoin (Retin-A), 333
Triadapin (doxepin), 416
Trialodine (trazodone), 416
Triamcinolone (Aristocort,
    Azmacort), 333
Triaminic Expectorant with
    Codeine (codeine,
    guaifenesin,
    phenylpropanolamine,
    alcohol), 416
Triamterene (Dyrenium), 32, 33,
    333
Triaphen-10. See *Aspirin (A.S.A.).*

Triavil (amitriptyline,
    perphenazine), 417
Triazolam (Halcion), 24–25, 333
  abuse of, 272–273
Trichlorex (trichlormethiazide),
    417
Trichlormethiazide (Diurese,
    Trichlorex), 32, 33, 333
Tricyclic antidepressants, 37–38
  activated charcoal and, 38
  antagonists for, 38, 196, 209
  butorphanol and, 80
  fosphenytoin and, 121
  meperidine and, 156
  racemic epinephrine and,
      116–117
  toxicity of, 37–38
Tridil. See *Nitroglycerin.*
Tridione (trimethadione), 417
Trifluoperazine, 333
Triflupromazine (Vesprin), 333
Trihexyphenidyl (Artane), 333
Trikacide (metronidazole), 417
Trilafon (perphenazine), 417
Tri-Levlen (estrogen and
    progestin), 417
Trimeprazine (Temaril), 23, 24,
    333
Trimethadione (Tridione), 333
Trimethobenzamide (Tigan), 334
Trimethoprim (Trimpex), 334
Trimetrexate (NeuTrexin), 334
Trimipramine (Surmontil),
    37–38, 334
Trimox (amoxicillin), 417
Trimpex (trimethoprim), 417
Trinalin (azatadine,
    pseudoephedrine), 417
Tri-Norinyl (estrogen and
    progestin), 417

Triostat (liothyronine), 417

Triphasil (estrogen and progestin), 417

Triprolidine (Myidyl), 23, 24, 334

Triptil (protriptyline), 37–38, 417

Triquilar (estrogen and progestin), 418

Troglitazone (Rezulin), 21, 22, 334

Trovafloxacin (Trovan), 334

Trovan (trovafloxacin), 418

Truphylline. See *Aminophylline*.

Tubex cartridges, 237, 240–241

Tuinal (amobarbital, secobarbital), 418

Turmeric, 429

Tussar DM (chlorpheniramine, dextromethorphan, pseudoephedrine), 418

Tussar SF (codeine, guaifenesin, pseudoephedrine), 418

Tussar-2 (codeine, guaifenesin, pseudoephedrine), 418

Tussend (hydrocodone, pseudoephedrine), 418

Tussend Expectorant (hydrocodone, guaifenesin, pseudoephedrine), 418

Tussigon (homatropine, hydrocodone), 418

Tussionex (hydrocodone, phenyltoloxamine), 418

Tussionex Pennkinetic, 34–35

Tussi-Organidin (codeine, glycerol), 34–35, 418

Tussi-Organidin DDMR (dextromethorphan, iodinated glycerol), 418

Twilite. See *Diphenhydramine (Benadryl)*.

Tycolet (acetaminophen, hydrocodone), 419

Tylenol with Codeine (acetaminophen, codeine), 419

Tylox (acetaminophen, oxycodone), 419

Ultracef (cefadroxil), 419

Ultralente Purified Beef. See *Insulin*.

Ultram (tramadol), 419

Uniphyl. See *Theophylline*.

Unipres (hydralazine, hydrochlorothiazide), 419

Unitensen (cryptenamine), 419

Urecholine (bethanechol), 419

Uridon (chlorthalidone), 419

Urine, drug excretion and, 4

Urispas (flavoxate), 419

Uritol. See *Furosemide (Lasix, Uritol)*.

Uroplus DS (sulfamethoxazole, trimethoprim), 419

Urozide (hydrochlorothiazide), 419

Ursodiol, 334

Uticillin VK (pencillin V), 419

Utimox (amoxicillin), 419

Valacyclovir (Valtrex), 334

Valdrene. See *Diphenhydramine (Benadryl)*.

Valisone (betamethasone), 420

Valium. See *Diazepam (Meval, Valium, Vivol)*.

Valmid (ethinamate), 420

Valproic acid (Depakene, Epival), 39, 334

Valsartan (Diovan), 334

Valtrex (valacyclovir), 420

Vancenase AQ (beclomethasone), 420

Vancenase Nasal Inhaler (beclomethasone), 420

Vanceril (beclomethasone), 296, 420

Vancocin (vancomycin), 420

Vancomycin (Vancocin), 334

Vantin (cefpodoxime), 420

Vapo-Iso. See Isoproterenol (Isuprel).

Vaponefrin (racemic epinephrine, racepinephrine), 116–118, 420
  contraindications to, 116
  dosage of, 117
  for anaphylaxis, 279
  for respiratory distress, 296
  interactions with, 116–117
  toxicity of, 117–118

Vaporole. See Amyl nitrite (Vaporole).

Vascor (bepridil), 29–30, 420

Vaseretic (enalapril, hydrochlorothiazide), 420

Vasocidin (prednisolone, sulfacetamide), 420

Vasoconstrictors, 474

Vasodilan (isoxsuprine), 421

Vasodilators, 474

Vasopressors. See also Vasoconstrictors.
  for hypotension, 30, 33, 67, 77, 93

Vasotec (enalapril), 19–20, 421

Vazepam. See Diazepam (Meval, Valium, Vivol).

V-cillin K (penicillin V), 421

VC-K 500 (penicillin V), 421

Vecuronium (Norcuron), 219–220
  benzodiazepines with, 220
  contraindications to, 219
  dosage of, 219
  interactions with, 219
  intubation with, 300
  narcotics with, 220
  toxicity of, 220

Veetids (penicillin V), 421

Velosef (cephradine), 421

Velosulin. See Insulin.

Venlafaxine (Effexor), 20–21, 334

Ventolin. See Albuterol (Proventil, Ventolin).

Ventricular dysrhythmias. See also Tachycardia algorithm.
  VF/VT algorithm for, 464–465

Verapamil (Calan, Isoptin, Verelan), 29–30, 220–223, 334
  contraindications to, 221
  dosage of, 221–222
  for atrial dysrhythmia, 283
  for paroxysmal supraventricular tachycardia, 285, 469
  interactions with, 221, 469, 470
  metoprolol and, 160
  propranolol and, 207
  toxicity of, 222

Verelan. See Verapamil (Calan, Isoptin, Verelan).

Vermox (mebendazole), 421

Versed. See Midazolam (Versed).

Vesprin (triflupromazine), 421

Viagra (sildenafil), 330
  amyl nitrite and, 68
  nitroglycerin and, 174
  nitroprusside and, 176

Vials, 237–239, 237–238

Vibramycin (doxycycline), 421

Vibra-Tabs (doxycycline), 421

Vicodin (acetaminophen, hydrocodone), 421

Vicoprofen (hydrocodone, ibuprofen), 421

Videx (didanosine), 422

Viracept (nelfinavir), 422

Virazole (ribavirin), 422

Visken (pindolol), 422

Vistacrom (cromolyn), 422

Vistaril (hydroxyzine), 422

Vitamin B₁ (thiamine), 217–218
  dosage of, 218
  for alcohol abuse, 274
  for diabetic emergency, 291
  for narcotic abuse, 270
  for seizure, 298
  poisoning and, 294
  toxicity of, 218

Vivactil (protriptyline), 422

Vivol. See Diazepam (Meval, Valium, Vivol).

Vivox (doxycycline), 422

Volmax. See Salbutamol (Volmax).

Voltaren (diclofenac), 35–36, 422

Vomiting, 300

Vontrol (diphenidol), 422

Warfarin (Coumadin, Sofarin), 334
  aspirin and, 70
  dextran and, 261

Warfarin (Coumadin, Sofarin) (Continued)
  tissue plasminogen activator and, 62

Warfilone. See Warfarin (Coumadin, Sofarin).

Weight conversion table, 435t–436t

Wellbutrin (bupropion), 422

Westcort. See Hydrocortisone (Solu-Cortef, Westcort).

Wigraine (caffeine, ergotamine), 422

Wigrettes (ergotamine), 422

Winpred (prednisone), 422

Winstrol (stanozolol), 423

Wyamycin. See Erythromycin.

Wycillin (penicillin V), 423

Wygesic (acetaminophen, propoxyphene), 423

Wymox (amoxicillin), 423

Wytensin (guanabenz), 423

Xanax (alprazolam), 24–25, 272–273, 423

Xylocaine. See Lidocaine (Xylocaine).

Yocon (yohimbine), 423

Yodoxin (iodoquinol), 423

Yohimbine, 334

Yohimex (yohimbine), 423

Yutopar (ritodrine), 423

Zafirlukast (Accolate), 334

Zalcitabine (Hivid), 334

Zantac. See Ranitidine.

Zarontin (ethosuximide), 423
Zaroxolyn (metolazone), 32, 33, 423
Zebeta (bisoprolol), 26–27, 423
Zefazone (cefmetazole), 423
Zenapax (dacliximab), 423
Zerit (stavudine), 424
Zestoretic (hydrochlorothiazide, lisinopril), 424
Zestril (lisinopril), 19–20, 424
Ziac (bisoprolol, hydrochlorothiazide), 424
Zidovudine (Retrovir), 335
Zithromax (azithromycin), 424
Zocor (simvastatin), 30–31, 424

Zofran (ondansetron), 424
Zoladex (goserelin), 424
Zolmitriptan (Zomig), 335
Zoloft (sertraline), 20–21, 424
Zolpidem (Ambien), 335
Zomig (zolmitriptan), 424
ZORprin. See Aspirin (A.S.A.).
Zostrix (capsaicin), 424
Zovirax (acyclovir), 424
Zurinol (allopurinol), 424
Zyban (bupropion), 424
Zydone (acetaminophen, hydrocodone), 424
Zyloprim (allopurinol), 424
Zyrtec (cetirizine), 424